Imaging the Failing Heart

Editor

MANI A. VANNAN

HEART FAILURE CLINICS

www.heartfailure.theclinics.com

Consulting Editor
EDUARDO BOSSONE

Founding Editor
JAGAT NARULA

April 2019 • Volume 15 • Number 2

RALUCA DULGHERU, MD
Department of Cardiology, Heart Valve Clinic,
University of Liege Hospital, GIGA
Cardiovascular Sciences, CHU Sart Tilman,
Liege, Belgium

IACOPO FABIANI, MD, PhD
Departments of Cardiac, Thoracic and
Vascular, Surgical, Medical and Molecular
Pathology and Critical Care Medicine,
University of Pisa, Pisa, Italy

DORA FABIJANOVIC, MD
Professor, Department of Cardiovascular
Diseases, University of Zagreb School of
Medicine, University Hospital Centre Zagreb,
Zagreb, Croatia

FRANCESCO FERRARA, MD, PhD
Cardiology Division, Cava de' Tirreni,
University Hospital of Salerno, Italy

GIAN GIACOMO GALEOTTI, MD
Cardiac, Thoracic and Vascular Department,
University of Pisa, Pisa, Italy

MADALINA GARBI, MD, PhD
King's Health Partners, King's College
Hospital NHS Foundation Trust,
King's College Hospital, London,
United Kingdom

LUNA GARGANI, MD, PhD
Cardiologist, Researcher, Institute of Clinical
Physiology, National Research Council, Pisa,
Italy

JONG-WON HA, MD, PhD
Division of Cardiology, Severance
Cardiovascular Hospital, Yonsei University
College of Medicine, Seoul, Republic of Korea

THURA T. HARFI, MD, MPH
Division of Cardiology, Department of
Medicine, The Ohio State University Wexner
Medical Center, The Ohio State University,
Columbus, Ohio, USA

GEU-RU HONG, MD, PhD
Division of Cardiology, Severance
Cardiovascular Hospital, Yonsei
University College of Medicine, Seoul,
Republic of Korea

RAMI KAHWASH, MD
Division of Cardiology, Department of
Medicine, The Ohio State University Wexner
Medical Center, The Ohio State University,
Columbus, Ohio, USA

DAVID M. KAYE, MBBS, PhD
Cardiologist, Department of Cardiology,
The Alfred, Head, Heart Failure
Research Laboratory, Baker Heart and
Diabetes Institute, Melbourne, Victoria,
Australia

KALIE Y. KEBED, MD
Advanced Cardiac Imaging Fellow,
Section of Cardiology, The University of
Chicago Medicine, The University of
Chicago Medical Center, Chicago, Illinois,
USA

IN-CHEOL KIM, MD, PhD
Division of Cardiology, Keimyung University
Dongsan Medical Center, Daegu, Republic of
Korea

PATRIZIO LANCELLOTTI, MD, PhD
Department of Cardiology, Heart Valve
Clinic, University of Liege Hospital,
GIGA Cardiovascular Sciences, CHU
Sart Tilman, Liege, Belgium; Gruppo Villa
Maria Care and Research, Anthea Hospital,
Bari, Italy

**ROBERTO M. LANG, MD, FASE, FACC,
FESC, FAHA, FRCP**
Professor of Medicine and Radiology,
Director Noninvasive Cardiac Imaging
Laboratories, Section of Cardiology,
Heart & Vascular Center, The University of
Chicago Medicine, The University of
Chicago Medical Center, Chicago, Illinois,
USA

STELLA MARCHETTA, MD
Department of Cardiology, Heart Valve Clinic,
University of Liege Hospital, GIGA
Cardiovascular Sciences, CHU Sart Tilman,
Liege, Belgium

ALBERTO M. MARRA, MD
IRCCS SDN, Naples, Italy

ELSEVIER

1600 John F. Kennedy Boulevard • Suite 1800 • Philadelphia, Pennsylvania, 19103-2899

http://www.theclinics.com

HEART FAILURE CLINICS Volume 15, Number 2
April 2019 ISSN 1551-7136, ISBN-13: 978-0-323-67797-4

Editor: Stacy Eastman
Developmental Editor: Laura Fisher

Heart Failure Clinics (ISSN 1551-7136) is published quarterly by Elsevier Inc., 360 Park Avenue South, New York, NY 10010-1710. Months of publication are January, April, July, and October. Business and editorial offices: 1600 John F. Kennedy Boulevard, Suite 1800, Philadelphia, PA 19103-2899. Periodicals postage paid at New York, NY, and additional mailing offices. Subscription prices are USD 261.00 per year for US individuals, USD 501.00 per year for US institutions, USD 100.00 per year for US students and residents, USD 300.00 per year for Canadian individuals, USD 580.00 per year for Canadian institutions, USD 315.00 per year for international individuals, USD 580.00 per year for international institutions, and USD 100.00 per year for Canadian and foreign students/residents. To receive student and resident rate, orders must be accompanied by name of affiliated institution, date of term, and the *signature* of program/residency coordinator on institution letterhead. Orders will be billed at individual rate until proof of status is received. Foreign air speed delivery is included in all *Clinics* subscription prices. All prices are subject to change without notice. **POSTMASTER:** Send address changes to *Heart Failure Clinics*, Elsevier Health Sciences Division, Subscription Customer Service, 3251 Riverport Lane, Maryland Heights, MO 63043. **Customer Service: 1-800-654-2452 (US and Canada). From outside of the US and Canada, call 314-447-8871. Fax: 314-447-8029. For print support, E-mail: JournalsCustomerService-usa@elsevier.com. For online support, E-mail: JournalsOnlineSupport-usa@elsevier.com.**

Reprints. For copies of 100 or more of articles in this publication, please contact the Commercial Reprints Department, Elsevier Inc., 360 Park Avenue South, New York, NY 10010-1710. Tel.: 212-633-3874; Fax: 212-633-3820; E-mail: reprints@elsevier.com.

Heart Failure Clinics is covered in *MEDLINE/PubMed (Index Medicus).*

Contributors

CONSULTING EDITOR

EDUARDO BOSSONE, MD, PhD, FCCP, FESC, FACC
Division of Cardiology, A. Cardarelli Hospital, Naples, Italy

EDITOR

MANI A. VANNAN, MBBS, FACC, FAHA, FASE, MRCP (UK), MRCP (I)
Co-Chief, Structural and Valvular Center of Excellence, Piedmont Heart Institute, Atlanta, Georgia, USA

AUTHORS

WILLIAM T. ABRAHAM, MD
Division of Cardiology, Department of Medicine, The Ohio State University Wexner Medical Center, The Ohio State University, Columbus, Ohio, USA

KARIMA ADDETIA, MD, FASE
Assistant Professor of Medicine, Section of Cardiology, The University of Chicago Medicine, The University of Chicago Medical Center, Chicago, Illinois, USA

MICHELE ARCOPINTO, MD
Emergency Department, A Cardarelli Hospital, Naples, Italy

TOR BIERING-SØRENSEN, MD, PhD, MPH
Department of Cardiology, Herlev and Gentofte Hospital, University of Copenhagen, Copenhagen, Denmark

BARRY A. BORLAUG, MD
Department of Cardiovascular Medicine, Mayo Clinic and Foundation, Rochester, Minnesota, USA

EDUARDO BOSSONE, MD, PhD, FCCP, FESC, FACC
Division of Cardiology, A. Cardarelli Hospital, Naples, Italy

MAJA CIKES, MD, PhD
Assistant Professor, Department of Cardiovascular Diseases, University of Zagreb School of Medicine, University Hospital Centre Zagreb, Zagreb, Croatia

ANTONIO CITTADINI, MD
Department of Translational Medical Sciences, Federico II University, Interdisciplinary Research Centre in Biomedical Materials (CRIB), Naples, Italy

CARLA CONTALDI, MD
Cardiology Division, Cava de' Tirreni, University Hospital of Salerno, Italy

ROBERTA D'ASSANTE, PhD
IRCCS SDN, Naples, Italy

FRANK LLOYD DINI, MD, FESC
Cardiac, Thoracic and Vascular Department, University of Pisa, Pisa, Italy

THOMAS H. MARWICK, MBBS, MPH, PhD
Cardiologist, Department of Cardiology,
The Alfred, Director, Baker Heart and
Diabetes Institute, Melbourne, Victoria,
Australia

DAVOR MILICIC, MD, PhD, FACC, FESC
Professor, Department of Cardiovascular
Diseases, University of Zagreb School of
Medicine, University Hospital Centre Zagreb,
Zagreb, Croatia

MICHAEL WESLEY MILKS, MD
Division of Cardiology, Department of
Medicine, The Ohio State University Wexner
Medical Center, The Ohio State University,
Columbus, Ohio, USA

SHANE NANAYAKKARA, MBBS
Cardiologist, Department of Cardiology, The
Alfred, Research Fellow, Baker Heart and
Diabetes Institute, Melbourne, Victoria,
Australia

MASARU OBOKATA, MD, PhD
Department of Cardiovascular Medicine, Mayo
Clinic and Foundation, Rochester, Minnesota,
USA

FLEMMING J. OLSEN, MD
Department of Cardiology, Herlev and Gentofte
Hospital, University of Copenhagen,
Copenhagen, Denmark

DAVID A. ORSINELLI, MD
Division of Cardiology, Department of
Medicine, The Ohio State University Wexner
Medical Center, The Ohio State University,
Columbus, Ohio, USA

CÉCILE OURY, PhD
Department of Cardiology, Heart Valve Clinic,
University of Liege Hospital, GIGA
Cardiovascular Sciences, CHU Sart Tilman,
Liege, Belgium

NICOLA RICCARDO PUGLIESE, MD
Departments of Cardiac, Thoracic
and Vascular, Surgical, Medical and
Molecular Pathology and Critical
Care Medicine, University of Pisa,
Pisa, Italy

SUBHA V. RAMAN, MD
Division of Cardiology, Department of
Medicine, The Ohio State University Wexner
Medical Center, The Ohio State University,
Columbus, Ohio, USA

KATE RANKIN, MBBS (Hons), FRACP
Division of Cardiology, Ted Rogers
Program in Cardiotoxicity Prevention,
Peter Munk Cardiac Center, Toronto
General Hospital, Toronto, Ontario,
Canada

YOGESH N.V. REDDY, MBBS, MSc
Department of Cardiovascular Medicine, Mayo
Clinic and Foundation, Rochester, Minnesota,
USA

ILARIA ROVAI, MD
Cardiac, Thoracic and Vascular Department,
University of Pisa, Pisa, Italy

ANDREA SALZANO, MD
Department of Cardiovascular Sciences,
NIHR Leicester Biomedical Research
Centre, University of Leicester, Glenfield
Hospital, Leicester, United Kingdom;
Department of Translational Medical
Sciences, Federico II University, Naples,
Italy

ERIK B. SCHELBERT, MD, MS
Director, UPMC Cardiovascular Magnetic
Resonance Center, Heart and Vascular
Institute, UPMC, Assistant Professor of
Medicine and Clinical and Translational
Science, Department of Medicine, University
of Pittsburgh School of Medicine, Clinical
and Translational Science Institute,
University of Pittsburgh, Pittsburgh,
Pennsylvania, USA

CHI YOUNG SHIM, MD, PhD
Division of Cardiology, Severance
Cardiovascular Hospital, Yonsei
University College of Medicine, Seoul,
Republic of Korea

TORU SUZUKI, MD, PhD
Department of Cardiovascular Sciences,
NIHR Leicester Biomedical Research Centre,
University of Leicester, Glenfield Hospital,
Leicester, United Kingdom

GIUSEPPE TERLIZZESE, MD
Cardiac, Thoracic and Vascular Department,
University of Pisa, Pisa, Italy

BABITHA THAMPINATHAN, RDCS
Division of Cardiology, Ted Rogers Program in
Cardiotoxicity Prevention, Peter Munk Cardiac
Center, Toronto General Hospital, Toronto,
Ontario, Canada

**PAALADINESH THAVENDIRANATHAN, MD,
SM, FRCPC, FASE**
Division of Cardiology, Ted Rogers Program in
Cardiotoxicity Prevention, Peter Munk Cardiac
Center, Toronto General Hospital, Toronto,
Ontario, Canada

XIAO ZHOU, MD, PhD
PLA Chinese Hospital, Beijing, China

Contents

  Video content accompanies this article at http://www.heartfailure.theclinics.com.

> Despite the rapid development of emerging imaging technologies, left ventricular ejection fraction represents the cornerstone of diagnosis, choice of treatment, and prognosis in heart failure. However, true myocardial function often remains underestimated or overestimated in different conditions underlying this heterogeneous syndrome. Changes in left ventricular size and left ventricular ejection fraction, termed reverse remodeling, are among the main goals of treatment in heart failure, aimed at halting or attenuating disease progression. The lack of effective therapeutic approaches in nearly one-half of the heart failure population highlights the need for integrating novel echocardiographic measures to better understand the underlying pathophysiologic mechanisms.

> Several left ventricular geometric patterns have been described both in healthy and pathologic hearts. Left ventricular mass, wall thickness, and the ratio of wall thickness to radius are important measures to characterize the spectrum of left ventricular geometry. For clinicians, an increase in left ventricular mass is the hallmark of left ventricular hypertrophy. Although pathologic hypertrophy initially can be compensatory, eventually it may become maladaptive and evolve toward progressive left ventricular dysfunction and heart failure. In particular, patients who show left ventricular dilation and hypertrophy in association with a low relative wall thickness are likely to carry the highest risk.

> Heart failure (HF) has evolved in an epidemic manner and constitutes a major public health issue. Currently, several prognostic markers and treatment options exist to guide treatment of HF with reduced ejection fraction, but echocardiographic deformation imaging suggests novel pathophysiologic aspects that could help optimize treatment further. Even though no formal treatment options currently exist for patients with HF with preserved ejection fraction, some HF medication does seem to attenuate strain measures. Speckle tracking has furthermore helped characterize this condition and to confer prognostic information. Thus, strain imaging could facilitate novel trials, and thereby hopefully introduce treatment opportunities.

is a need to better understand noninvasive measures. Echocardiography and cardiac MRI offer promising modalities to quantify ventriculo-vascular interactions. Significant heterogeneity exists around exercise protocols, and there is a need to develop consensus methodology and to validate these noninvasive measures in all forms of heart failure.

Noninvasive imaging, particularly echocardiography, plays a central role in the evaluation for heart failure with preserved ejection fraction (HFpEF). Echocardiography helps to rule in HFpEF among patients with unexplained dyspnea when the diagnosis is uncertain. In established HFpEF, echocardiography provides important insights into pathophysiology and phenotyping, such as isolated left ventricular diastolic dysfunction, left atrial dysfunction, abnormal right ventricular-pulmonary artery coupling, ischemia, or obesity phenotypes. In addition, imaging enables risk stratification for HFpEF. This article provides a critical appraisal of the role of echocardiography in the diagnosis and evaluation of HFpEF.

Patients with heart failure show myocardial, valvular, and electrical dysfunction, which results in enlarged cardiac chambers and increased intracardiac volume and pressure. Intracardiac flow analysis can provide information regarding the shape and wall properties, chamber dimensions, and flow efficiency throughout the cardiac cycle. There is increasing interest in vortex flow analysis for patients with heart failure to overcome limitations of conventional parameters. In conjunction with the conventional structural and functional parameters, vortex flow analysis–guided treatment in heart failure might be a novel option for cardiac physicians.

The heart and blood vessels are constantly interfering with each other in a closed system. For a few decades, the concept of ventricular-arterial coupling has been considered as a key pathogenesis of heart failure especially in heart failure with preserved ejection fraction.

Heart failure is a clinical syndrome with a broad spectrum of presentations. Cardiovascular imaging techniques such as echocardiography, cardiovascular magnetic resonance, computed tomography, and nuclear imaging play a crucial role in diagnosis, guiding management, and providing prognostic information. Each of these imaging modalities has their own respective strengths and weaknesses. Cardiac imaging can help differentiate between ischemic and nonischemic cardiomyopathies. Additionally, imaging techniques can display disease-specific findings, aiding in diagnosis of nonischemic cardiomyopathies and can provide a means to monitor response to therapy. The choice of imaging modality in the workup of cardiomyopathy should be based on the specific clinical question and the knowledge of the strengths and limitations of each imaging modality.

Lung ultrasound B-lines are the sonographic pattern of partial deaeration of the lung. In patients with pulmonary edema they are detected as multiple, diffuse, and bilateral, by placing the ultrasound probe in the intercostal spaces. B-lines can be used for bedside monitoring of pulmonary decongestion, and can guide diuretic therapy. Persistent pulmonary congestion after hospitalization for acute heart failure increases the risk of being rehospitalized in the following months. Adding B-lines assessment to echocardiography in an integrated cardiopulmonary ultrasound is of great value in establishing the kind and degree of myocardial and valvular impairment, and their hemodynamic consequences as pulmonary edema.

 Video content accompanies this article at http://www.heartfailure.theclinics.com.

Treatment of patients with heart failure with reduced ejection fraction has evolved. Recently, a fully implantable remote hemodynamic monitoring sensor in the pulmonary artery was approved in the treatment of patients at risk of heart failure readmissions. Several novel devices designed to offload the left atrium by creating a small interatrial shunt are being investigated. Cardiac imaging plays a vital role in the selection process, implantation, and monitoring of individuals with such devices. This article discusses in detail various imaging techniques and key clinical points relating to several cardiac devices used in the treatment of patients with heart failure.

Heart failure is a life-threatening disease. Its prevalence is characterized by a slow, steady increase, with unacceptable high mortality. Slowing disease progression is imperative. One of the most active field is the development of novel biomarkers. Biomarkers are used in routine clinical care for diagnosis, monitoring (response to treatment), and risk stratification of patients with heart failure. In this review, we consider in 2 different sections: blood-derived and imaging biomarkers. Finally, we analyze the effect of combining these 2 categories of biomarkers available in heart failure, aiming at understanding whether their role is complementary or subtractive.

HEART FAILURE CLINICS

SERIES OF RELATED INTEREST

Cardiology Clinics
http://www.cardiology.theclinics.com/

THE CLINICS ARE AVAILABLE ONLINE!
Access your subscription at:
www.theclinics.com

Preface

Imaging Heart Failure

Beyond Modalities of Pathophysiology, Prognosis, Therapy, and Practice

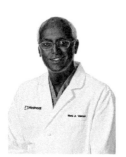 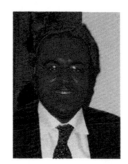

Mani A. Vannan, MBBS, FACC, FAHA, FASE, MRCP (UK), MRCP (I)   Eduardo Bossone, MD, PhD, FCCP, FESC, FACC

Editors

Imaging heart failure (HF) syndrome continues to be a hot topic because it challenges the imager to provide the best diagnostic and prognostic information in a cost-effective manner. The most common indication for an imaging test in the hospitalized patient is HF. In the ambulatory population, HF is either a close second or equals chest pain syndrome (including coronary artery disease) as the most indication for an imaging test. The increasing use of device therapy in HF has further tasked the imager to formulate an integrated pathway that yields comprehensive data relevant not only to diagnosis and prognosis but also to aid in selection and timing of appropriate device therapy.

This issue is deliberately formatted to address the key pathophysiologic and clinical questions in HF without focusing on the role of each imaging modality. The goal was to tackle the issue of how best to image each of these key issues agnostic to the imaging modality, and why. While Echocardiography remains the cornerstone of imaging HF, the emergence of myocardial structure and dysfunction as an independent and early marker of the disease has increased the role of cardiovascular magnetic resonance and biomarkers. Similarly, the focus of

imaging HF is not just the left ventricle anymore, the prognostic and predictive value of left atrial and right ventricular function is now routinely included in the standard evaluation of the HF syndrome. Also, the resting and exercise hemodynamic profile of the disease is a crucial determinant of symptoms, selection of drug or device therapy, and response to therapy. Thus, the contemporary best-practice approach of imaging HF requires the paradigm to be one which is able to deliver all of the data accurately and reliably. The sheer numbers of patients with HF tested each day, not only the duplicate testing of the newly diagnosed but also repeat testing of decompensated HF, place an enormous burden on resources and cost. The increasing role of biomarkers may reduce some of this burden in the future, but at the present time imaging is necessary for the confirmation and decision making once the clinical diagnosis of HF is made.

It is both a challenging and exciting time for the role of imager and imaging in HF syndrome. A clear understanding of the current and emerging concepts of risk-profiling and advances in therapy is central to a quality imaging approach in the care

Heart Failure Clin 15 (2019) xiii–xiv
https://doi.org/10.1016/j.hfc.2019.02.001
1551-7136/19/© 2019 Published by Elsevier Inc.

of the patient with HF. This issue is a valuable read for every imager involved in care of the HF patient.

Mani A. Vannan, MBBS, FACC, FAHA, FASE, MRCP (UK), MRCP (I)
Structural and Valvular Center of Excellence
Piedmont Heart Institute
95 Collier Road
Suite 2065
Atlanta, GA 30305, USA

Eduardo Bossone, MD, PhD, FCCP, FESC, FACC
Division of Cardiology
A. Cardarelli Hospital
Via A. Cardarelli, 9 – 80131 Naples, Italy

E-mail addresses:
mvannan2560@gmail.com (M.A. Vannan)
ebossone@hotmail.com (E. Bossone)

Left Ventricular Size and Ejection Fraction
Are They Still Relevant?

Dora Fabijanovic, MD, Davor Milicic, MD, PhD,
Maja Cikes, MD, PhD*

KEYWORDS

- Left ventricular volumes • Left ventricular ejection fraction • Cardiac remodeling
- Echocardiography • Heart failure

KEY POINTS

- Changes in left ventricular volumes are highly load dependent and are the result of overall left ventricular function, amalgamating different components of left ventricular deformation.
- Ventricular remodeling represents changes in ventricular architecture, paralleled by changes in ventricular volumes and mass, occurring as a compensatory reaction to changes in myocardial contractility or loading conditions.
- One of the main purposes of the remodeling process is preservation of stroke volume despite a potential impairment in left ventricular ejection fraction.
- The left ventricular ejection fraction is a powerful predictor of adverse outcomes and the effects of heart failure treatments when less than 45%, but its correlation with severity of heart failure symptoms is poor.
- Important pitfalls of left ventricular ejection fraction should be acknowledged; other components of left ventricular geometry and function as well as loading conditions of the heart should be taken into account when assessing cardiac function and risk in heart failure.

 Video content accompanies this article at http://www.heartfailure.theclinics.com.

INTRODUCTION

Chronic heart failure (CHF), one of the fastest growing global public health burdens, is a clinical syndrome characterized by symptoms (shortness of breath, ankle swelling, and fatigue) and signs (elevated jugular venous pressure, pulmonary crackles, third heart sound) caused by a structural and/or functional cardiac abnormality.[1] The incidence of CHF in the adult population of developed countries is 5 to 10 cases per 1000 persons per year, and more than 10% of the population older than 70 years suffer from CHF.[1] The central role of left ventricular ejection fraction (LVEF), the most commonly used indicator of left ventricular (LV) systolic function and the principal diagnostic parameter in heart failure (HF), was emphasized in the most recent Guidelines of the European Society of Cardiology for the Diagnosis and Treatment of Acute and Chronic Heart Failure, by a further subcategorization of patients with HF in respect to this parameter; in

Disclosure Statement: M. Cikes has received speaker fees from GE Healthcare. The other authors have nothing to disclose.
Department of Cardiovascular Diseases, University of Zagreb School of Medicine, University Hospital Centre Zagreb, Kispaticeva 12, Zagreb 10000, Croatia
* Corresponding author.
E-mail address: maja.cikes@gmail.com

Heart Failure Clin 15 (2019) 147–158
https://doi.org/10.1016/j.hfc.2018.12.012

addition to patients with HF with reduced EF (HFrEF) and HF with preserved EF (HFpEF), the term HF with midrange EF (HFmrEF) was introduced.[1] The main reasons leading to this new classification were heterogeneous etiologies and comorbidities and, importantly, different response to available therapies.[2] In addition to the very important prognostic role of LVEF, mainly observed in patients with HFrEF, the LVEF still determines the availability of effective therapies for HF; although disease-modifying therapeutic approaches have been proven effective in patients with HFrEF, treatment of patients with HFpEF (and partially those with HFmrEF) remains limited to symptomatic treatment with diuretics and the treatment of comorbidities.[1]

In this review, we aimed to summarize the pathophysiological implications of changes in LV size and LVEF, as well as their implications for patient management across the EF spectrum of patients with HF.

THE QUANTIFICATION OF LEFT VENTRICULAR VOLUMES AND EJECTION FRACTION

The LVEF represents the result of the overall LV deformation and is calculated as the difference between the end-diastolic volume (EDV) and end-systolic volume (ESV) divided by the EDV.[3–5] LV volumes also determine the stroke volume (SV), calculated as the difference between the EDV and ESV, and, if multiplied by the heart rate, the SV provides measurements of cardiac output. LV volumes can be quantified by echocardiography using 2-dimensional or 3-dimensional (3D) approaches.[6] Volume calculations based on linear measurements (M-mode echocardiography) are inaccurate in the setting of LV shape changes and its clinical use is thus discouraged.[6] In addition to echocardiography, 3D quantification of LV volumes and LVEF can also be obtained by cardiac MRI (cMRI) and gated single-photon emission computed tomography scans. Recently, newer echocardiographic techniques such as 3D and contrast echocardiography were found to provide improved reproducibility and agreement with cMRI[7–9]**Fig. 1**). However, striking variability in LVEF measurements performed by the Surgical Treatment for Ischemic Heart Failure (STICH) trail echocardiography, cMRI and single-photon emission computed tomography scanning core laboratories were recently published: values within a 5% LVEF range were represented in only 43% to 54% of the observations between these imaging modalities.[7] Nonetheless, LVEF remained significantly associated with mortality risk, regardless of the modality used.[7]

LEFT VENTRICULAR REMODELING IN CHRONIC HEART FAILURE: THE RELEVANCE OF ASSESSING LEFT VENTRICULAR GEOMETRY

Volume-based parameters of cardiac size and function are highly dependent on the loading conditions of the heart. The alterations of LV volumes occurring in response to loading changes will define the SV and cardiac output of the heart, independent of the intrinsic contractility of the LV.[5] Namely, a larger ventricle can generate a larger SV compared with a smaller one; more important, a larger ventricle with a reduced amount of deformation/contractility could produce the same amount of SV as a smaller one with normal contractility[5,10] (**Fig. 2**). Such compensatory responses are the hallmark of ventricular remodeling—changes in ventricular architecture, paralleled by changes in ventricular volumes and mass, occurring as a compensatory reaction to changes in myocardial contractility or loading conditions. In the setting of chronic loading changes, remodeling is initiated at the cellular level by pathologic myocyte hypertrophy and apoptosis, myofibroblast proliferation, and interstitial fibrosis, which develop as a response to myocardial injury and increased LV wall stress.[11–16] In addition to hemodynamic load, neurohormonal activation is another relevant determinant of cardiac remodeling.

The etiology of cardiac remodeling is heterogeneous; it can represent physiologic adaptation as seen in professional athletes, but is predominantly caused by pathologic conditions that lead to pressure or volume overload (such as arterial hypertension or aortic stenosis and valvular regurgitation, respectively) as well as conditions leading to primary myocardial involvement, such as myocardial infarction, inflammatory or infiltrative heart muscle diseases, or idiopathic dilated cardiomyopathy.[12] The main purpose of the remodeling process achieved by gradual LV dilatation is preservation of the SV despite a significantly impaired LVEF.[17] Although this pathophysiologic adaptation is ultimately associated with an increased risk of adverse events and death, decreased filling pressures within the dilated LV contribute to a delayed occurrence of HF symptoms.[17,18]

In volume overload (eg, valvular regurgitation), an increase in end-diastolic wall stress induces serial myocyte hypertrophy, leading to eccentric LV hypertrophy and LV cavity dilatation, thus enabling the preservation of SV.[19] With sustained volume overload, as a result of excessive LV enlargement, LV geometry changes from an elongated shape to a more globular one, thus causing further increase in local wall stress, ultimately leading to LV fibrosis

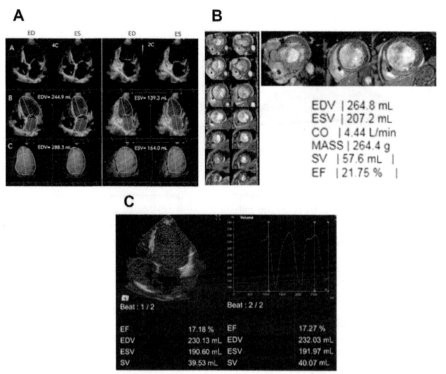

Fig. 1. (*A–C*) Comparison of 2-dimensional (2D), contrast, and 3-dimensional (3D) echocardiography with cardiac magnetic resonance (CMR) measured left ventricular (LV) volumes and ejection fraction (EF). (*A*). Two-dimensional echocardiography of left ventricular volumes and EF. 2D of echocardiographic apical 4-chamber and 2-chamber views in end diastole (ED) and end systole (ES). The noncontrast ED and ES volumes in (*B*) are smaller than the corresponding volumes in (*C*), which shows contrast echocardiography. The contrast fills the LV trabeculations so that the calculated volumes are closer to the CMR volumes. The LV EF in noncontrast and contrast was 25.3% and 17.1%, respectively. (*B*) CMR volumes from the patient in (*A*). The LV volumes using serial short axis cut planes of the LV (*left*) showed greater volumes than noncontrast 2D echocardiography and contrast echocardiography (although this was closer to CMR volumes). The LV EF was comparable by all 3 methods. The exclusion of papillary muscles, variable inclusion of LV outflow tract and inclusion of the trabeculae in the CMR approach all contribute to the differences in volumes by echocardiography and CMR. (*C*) A 3D echocardiographic image of the LV from the patient in (*A*). The volumes are bigger than 2D noncontrast volumes but smaller than contrast volumes, because 3D echocardiography tracks the trabeculated endocardium in the absence of contrast. The 3D volumes have been shown to better correlate with CMR volumes, although the use of contrast with 3D imaging may further improve this correlation. CO, cardiac output; EDV, ED volume; ESV, ES volume; EF, ejection fraction; SV, stroke volume.

and a decrease in the SV.[5,10] In pressure overload conditions (eg, arterial hypertension, aortic stenosis), an increase in peak systolic wall stress induces parallel sarcomere replication, leading to concentric LV hypertrophy, thus decreasing systolic wall stress at early stages of LV remodeling and preserving cardiac output.[15,19] Pathologic LV remodeling process in patients after myocardial infarction represent a combination of volume (infarcted zone) and pressure (noninfarcted zone) load, which results in the combination of concentric and eccentric hypertrophy.[15] In response to pressure load and loss of contractile elements within the infarcted zone, the later phase of LV dilatation and hypertrophy can continue for months and even years.[17,20,21] Beside routinely

used echocardiographic parameters of LV remodeling, such as LV volumes, size, and mass, the initial impairment in systolic function described as a decrease in the longitudinal systolic function, most often observed in pressure overload conditions, is frequently underestimated owing to increased compensatory circumferential contraction, which may ultimately result in a normal LVEF[5,19] (**Fig. 3**).

SHORTCOMINGS OF VOLUME-BASED QUANTIFICATION OF LEFT VENTRICULAR SIZE AND EJECTION FRACTION

Several main limitations of volume-based parameters of LV size and function should be pointed out

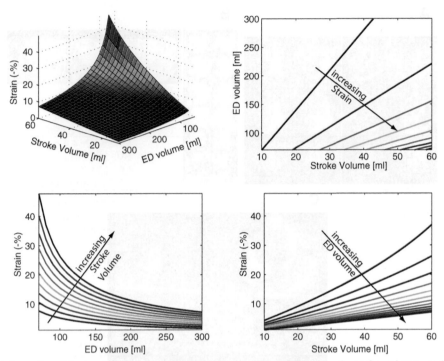

Fig. 2. Relation of ventricular size expressed as end-diastolic volume (ED volume), stroke volume, and deformation expressed as strain. (*From* Bijnens B, Cikes M, Butakoff C, et al. Myocardial motion and deformation: what does it tell us and how does it relate to function? Fetal Diagn Ther 2012;32(1–2):10; with permission.)

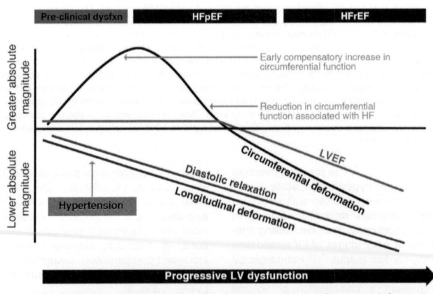

Fig. 3. The interplay of different components of cardiac function and their influence on left ventricular ejection fraction (LVEF). In the example of untreated arterial hypertension as underlying etiology of heart failure, the transition from heart failure with preserved ejection fraction (HFpEF) to heart failure with reduced ejection fraction (HFrEF) is described through the onset of LV dysfunction recognized as reduced longitudinal shortening with a compensatory increase in circumferential shortening with still preserved LVEF. An impairment in LVEF and the concurrent transition from HFpEF to HFrEF occurs upon impairment in circumferential deformation. (*From* Cikes M, Solomon SD. Beyond ejection fraction: an integrative approach for assessment of cardiac structure and function in heart failure. Eur Heart J 2016;37(21):1647; with permission.)

and taken into consideration when using these measurements. Unlike tomographic techniques such as cMRI or 3D echocardiography, 2-dimensional echocardiography is based on postulations on LV shape according to which it attempts to estimate a 3D volume.[22] One of the shortcomings closely bound to this limitation is that of LV foreshortening; others include poor image quality, and in particular high intraobserver and interobserver variability, even between different imaging modalities.[7,22]

Changes in LV volumes are the result of the overall LV deformation, thus representing global LVEF, amalgamating different components of LV deformation (such as longitudinal and circumferential deformation). This implies that any regional variability is averaged out in measurements of the LVEDV and the LVESV, and that different components of LV deformation cannot be assessed individually, nor can information on the mechanism of changes in volumes be obtained.[5] Moreover, it should be kept in mind that changes in the LVEF are not always related to changes in contractility (**Table 1**).

Finally, although LVEF represents a very powerful predictor of adverse outcomes as well as a predictor of the effects of HF treatments when less than 45%,[3,4,23] it was not shown to be useful as a prognosticator in patients with higher LVEF values[23,24] (**Fig. 4**). Furthermore, its correlation with the severity of HF symptoms is poor.[3–5] For example, a patient with HFpEF can have much more pronounced HF symptoms than one with HFrEF; even within the HFrEF population, symptom severity can vary by several New York Heart Association functional classes, irrespective of similar LVEF values (**Fig. 5**, Video 1).

THE IMPLICATIONS OF LEFT VENTRICULAR SIZE AND EJECTION FRACTION FOR THE MANAGEMENT OF HEART FAILURE PATIENTS
Heart Failure with Reduced Ejection Fraction

Despite heterogeneous etiologies of LV dysfunction in HFrEF, LV volumes and particularly LVEF are often used as robust diagnostic and prognostic variables. Importantly, the availability of

Table 1
Relationship between LV volumes, LVEF, and contractility in several clinical examples

LVEDV	LVESV	LVEF	Contractility	Clinical Example
←→/↑	↑/↑↑	↘	↑	Athletes (some cases)
↘	↘	↘	↑	Tachycardia, dobutamine
↑↑	←→/↑	↑	↘	Volume overload (mitral regurgitation, aortic regurgitation)
↘	↘↘	↑	↘	Pressure overload (hypertension, aortic stenosis), HCM
↘	↘	↘	←→	RV failure (decreased LV preload)
←→	←→	←→	↘	Acute MI (some cases)
↑↑	↑↑	↘↘	↘↘	Ischemic/dilated cardiomyopathy

As a ratio of LV volumes, the LVEF reflects the changes in these load-sensitive parameters, but does not always reflect change in LV contractility.

Abbreviations: HCM, hypertrophic cardiomyopathy; LV, left ventricular; LVEDV, left ventricular end-diastolic volume; LVEDV, left ventricular end-systolic volume; LVEF, left ventricular ejection fraction; MI, myocardial infarction; RV, right ventricular.

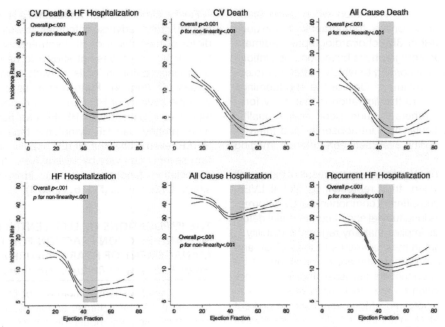

Fig. 4. The association between ejection fraction as a continuous variable and the outcomes of the CHARM trial. CV, cardiovascular; HF, heart failure. (*From* Lund LH, Claggett B, Liu J, et al. Heart failure with mid-range ejection fraction in CHARM: characteristics, outcomes and effect of candesartan across the entire ejection fraction spectrum. Eur J Heart Fail 2018;20(8):1234; with permission.)

evidence-based therapies for CHF is still determined by LVEF cutoff values; clinically proven treatments are shown to decrease morbidity and mortality only in HFrEF, but not in patients with HFpEF.[1,16,25,26] Beside improvement in survival rates and reduced incidence of adverse cardiovascular events, reverse remodeling in HFrEF is considered as one of the goals of CHF treatment, as well as a safe guide for investigation of novel HF treatments.[12,16,26–33] Relevant knowledge on LV remodeling and its reversal in HFrEF stems from numerous randomized, controlled trials of medications established as disease-modifying agents in this patient population.

The echocardiographic substudy of the Studies of Ventricular Enlargement (SAVE) trial assessed the effect of captopril on LV enlargement and its influence on clinical outcomes in patients with LV dysfunction after acute myocardial infarction. LV systolic area and percent of change in LV area were strong predictors of cardiovascular mortality and adverse cardiovascular events, regardless of the treatment arm.[12,20] Interestingly, although diabetic patients within the same study population developed HF significantly more often than nondiabetic patients, after adjusting for history of hypertension, prior myocardial infarction, age, treatment group, and smoking, diabetes was not associated with greater LV enlargement 2 years after

myocardial infarction.[18] On the contrary, diabetic patients had higher LV wall thickness and consequently higher LV filling pressures, leading to a faster onset of symptoms of HF.[18] Long-term treatment with angiotensin-converting enzyme inhibitors in patients with HFrEF with asymptomatic LV systolic dysfunction investigated in the Studies of Left Ventricular Dysfunction (SOLVD) Prevention Trial showed significant reduction in LV volumes together with lower incidence of symptomatic HF, thus further emphasizing the importance of reversing the remodeling process by timely initiation of HF treatment.[27,34]

In the VALsartan In Acute myocardial iNfarcTion (VALIANT) echocardiographic substudy, in patients with an LVEF 35% or less, symptomatic HF, or both after myocardial infarction, the impact of abnormal LV geometry, defined by an interplay between the LV mass index (LVMi) and relative wall thickness (RWT), on clinical outcomes was established. Patients with concentric remodeling (normal LVMi, increased RWT), eccentric hypertrophy (increased LVMi, normal RWT), and particularly those with concentric hypertrophy (increased LVMi and RWT) were all at increased risk of cardiovascular morbidity and mortality, even after adjusting for relevant covariates.[35]

Multiple randomized clinical trials have demonstrated additional benefits of beta-blockers when

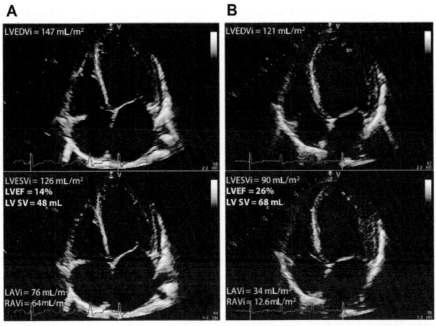

Fig. 5. Apical 4-chamber views from 2 patients with dilated cardiomyopathy (DCM) and low left ventricular ejection fractions (LVEFs), but different stroke volumes (SVs) and symptoms. (*A*) End-diastolic frame (*top*) and end-systolic frame (*bottom*) from a patient with DCM, New York Heart Association functional class IV, referred for left ventricular assist device implantation. The LV volume indices, measured by the biplane method, indicate severe LV dilation. The calculated SV is reduced, as is the LV ejection fraction. Both atria are also severely enlarged, and the LV filling pattern suggested restrictive hemodynamics. (*B*) End-diastolic (*top*) and end-systolic (*bottom*) frames from a patient with DCM and New York Heart Association functional class II, in regular outpatient follow-up for chronic heart failure. The LV volume indices, measured by the biplane method, also indicate severe LV dilation. The calculated SV, however, is preserved, while the ejection fraction by Simpson's biplane method is reduced. In this patient, there was only mild to moderate left atrial enlargement and second-grade diastolic dysfunction. See Video 1 for the corresponding moving images. LAVi, left atrial volume index; LVEDVi, left ventricular end diastolic volume index; LVESVi, left ventricular end systolic volume index; RAVi, right atrial volume index. (*Modified from* Cikes M. Dilated cardiomyopathies. In: Solomon SD, Wu J, Gillam L, editors. Essential echocardiography: a companion to Braunwald's heart disease. Philadelphia, PA: Elsevier; 2018. p. 220; with permission.)

added to standard chronic HF therapy.[36–40] The reduction in all-cause mortality has been proven both by bisoprolol and metoprolol in patients with CHF. More insight on LV remodeling has been based on combination treatment by angiotensin-converting enzyme inhibitors and carvedilol: a significant decrease in LVEDVi and LVESVi and improvement in LVEF has been shown, compared with angiotensin-converting enzyme inhibitor treatment alone.[41]

Although an animal model of the effects of the mineralocorticoid receptor antagonist eplerenone in the postinfarction setting suggested a significant increase in LVEF and decrease in LV volumes after 3 months of treatment,[42] prospective randomized trials provided inconsistent data on the effects of mineralocorticoid receptor antagonists on LV remodeling.[43] One of the more recent trials (Eplerenone Post-acute myocardial infarction Heart failure Efficacy and SUrvival Study [EPHESUS]) did not confirm the occurrence of reverse LV remodeling after 36 weeks of eplerenone treatment.[44]

Heart Failure with Preserved Ejection Fraction

Owing to the distinct limitation of LVEF as a measure of cardiac remodeling, as well as a predictor of adverse outcomes in HFpEF,[45] LV geometry has been investigated as a possible predictor of adverse cardiovascular outcomes in patients with preserved LVEF.[35,46,47] In 935 patients with HFpEF with a LVEF of 45% or greater enrolled in Treatment of Preserved Cardiac Function Heart Failure with an Aldosterone Antagonist Trial (TOPCAT), a high prevalence of concentric LV remodeling and hypertrophy, LA enlargement, and pulmonary hypertension was observed, although neither LV volumes nor LVEF were associated with higher risk for the primary composite end point (HF hospitalization, aborted sudden death, or cardiovascular death) in the univariable Cox model analysis.[47] Furthermore, a significant association between LV mass, LV geometry, left atrial area, diastolic dysfunction, right ventricular systolic pressure, and the occurrence of the primary composite end point of all-cause death or cardiovascular hospitalization was reported in the univariate analysis among patients included in the echocardiographic substudy of the Irbesartan in Heart Failure With Preserved Ejection Fraction (I-PRESERVE) trial.[46] However, only LV mass and left atrial size remained independently related to an increased risk of morbidity and mortality.[46]

Heart Failure with Midrange Ejection Fraction

HFmrEF, a recently introduced subgroup of patients with an LVEF between 40% and 49%, accounts for nearly 20% of the HF population.[48] Stimulating research into the underlying characteristics, pathophysiology and treatment was pointed out as the main aim of identifying HFmrEF as a separate subgroup of patients with HF.[1] However, the high variability of LVEF measurements, even more pronounced when assessed by different imaging modalities (>5% in approximately 50% of patients),[7] raises concern about the need for further subclassification of the HF population based on LVEF, particularly with such narrow boundaries.

Although the pathophysiological and etiologic differences between HFpEF and HFrEF are well-established,[49] patients with HFmrEF seem to be similar to those with HFrEF with respect to ischemic etiology, as demonstrated in the analysis of the 42,987 patients with HF included in the Swedish Heart Failure registry, in which the percentage of ischemic heart disease was 60% for HFrEF, 61% for HFmrEF, and 52% for HFpEF.[50] Likewise, in 9134 patients in the European Society of Cardiology Heart Failure Long-Term Registry, ischemic etiology was confirmed in 48.6% of patients with HFrEF, 41.8% of patients with HFmrEF, but only in 23.7% of patients with HFpEF.[51] Ischemic heart disease is also relevant in mediating the transition of patients with HF across the LVEF spectrum—an accelerated transition of those with HFpEF to lower LVEF categories and lack of significant LVEF recovery in patients with HFrEF.[52] Indeed, these dynamic transitions among the HF subgroups have been documented: in an analysis of 3480 consecutive patients with HF included in Chronic Heart Failure Analysis and Registry in the Tohoku District-2 (CHART-2), patients with HFmrEF transitioned to HFpEF and HFrEF by 44% and 16% at 1 year, and 45% and 21% at 3 years.[53] The changes in LV geometry in

HFmrEF seem to be intermediate between the other 2 HF subgroups, that is, lying between eccentric remodeling more typical for patients with HFrEF and concentric remodeling mainly occurring in HFrEF.[54]

The efficacy of pharmacotherapies in HFmrEF was observed through secondary analyses of several major clinical trials.[53,55–57] The Candesartan in Heart Failure: Assessment of Reduction in Mortality and Morbidity (CHARM) trial and showed a significant reduction in cardiovascular death or HF hospitalization in patients with an LVEF up to around 50%.[55] In the observational CHART-2 study, therapy with beta-blockers was associated with improved survival in patients with HFmrEF and patients with HFrEF, but not in patients with HFpEF.[53] Although the effect of spironolactone in patients with an LVEF of 45% or greater enrolled in the TOPCAT trial did not decrease the incidence of primary outcome of HF hospitalization, cardiovascular death, or aborted cardiac arrest,[56] patients at the lower end of the EF spectrum (LVEF between 45% and 50%) were more likely to benefit from spironolactone with respect to the primary end point and HF hospitalization.[57]

NOVEL MEASURES OF CARDIAC FUNCTION AND THEIR USEFULNESS IN THE MANAGEMENT OF HEART FAILURE

Normal myocardial deformation is defined by balanced contraction of 3 main myocardial layers: endocardial and epicardial longitudinal fibers, and the midmyocardial circumferential fibers.[19,22] In various conditions, most typically LV remodeling owing to pressure overload and HFpEF, early myocardial dysfunction manifests as a decrease in longitudinal function, whereas increased circumferential function often serves as compensatory mechanism thus maintaining a normal global LV function, predominantly defined by LVEF[19,22,58] (see Fig. 3). Paralleling the increasing awareness of multiple limitations of LVEF, additional echocardiographic modalities, such as Doppler myocardial imaging or speckle-tracking echocardiography, are entering the clinical arena, enabling the assessment of specific components of LV deformation and regional myocardial dysfunction, which is particularly suited for the detection of early stages of HF.[58,59]

In the VALIANT echocardiography substudy of patients with high-risk myocardial infarction, circumferential strain rate was predictive of reverse remodeling (defined as a ≥15% increase in the ESV from baseline to 20 months), thus highlighting its compensatory function in maintaining normal cardiac output and LVEF, whereas both

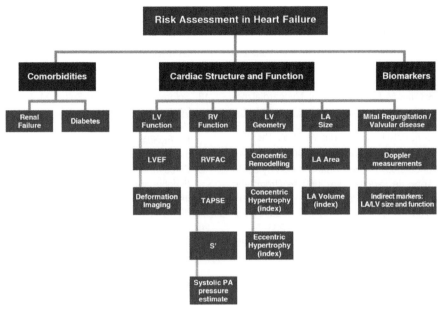

Fig. 6. An integrated approach to the assessment of risk in heart failure, beyond LVEF alone. LA, left atrial; LV, left ventricular; LVEF, left ventricular ejection fraction; PA, pulmonary artery; RV, right ventricular; RVFAC, right ventricular fractional area change; S', tissue Doppler-derived tricuspid lateral annular systolic velocity; TAPSE, tricuspid annular plane systolic excursion.

longitudinal and circumferential strain rate were predictors of adverse outcomes after myocardial infarction, independent of LVEF.[59]

Data from the PARAMOUNT trial showed high prevalence of reduced longitudinal strain (in 66.7% of patients) and circumferential strain (in 40.4% patients) among patients with HFpEF, with significantly decrease values of longitudinal strain and circumferential strain compared with normal controls and age- and sex-matched patients with diagnosis of arterial hypertension, accompanied by the evidence of diastolic dysfunction.[58] Decreased longitudinal strain was independently associated with higher LVESVi, LVEDVi, and LVMi, and higher N-terminal pro b-type natriuretic peptide levels, thus emphasizing its negative predictive value in this subgroup of patients with HF.[58]

SUMMARY

Despite the rapid development of emerging imaging technologies, LVEF still represents the cornerstone of diagnosis, choice of treatment, and prognosis in patients with HF. However, predominantly owing to its high load dependence, true myocardial function often remains underestimated or overestimated in different conditions underlying the heterogeneous syndrome of HF.

Reverse remodeling is one of the main goals of treatment in HF, aimed at halting or attenuating

the progression of the disease. The lack of effective therapeutic approaches in nearly one-half of the HF population (those with preserved LVEF) highlights the need for the integration of novel echocardiographic measures to better understand the underlying pathophysiological mechanism, whereas an integrated approach to the assessment of risk in patients with HF requires an integration of various echocardiographic attributes of cardiac structure and function with relevant clinical parameters (**Fig. 6**).

SUPPLEMENTARY DATA

Supplementary data related to this article can be found online at https://doi.org/10.1016/j.hfc. 2018.12.012.

REFERENCES

1. Ponikowski P, Voors AA, Anker SD, et al. ESC Guidelines for the diagnosis and treatment of acute and chronic heart failure. Eur J Heart Fail 2016;18(8): 891–975.
2. Butler J, Fonarow GC, Zile MR, et al. Developing therapies for heart failure with preserved ejection fraction: current state and future directions. JACC Heart Fail 2014;2:97–112.
3. Kramer DG, Trikalinos TA, Kent DM, et al. Quantitative evaluation of drug or device effects on Ventricular remodeling as predictors of therapeutic effects

on mortality in patients with heart failure and reduced ejection fraction: a meta-analytic approach. J Am Coll Cardiol 2010;56(5):392–406.

4. Konstam MA, Udelson JE, Anand IS, et al. Ventricular remodeling in heart failure: a credible surrogate end point. J Card Fail 2003;9:350–3.

5. Bijnens B, Cikes M, Butakoff C, et al. Myocardial motion and deformation: what does it tell us and how does it relate to function? Fetal Diagn Ther 2012; 32(1–2):5–16.

6. Lang RM, Badano LP, Mor-Avi V, et al. Recommendations for cardiac chamber quantification by echocardiography in adults: an update from the American Society of Echocardiography and the European Association of Cardiovascular Imaging. Eur Heart J Cardiovasc Imaging 2015;16(3):233–70.

7. Pellikka PA, She L, Holly TA, et al. Variability in ejection fraction measured by echocardiography, gated single-photon emission computed tomography, and cardiac magnetic resonance in patients with coronary artery disease and left ventricular dysfunction. JAMA Netw Open 2018;1(4):e181456.

8. Dorosz JL, Lezotte DC, Weitzenkamp DA, et al. Performance of 3-dimensional echocardiography in measuring left ventricular volumes and ejection fraction: a systematic review and metaanalysis. J Am Coll Cardiol 2012;59(20):1799–808.

9. Wood PW, Choy JB, Nanda NC, et al. Left ventricular ejection fraction and volumes: it depends on the imaging method. Echocardiography 2014;31(1): 87–100.

10. Cikes M. Dilated cardiomyopathies. In: Solomon SD, Wu J, Gillam LD, editors. Braunwald's heart disease essential echocardiography: a companion to Braunwald's heart disease. 1st edition. Philadelphia: Elsevier Health Science; 2018. p. 223–33.

11. Cohn JN, Johnson G, Ziesche S, et al. A comparison of enalapril with hydralazine-isosorbide dinitrate in the treatment of chronic congestive heart failure. N Engl J Med 1991;325(5):303–10.

12. Cohn JN, Ferrari R, Sharpe N. Cardiac remodeling–concepts and clinical implications: a consensus paper from an international forum on cardiac remodeling. Behalf of an International Forum on Cardiac Remodeling. J Am Coll Cardiol 2000;35(3):569–82.

13. McKay RG, Pfeffer MA, Pasternak RC, et al. Left ventricular remodeling after myocardial infarction: a corollary to infarct expansion. Circulation 1986; 74(4):693–702.

14. Patten RD, Konstam MA. Ventricular remodeling and the renin angiotensin aldosterone system. Congest Heart Fail 2000;6(4):187–92.

15. Opie LH, Commerford PJ, Gersh BJ, et al. Controversies in ventricular remodelling. Lancet 2006; 367(9507):356–67.

16. Konstam MA, Kramer DG, Patel AR, et al. Left ventricular remodeling in heart failure: current concepts in clinical significance and assessment. JACC Cardiovasc Imaging 2011;4(1):98–108.

17. Pfeffer MA, Braunwald E. Ventricular remodeling after myocardial infarction. Experimental observations and clinical implications. Circulation 1990;81(4): 1161–72.

18. Solomon SD, St John Sutton M, Lamas GA, et al. Ventricular remodeling does not accompany the development of heart failure in diabetic patients after myocardial infarction. Circulation 2002;106(10): 1251–5.

19. Cikes M, Sutherland GR, Anderson LJ, et al. The role of echocardiographic deformation imaging in hypertrophic myopathies. Nat Rev Cardiol 2010;7(7): 384–96.

20. St John Sutton M, Pfeffer MA, Plappert T, et al. Quantitative two-dimensional echocardiographic measurements are major predictors of adverse cardiovascular events after acute myocardial infarction. The protective effects of captopril. Circulation 1994;89(1):68–75.

21. Olivetti G, Capasso JM, Sonnenblick EH, et al. Side-to-side slippage of myocytes participates in ventricular wall remodeling acutely after myocardial infarction in rats. Circ Res 1990;67(1):23–34.

22. Cikes M, Solomon SD. Beyond ejection fraction: an integrative approach for assessment of cardiac structure and function in heart failure. Eur Heart J 2016;37(21):1642–50.

23. Solomon SD, Anavekar N, Skali H, et al. Influence of ejection fraction on cardiovascular outcomes in a broad spectrum of heart failure patients. Circulation 2005;112(24):3738–44.

24. Udelson JE, Konstam MA. Relation between left ventricular remodeling and clinical outcomes in heart failure patients with left ventricular systolic dysfunction. J Card Fail 2002;8(Suppl):465–71.

25. Granger CB, McMurray JJ, Yusuf S, et al. Effects of candesartan in patients with chronic heart failure and reduced left-ventricular systolic function intolerant to angiotensin-converting-enzyme inhibitors: the CHARM- Alternative trial. Lancet 2003;362: 772–6.

26. McMurray JJ, Ostergren J, Swedberg K, et al. Effects of candesartan in patients with chronic heart failure and reduced left-ventricular systolic function taking angiotensin-converting- enzyme inhibitors: the CHARM-Added trial. Lancet 2003;362:767–71.

27. Konstam MA, Kronenberg MW, Rousseau MF, et al. Effects of the angiotensin converting enzyme inhibitor enalapril on the long-term progression of left ventricular dilatation in patients with asymptomatic systolic dysfunction. SOLVD (Studies of Left Ventricular Dysfunction) Investigators. Circulation 1993;88: 2277–83.

28. Solomon SD, Skali H, Anavekar NS, et al. Changes in ventricular size and function in patients treated

with valsartan, captopril, or both after myocardial infarction. Circulation 2005;111:3411–9.

29. Greenberg B, Quinones MA, Koilpillai C, et al. Effects of long-term enalapril therapy on cardiac structure and function in patients with left ventricular dysfunction. Results of the SOLVD echocardiography substudy. Circulation 1995;91:2573–81.

30. Pfeffer MA, Braunwald E, Moye LA, et al. Effect of captopril on mortality and morbidity in patients with left ventricular dysfunction after myocardial infarction. Results of the survival and ventricular enlargement trial. The SAVE Investigators. N Engl J Med 1992;327:669–77.

31. Wong M, Johnson G, Shabetai R, et al. Echocardiographic variables as prognostic indicators and therapeutic monitors in chronic congestive heart failure. Veterans Affairs cooperative studies V-HeFT I and II. V-HeFT VA Cooperative Studies Group. Circulation 1993;87(Suppl):VI65–70.

32. Wong M, Staszewsky L, Latini R, et al. Severity of left ventricular remodeling defines outcomes and response to therapy in heart failure: Valsartan Heart Failure Trial (Val-HeFT) echocardiographic data. J Am Coll Cardiol 2004;43:2022–7.

33. Shah AM, Shah SJ, Anand IS, et al. Cardiac structure and function in heart failure with preserved ejection fraction: baseline findings from the echocardiographic study of the Treatment of Preserved Cardiac Function Heart Failure with an Aldosterone Antagonist trial. Circ Heart Fail 2014;7(1):104–15.

34. SOLVD Investigators, Yusuf S, Pitt B, Davis CE, et al. Effect of enalapril on mortality and the development of heart failure in asymptomatic patients with reduced left ventricular ejection fractions. N Engl J Med 1992;327(10):685–91.

35. Verma A, Meris A, Skali H, et al. Prognostic implications of left ventricular mass and geometry following myocardial infarction: the VALIANT (VALsartan In Acute myocardial iNfarcTion) Echocardiographic Study. JACC Cardiovasc Imaging 2008;1(5):582–91.

36. Packer M, Bristow MR, Cohn JN, et al. The effect of carvedilol on morbidity and mortality in patients with chronic heart failure. U.S. Carvedilol Heart Failure Study Group. N Engl J Med 1996;334(21):1349–55.

37. The Cardiac Insufficiency Bisoprolol Study II (CIBIS-II): a randomised trial. Lancet 1999;353(9146):9–13.

38. Effect of metoprolol CR/XL in chronic heart failure: Metoprolol CR/XL Randomised Intervention Trial in Congestive Heart Failure (MERIT-HF). Lancet 1999;353(9169):2001–7.

39. A randomized trial of beta-blockade in heart failure. The Cardiac Insufficiency Bisoprolol Study (CIBIS). CIBIS Investigators and Committees. Circulation 1994;90(4):1765–73.

40. Bristow MR, Gilbert EM, Abraham WT, et al. Carvedilol produces dose-related improvements in left ventricular function and survival in subjects with chronic heart failure. Circulation 1996;94:2807–16.

41. Australia/New Zealand Heart Failure Research Collaborative Group. Randomised, placebo-controlled trial of carvedilol in patients with congestive heart failure due to ischaemic heart disease. Lancet 1997;349(9049):375–80.

42. Suzuki G, Morita H, Mishima T, et al. Effects of long-term monotherapy with eplerenone, a novel aldosterone blocker, on progression of left ventricular dysfunction and remodeling in dogs with heart failure. Circulation 2002;106:2967–72.

43. Zannad F, Gattis Stough W, Rossignol P, et al. Mineralocorticoid receptor antagonists for heart failure with reduced ejection fraction: integrating evidence into clinical practice. Eur Heart J 2012;33(22):2782–95.

44. Udelson JE, Feldman AM, Greenberg B, et al. Randomized, double-blind, multicenter, placebo-controlled study evaluating the effect of aldosterone antagonism with eplerenone on ventricular remodeling in patients with mild-to-moderate heart failure and left ventricular systolic dysfunction. Circ Heart Fail 2010;3:347–53.

45. Solomon SD, Wang D, Finn P, et al. Effect of candesartan on cause-specific mortality in heart failure patients: the Candesartan in Heart failure Assessment of Reduction in Mortality and morbidity (CHARM) Program. Circulation 2004;110:2180–3.

46. Zile MR, Gottdiener JS, Hetzel SJ, et al. Prevalence and significance of alterations in cardiac structure and function in patients with heart failure and a preserved ejection fraction. Circulation 2011;124(23):2491–501.

47. Shah AM, Claggett B, Sweitzer NK, et al. Cardiac structure and function and prognosis in heart failure with preserved ejection fraction: findings from the echocardiographic study of the Treatment of Preserved Cardiac Function Heart Failure with an Aldosterone Antagonist (TOPCAT) Trial. Circ Heart Fail 2014;7(5):740–51.

48. Nauta JF, Hummel YM, van Melle JP, et al. What have we learned about heart failure with mid-range ejection fraction one year after its introduction? Eur J Heart Fail 2017;19(12):1569–73.

49. Paulus WJ, Tschöpe C. A novel paradigm for heart failure with preserved ejection fraction: comorbidities drive myocardial dysfunction and remodeling through coronary microvascular endothelial inflammation. J Am Coll Cardiol 2013;62:263–71.

50. Vedin O, Lam CS, Koh AS, et al. Significance of ischemic heart disease in patients with heart failure and preserved, midrange, and reduced ejection fraction: a nationwide cohort study. Circ Heart Fail 2017;10(6) [pii:e003875].

51. Chioncel O, Lainscak M, Seferovic PM, et al. Epidemiology and one-year outcomes in patients with

chronic heart failure and preserved, mid-range and reduced ejection fraction: an analysis of the ESC Heart Failure Long-Term Registry. Eur J Heart Fail 2017;19(12):1574–85.

52. Dunlay SM, Roger VL, Weston SA, et al. Longitudinal changes in ejection fraction in heart failure patients with preserved and reduced ejection fraction. Circ Heart Fail 2012;5:720–6.

53. Tsuji K, Sakata Y, Nochioka K, et al. Characterization of heart failure patients with mid-range left ventricular ejection fraction-a report from the CHART-2 Study. Eur J Heart Fail 2017;19(10):1258–69.

54. Rickenbacher P, Kaufmann BA, Maeder MT, et al. Heart failure with mid-range ejection fraction: a distinct clinical entity? Insights from the Trial of Intensified versus standard Medical therapy in Elderly patients with Congestive Heart Failure (TIME-CHF). Eur J Heart Fail 2017;19(12):1586–96.

55. Lund LH, Claggett B, Liu J, et al. Heart failure with mid-range ejection fraction in CHARM: characteristics, outcomes and effect of candesartan across the entire ejection fraction spectrum. Eur J Heart Fail 2018; 20(8):1230–9.

56. Pitt B, Pfeffer MA, Assmann SF, et al. Spironolactone for heart failure with preserved ejection fraction. N Engl J Med 2014;370:1383–92.

57. Solomon SD, Claggett B, Lewis EF, et al. Influence of ejection fraction on outcomes and efficacy of spironolactone in patients with heart failure with preserved ejection fraction. Eur Heart J 2016;37(5): 455–62.

58. Kraigher-Krainer E, Shah AM, Gupta DK, et al. Impaired systolic function by strain imaging in heart failure with preserved ejection fraction. J Am Coll Cardiol 2014;63(5):447–56.

59. Hung CL, Verma A, Uno H, et al. Longitudinal and circumferential strain rate, left ventricular remodeling, and prognosis after myocardial infarction. J Am Coll Cardiol 2010;56(22): 1812–22.

Left Ventricular Mass and Thickness: Why Does It Matter?

Frank Lloyd Dini, MD, FESC[a],*, Gian Giacomo Galeotti, MD[a], Giuseppe Terlizzese, MD[a], Iacopo Fabiani, MD, PhD[a,b], Nicola Riccardo Pugliese, MD[a,b], Ilaria Rovai, MD[a]

KEYWORDS

- Hypertrophy • Left ventricular mass • Heart failure • Ventricular dysfunction

KEY POINTS

- In nondilated ventricles, left ventricular geometric patterns are classified according to whether left ventricular mass is normal or increased and whether relative wall thickness is above or below 0.42.
- In dilated ventricles, eccentric remodeling is characterized by normal left ventricular mass and reduced relative wall thickness (<0.32), whereas eccentric hypertrophy is depicted by an increased left ventricular mass and a reduced relative wall thickness (<0.32).
- In nondilated ventricles, the highest risk of adverse outcome is in patients with left ventricular concentric hypertrophy.
- Among patients with heart failure, dilated ventricles, and reduced ejection fraction, eccentric hypertrophy portends the worst prognosis.

BACKGROUND

Myocardial hypertrophy has been considered a compensatory mechanism that allows the heart to adapt to increased workload. The adaptive nature of this response was clearly shown in the 1960s, when overload-induced hypertrophy was found to normalize wall stress in the hearts of patients with cardiac valve disease.[1–3] Physiologic left ventricular (LV) hypertrophy (LVH) typically occurs in the athlete's heart and regresses on reduction or cessation of physical activity, whereas pathologic LVH may be the result of a variety of cardiac disease states. The development of pathologic LVH, although initially beneficial, because it permits the heart to maintain cardiac pump function normal despite abnormal pressure or volume load, ultimately may be associated with a depression of the intrinsic contractile state of the myocardium.[4,5]

Pathologic hypertrophy initially was divided into 2 phenotypes: concentric hypertrophy, where LV wall thickness is increased without a corresponding increase in ventricular size, and eccentric hypertrophy, where the ventricle is enlarged and wall thickness is normal or reduced. Subtypes of hypertrophy are very much influenced by the manner in which the overload has occurred. Concentric hypertrophy typically develops when the left ventricle is submitted to a sustained and increased pressure overload, such as occurs in aortic stenosis. Eccentric LVH is seen characteristically in volume-overloaded hearts.[6] After myocardial infarction, there may be hypertrophy of the viable myocardium.[7,8]

The concept of LV remodeling was defined in the early 1990s as the changes in LV structure and volume occurring both acutely and chronically after myocardial infarction.[9,10] Since then, the concept has expanded to include all patients in whom the alterations in LV structure and geometry evolve after myocardial injury or primary or secondary myocardial disease and may comprise alterations in LV shape, LV dilation, and/or LVH.[11]

Disclosure: The authors have nothing to disclose.
Conflict of interest: none declared.
[a] Cardiac, Thoracic and Vascular Department, University of Pisa, Pisa, Italy; [b] Department of Surgical, Medical and Molecular Pathology and Critical Care Medicine, University of Pisa, Pisa, Italy
* Corresponding author. Cardiovascular Diseases Unit 1, Cardiac, Thoracic and Vascular Department, Azienda Universitaria Ospedaliera Pisana, Via Paradisa 2, Pisa 56124, Italy.
E-mail address: f.dini@ao-pisa.toscana.it

LVH is an integral constituent of the remodeling process, because it provides a basic mechanism that permits the heart to maintain cardiac pump function normal despite abnormal pressure or volume load. Nevertheless, it is also a marker for increased risk, suggesting that LVH may have maladaptive features.[12,13] In this clinical scenario, the adaptation is often incomplete, and, after variable periods, ventricular dilation occurs, resulting in a secondary increase in wall stress that seems to be a critical factor affecting development and progression of heart failure (HF).[14,15] As a result, an accurate determination of LV mass and wall thickness and their relationship with the remodeling process is crucial for the management of HF patients, given the clinical significance of these measures.

This review, therefore, addresses the following questions: (1) how to measure wall thickness, relative wall thickness (RWT), and LV mass and (2) the hemodynamic and prognostic impact of these measures in HF.

HOW TO MEASURE WALL THICKNESS, RELATIVE WALL THICKNESS, AND LEFT VENTRICULAR MASS

For the clinician, an increase in LV mass is the hallmark of LVH.[16] It can be estimated by measurements of LV dimension and wall thickness made with 2-D or M-mode echocardiograms, according to the formula of Devereux and colleagues.[17] The geometric patterns of LVH are traditionally classified based on ventricular weight (LV mass) and on the relation of wall thickness to chamber dimension (RWT).[18–20] LV mass is generally indexed for body surface area or height (LV mass index [LVMi]).[21]

3-D echocardiographic estimation of LV mass is the most accurate way to measure LV mass.[22] It has both a better correlation with cardiac magnetic resonance measurements and a better interobserver and intraobserver variability than 2-D and M-mode echocardiographic measurements (7% and 8% vs 37% and 19%, respectively).[23–26] The greatest limitations of this theoretically more accurate echocardiographic method are the need for high-quality images and the strong dependence on the equipment used (Fig. 1). The American Society of Echocardiography and the European Association of Cardiovascular Imaging recommendations define 3-D assessment of the LV mass as a promising technique, especially in remodeled, abnormally shaped ventricles and in cases of asymmetric or localized hypertrophy, but the available data are still insufficient to provide affordable reference values.[27]

RWT is calculated at end-diastole as the ratio of posterior wall thickness $\times$ 2 to LV end-diastolic diameter. Another formula used to assess RWT is the sum of interventricular septum thickness and posterior wall thickness in diastole divided by the end-diastolic diameter, also known as LV wall thickness–to–cavity radius, but the previously discussed method has been regarded as most reliable in case of asymmetric hypertrophy with a septal bulge.[21] The RWT allows categorization of 4 different LV geometric patterns: normal, concentric remodeling (normal LVMi and increased RWT), eccentric hypertrophy (increased LVMi and normal RWT), and concentric hypertrophy (increased LVMi and increased RWT).

The is no general agreement about the degree of LV mass that should indicate presence of LVH. Allocation of patients into categories of LV geometry can be made by reference to the new guidelines for the management of arterial hypertension, where LVH is assigned for values greater than or equal to 115 g/m^2 for men and greater than or equal to 95 g/m^2 for women.[28] A cutoff value for RWT of 0.42 generally is used to categorize geometric patterns,[29] even though the original cutoff used by Ganau and colleagues[20] was 0.44. Patients with normal LV mass can have either concentric remodeling (normal LV mass with increased RWT >0.42) or normal geometry (RWT <0.42), whereas patients with increased LV mass can have either concentric (RWT >0.42) or eccentric (RWT <0.42) hypertrophy.

Most of the initial studies on echocardiographic assessment of LVH have been performed predominantly in hypertensive patients in whom changes in LV shape and volume were limited.[20,30–32] The development of LVH is a complex process that can vary significantly in various cardiac conditions, resulting in different and more complex patterns of geometric remodeling. More recently, it has become apparent that LVH could exist in dilated and nondilated forms, regardless of LV geometry. The hallmarks of many cardiac diseases, especially ischemic or nonischemic dilated cardiomyopathies, are the presence of increased LV end-systolic and end-diastolic volumes in association with depressed LV ejection fraction (EF) and increased LV mass.

Trying to go beyond the simple but limitative classification of LV geometric patterns, discussed previously, Gaasch and Zile[33] have developed a new classification that is more inclusive of different geometric phenotypes that can be seen in both healthy and pathologic hearts. Their categorization of geometric abnormalities was based not only on RWT and mass but also on LV end-diastolic volume. Therefore, a normal end-diastolic volume

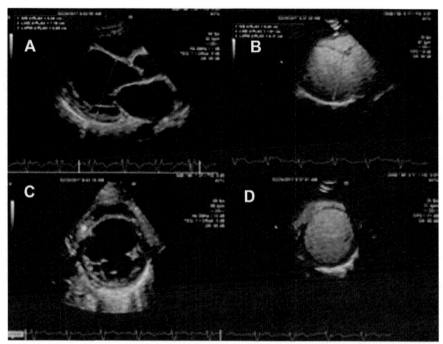

Fig. 1. Echocardiography for wall thickness measurement. (*A*) and (*C*) show parasternal long-axis and short-axis views of the LV in a patient with HF. These views are conventionally used to measure wall thickness (WT) and/or visually assess WT. Also, (*A*) is used to measure LV internal dimension in diastole (LVIDD) and systole. (*A*) The RWT is 0.89 × 2/7 .16 = 0.25. The same patient in (*B*) and (*D*) with contrast. The RWT is 0.37 × 2/7.61 = 0.01, a significant difference because of changes WT and LVIDD measurements. Contrast echo provides LV cavity measurements, which are much closer to CMR measurements, and this applies even to so-called good-quality echocardiograms.

and an increased RWT would be classified as concentric hypertrophy if LV mass is increased and as concentric remodeling if LV mass is normal. The term, *eccentric*, is applied exclusively to patterns with enlarged ventricles. Thus, eccentric phenotypes include those with physiologic hypertrophy, eccentric hypertrophy, and eccentric remodeling. Identification of patients with LV dilation and low RWT (<0.32 or <0.34) is also useful to further characterize patients with normal or hypertrophied ventricles into LV geometric patterns of eccentric LVH and eccentric remodeling.

THE HEMODYNAMIC AND PROGNOSTIC IMPACT OF HYPERTROPHY IN HEART FAILURE

It is well known that increased LV mass, dilation, and abnormal LV geometry are important markers of cardiovascular risk; however, although concentric hypertrophy carries the worst prognosis in hypertensive subjects[34–37] and in those with coronary artery disease,[35,38] there are strong data showing that an increase in LV mass is associated with increased mortality rates in patients with HF, LV enlargement, and low EF. In patients with LV dysfunction enrolled in the SOLVD

Registry and Trials, increasing levels of LVH were associated with adverse outcomes.[39]

The changes in ventricular size, shape, and volume taking place in HF have long been studied. Patients with HF and reduced EF (LVEF ≤40%) generally exhibit a remarkable LV enlargement. LVH is often present, typically eccentric, and frequently associated with a normal or lower than normal LV wall thickness. As LV volume increases, LV mass increases proportionally.[40] LV volume overload (eccentric) hypertrophy occurring with postinfarction LV remodeling is frequently indistinguishable from the geometric patterns that come about in other cardiac diseases, like dilated cardiomyopathy or advanced hypertensive heart disease.[11,41]

LV dysfunction and remodeling usually are the result of a progressive process that starts with a myocardial damage or excessive LV overload. In this setting, the LV chamber frequently dilates and becomes more spherical, with the development of a pattern of eccentric LVH in most of the cases. Chronic LV dilation may be temporarily compensatory because is a useful response to maintain stroke volume.[42,43] Augmenting cavity size may permit the ventricle to propel a much

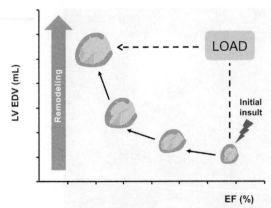

Fig. 2. LV dilation may be temporarily compensatory because it is a useful response to maintain stroke volume. This mechanism is especially apparent in a large spherical ventricle with poor EF, whose capacity of preserving stroke volume as well as CO depends on the size and shape of the ventricle. EDV, end-diastolic volume.

greater fraction of diastolic volume with the same amount of fiber shortening or to eject the same volume with a reduced degree of shortening (**Fig. 2**). This mechanism is especially apparent in large spherical ventricles with poor LVEF, whose capacity of preserving stroke volume as well as cardiac output (CO) depends on the size and shape of the ventricle. Because LV overload is initially matched by an adequate growth of cardiac myocytes, the chamber radius is increased and the wall thickness is increased moderately, but as the left ventricle further dilates this adaptive mechanism may progress to maladaptive eccentric (high-stress) LVH. Progressive ventricular dilatation may occur especially when hypertrophy cannot restore LV wall stress to normal.[44] Transition to failure is accompanied by progressive cavity enlargement and decline in wall thickness–to–cavity radius or RWT.[45] The association of increased LVMi and reduced RWT seems to represent an advanced stage of the disease, where maladaptive LV remodeling and wall thinning result from loss of contractile myocardium as a consequence of volume overload and energy starvation.[44] As the heart becomes no longer able to maintain its pumping function, CO finally declines. These considerations led the authors to investigate the prognostic significance of a geometric pattern characterized by a diminished RWT and an increased LVMi in patients (n = 536) with chronic HF, EF less than 50%, and LV end-diastolic volume greater than 91 mL/m². LVH was defined according to the cutoff values of severely increased LVMi: 148 g/m² in men and 122 g/m² in women.[22] As far as RWT is concerned, the cutoff value of 0.34 not only reflected the optimal threshold level for outcome prediction but also was closely associated with increased LV wall stress (**Fig. 3**). The results of this study showed an independent and incremental risk of adverse

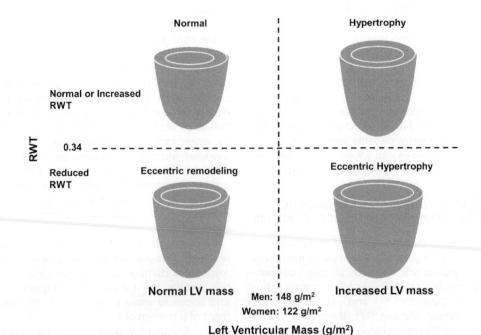

Fig. 3. Classification of geometric patterns in patients with HF, dilated left ventricle and reduced EF: normal mass with normal or increased RWT (normal), increased mass with normal or increased RWT (hypertrophy), normal mass with reduced RWT (eccentric remodeling), and increased mass with reduced RWT (eccentric hypertrophy).

outcome was associated with increased LVMi and decreased RWT.[46]

The lack of appropriate adaptation of the coronary circulation in patients with LVH may be an important factor in the fall of coronary reserve.[47] It has been proved that ventricular systolic wall stress and myocardial mass are 2 major determinants of myocardial oxygen consumption (MVO$_2$).[48] When maladaptive eccentric LVH occurs, because of an elevation in ventricular wall stress, MVO$_2$ rises and this may lead to the exhaustion of coronary blood flow reserve.[49] This underperfusion may be responsible for the development of subendomyocardial ischemia.[50–52] Coronary hemodynamic changes in the microcirculation may contribute to the onset of myocyte loss and to the formation of myocardial fibrosis.[53,54] The progressive mechanical overload of the spared hypertrophied myocytes could explain the initiation of a vicious circle, which perpetuates myocardial perfusion impairment, ischemia, and extracellular derangement, finally causing myocyte deaths and fibrous tissue proliferation.[55] These structural alterations and their pathophysiologic counterparts seem closely related to the evolution from compensatory LVH to myocardial failure (**Table 1**).[56]

Whatever the underlying cause of myocardial tissue structural and functional abnormalities, there is commonly a prolonged period before the occurrence of clinically manifest HF. Initially, there is an adaptive compensatory process with varying degrees of ventricular dilation and LVH, which is followed by progressive ventricular dysfunction. Hence, it is important to establish early to which degree LV remodeling may be considered compensatory or maladaptive.

A fundamental question that must be addressed before embarking on a strategy of treatment to reverse structural abnormalities is whether changes in LV geometry and thickness are adaptive or maladaptive. The ability of imaging techniques to investigate the progression of LV dysfunction to failure is rather limited when the examinations are carried out at rest, whereas they can provide useful information when they are performed during stress, either physical or pharmacologic.

Evaluating global myocardial function by stress echocardiography may be useful to distinguish between adaptive or maladaptive LVH and remodeling in patients with LV dysfunction. Cardiac power output is the product of mean arterial pressure (MAP) and CO.[57] Echo-derived peak cardiac power output–to–mass (CPOM), which is a variable that couples cardiac power output with LV mass at peak exercise or during maximal inotropic stimulation, can be calculated as the product of a constant (K=2.22 x 10-1), with CO and MAP divided by LV

Table 1
Transition to myocardial failure: the ventricular responses to injury and/or increased workload
Phase 1   Cardiac injury, pressure, and/or volume overload
Systolic and diastolic variables: reduced EF, normal or reduced CO, and normal or increased LV filling pressure Morphologic changes: LV remodeling (early) with or without dilation Pathophysiology: myocyte stunning and cell death
Phase 2   Compensation
Systolic and diastolic variables: reduced EF, LV dilation, maintained CO, and normal filling pressure Morphologic changes: LV remodeling (late), established LVH, and normal RWT Pathophysiology: myocyte hypertrophy, hibernation, increased energy expenditure, and normal coronary reserve
Phase 3   Progressive dysfunction
Systolic and diastolic variables: reduced EF, LV dilation, reduced CO, and increased LV filling pressure Morphologic changes: LV remodeling (late), eccentric LVH, and reduced RWT Pathophysiology: energy starvation, myocyte loss, reduced coronary reserve and subendocardial ischemia, reparative and interstitial fibrosis

mass (M): CPOM = K × CO (L/min) × MAP (mm Hg) × M^{-1} (g). It reflects the maximal rate at which cardiac work (watts) is delivered with respect to the potential energy stored in LV mass and is measured per 100 g of LV mass: 100 × LV power output divided by LV mass (W/100 g).

Because normal heart muscle grows to match the workload imposed on it, the mass of the LV wall depends on the chronic load with which it is confronted. Therefore, in normal hearts, a stronger ventricle with a greater muscular mass contracts to a higher LV power output under stimulation. The physiologic example of the former is the increase of peak COPM in athletes, which frequently exceeds 2.0 W/100 g. When the integrity of myocardial structure is compromised due to myocyte loss, interstitial fibrosis, and scar, a disproportion becomes apparent between maximal cardiac power output and LV mass, which leads to a decrease of peak CPOM. The inadequacy of

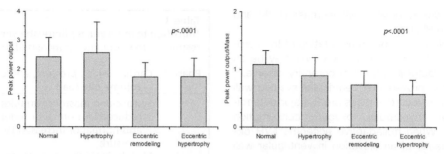

Fig. 4. Comparison of peak cardiac power output (watts) and of peak CPOM (W/100 g) in patients with HF, LV dysfunction, and dilation categorized according to geometric patterns: normal mass with normal or increased RWT (normal), increased mass with normal or increased RWT (hypertrophy), normal mass with reduced RWT (eccentric remodeling), and increased mass with reduced RWT (eccentric hypertrophy). These observations suggest that RWT is a critical determinant of ventricular performance in patients with LVH, dilated left ventricle and reduce EF.

eccentric LVH to perform external work during exercise is apparent in **Fig. 4**, in which peak cardiac power output and peak CPOM were compared in HF patients (n = 137) with different geometric patterns. The prognostic significance of CPOM during exercise or dobutamine stress echocardiography has been recently demonstrated.[58,59] This test also seems useful to distinguish between physiologic hypertrophy and pathologic hypertrophy.

SUMMARY

Although LVH initially can be compensatory to sustain increased workload, eventually it may become maladaptive. In particular, patients who show increased LV dimensions with the presence of LVH and low RWT are likely to carry the highest risk. Maladaptive eccentric LVH seems a critical factor capable of affecting the evolution toward end-stage HF. These considerations lead to the conclusion that acquisition of data on LV mass and thickness matters and that the assessment of relationship between LVH and ventricular performance also is important.

REFERENCES

1. Sandler H, Dodge HT. Left ventricular tension and stress in man. Circ Res 1963;13:91–104.
2. Hood WP Jr, Rackley CE, Rolett EL. Wall stress in the normal and hypertrophied human left ventricle. Am J Cardiol 1968;22(4):550–8.
3. Grossman W, Jones D, McLaurin LP. Wall stress and patterns of hypertrophy in the human left ventricle. J Clin Invest 1975;56(1):56–64.
4. Grossman W. Cardiac hypertrophy: useful adaptation or pathologic process? Am J Med 1980;69(4):576–84.
5. Strauer BE. Structural and functional adaptation of the chronically overloaded heart in arterial hypertension. Am Heart J 1987;114(4 Pt 2):948–57.
6. Lorell BH, Carabello BA. Left ventricular hypertrophy: pathogenesis, detection, and prognosis. Circulation 2000;102(4):470–9.
7. Anversa P, Beghi C, Kikkawa Y, et al. Myocardial infarction in rats. Infarct size, myocyte hypertrophy, and capillary growth. Circ Res 1986;58(1):26–37.
8. Anversa P, Loud AV, Levicky V, et al. Left ventricular failure induced by myocardial infarction. I. Myocyte hypertrophy. Am J Physiol 1985;248(6 Pt 2):H876–82.
9. Pfeffer MA, Braunwald E. Ventricular remodeling after myocardial infarction. Experimental observations and clinical implications. Circulation 1990;81(4):1161–72.
10. Cohn JN. Structural basis for heart failure. Ventricular remodeling and its pharmacological inhibition. Circulation 1995;91(10):2504–7.
11. Opie LH, Commerford PJ, Gersh BJ, et al. Controversies in ventricular remodelling. Lancet 2006;367(9507):356–67.
12. Barsotti A, Dini FL, Nardini V, et al. [From myocardial hypertrophy to heart failure: role of the interstitium]. Cardiologia 1993;38(12 Suppl 1):67–77.
13. Meerson FZ. The myocardium in hyperfunction, hypertrophy and heart failure. Circ Res 1969;25 (1): Suppl 2:1-163.
14. Katz AM. Cardiomyopathy of overload. A major determinant of prognosis in congestive heart failure. N Engl J Med 1990;322(2):100–10.
15. Katz AM. The "modern" view of heart failure: how did we get here? Circ Heart Fail 2008;1(1):63–71.
16. Gaasch WH, Delorey DE, St John Sutton MG, et al. Patterns of structural and functional remodeling of the left ventricle in chronic heart failure. Am J Cardiol 2008;102(4):459–62.
17. Devereux RB, Alonso DR, Lutas EM, et al. Echocardiographic assessment of left ventricular hypertrophy: comparison to necropsy findings. Am J Cardiol 1986;57(6):450–8.
18. Levy D, Savage DD, Garrison RJ, et al. Echocardiographic criteria for left ventricular hypertrophy: the

Framingham Heart Study. Am J Cardiol 1987;59(9): 956–60.

19. Gaasch WH. Left ventricular radius to wall thickness ratio. Am J Cardiol 1979;43(6):1189–94.

20. Ganau A, Devereux RB, Roman MJ, et al. Patterns of left ventricular hypertrophy and geometric remodeling in essential hypertension. J Am Coll Cardiol 1992;19(7):1550–8.

21. Marwick TH, Gillebert TC, Aurigemma G, et al. Recommendations on the use of echocardiography in adult hypertension: a report from the European Association of Cardiovascular Imaging (EACVI) and the American Society of Echocardiography (ASE). J Am Soc Echocardiogr 2015;28(7):727–54.

22. Lang RM, Badano LP, Mor-Avi V, et al. Recommendations for cardiac chamber quantification by echocardiography in adults: an update from the American Society of Echocardiography and the European Association of Cardiovascular Imaging. Eur Heart J Cardiovasc Imaging 2015;16(3):233–70.

23. Park SH, Shub C, Nobrega TP, et al. Two-dimensional echocardiographic calculation of left ventricular mass as recommended by the American Society of Echocardiography: correlation with autopsy and M-mode echocardiography. J Am Soc Echocardiogr 1996;9(2):119–28.

24. Chuang ML, Beaudin RA, Riley MF, et al. Three-dimensional echocardiographic measurement of left ventricular mass: comparison with magnetic resonance imaging and two-dimensional echocardiographic determinations in man. Int J Card Imaging 2000;16(5):347–57.

25. Mor-Avi V, Sugeng L, Weinert L, et al. Fast measurement of left ventricular mass with real-time three-dimensional echocardiography: comparison with magnetic resonance imaging. Circulation 2004; 110(13):1814–8.

26. Armstrong AC, Gidding S, Gjesdal O, et al. LV mass assessed by echocardiography and CMR, cardiovascular outcomes, and medical practice. JACC Cardiovasc Imaging 2012;5(8):837–48.

27. Lang RM, Badano LP, Tsang W, et al. EAE/ASE recommendations for image acquisition and display using three-dimensional echocardiography. Eur Heart J Cardiovasc Imaging 2012;13(1):1–46.

28. Lurbe E, Agabiti-Rosei E, Cruickshank JK, et al. European Society of Hypertension guidelines for the management of high blood pressure in children and adolescents. J Hypertens 2016;34(10):1887–920.

29. Konstam MA, Kramer DG, Patel AR, et al. Left ventricular remodeling in heart failure: current concepts in clinical significance and assessment. JACC Cardiovasc Imaging 2011;4(1):98–108.

30. Koren MJ, Devereux RB, Casale PN, et al. Relation of left ventricular mass and geometry to morbidity and mortality in uncomplicated essential hypertension. Ann Intern Med 1991;114(5):345–52.

31. Verdecchia P, Schillaci G, Borgioni C, et al. Prognostic value of left ventricular mass and geometry in systemic hypertension with left ventricular hypertrophy. Am J Cardiol 1996;78(2):197–202.

32. Muiesan ML, Salvetti M, Rizzoni D, et al. Persistence of left ventricular hypertrophy is a stronger indicator of cardiovascular events than baseline left ventricular mass or systolic performance: 10 years of follow-up. J Hypertens Suppl 1996;14(5):S43–9.

33. Gaasch WH, Zile MR. Left ventricular structural remodeling in health and disease: with special emphasis on volume, mass, and geometry. J Am Coll Cardiol 2011;58(17):1733–40.

34. Vakili BA, Okin PM, Devereux RB. Prognostic implications of left ventricular hypertrophy. Am Heart J 2001;141(3):334–41.

35. Brown DW, Giles WH, Croft JB. Left ventricular hypertrophy as a predictor of coronary heart disease mortality and the effect of hypertension. Am Heart J 2000;140(6):848–56.

36. de Simone G, Izzo R, Aurigemma GP, et al. Cardiovascular risk in relation to a new classification of hypertensive left ventricular geometric abnormalities. J Hypertens 2015;33(4):745–54 [discussion: 754].

37. Fabiani I, Pugliese NR, La Carrubba S, et al. Incremental prognostic value of a complex left ventricular remodeling classification in asymptomatic for heart failure hypertensive patients. J Am Soc Hypertens 2017;11(7):412–9.

38. Verma A, Meris A, Skali H, et al. Prognostic implications of left ventricular mass and geometry following myocardial infarction: the VALIANT (VALsartan In Acute myocardial iNfarcTion) Echocardiographic Study. JACC Cardiovasc Imaging 2008; 1(5):582–91.

39. Quinones MA, Greenberg BH, Kopelen HA, et al. Echocardiographic predictors of clinical outcome in patients with left ventricular dysfunction enrolled in the SOLVD registry and trials: significance of left ventricular hypertrophy. studies of left ventricular dysfunction. J Am Coll Cardiol 2000;35(5):1237–44.

40. Woythaler JN, Singer SL, Kwan OL, et al. Accuracy of echocardiography versus electrocardiography in detecting left ventricular hypertrophy: comparison with postmortem mass measurements. J Am Coll Cardiol 1983;2(2):305–11.

41. McCrohon JA, Moon JC, Prasad SK, et al. Differentiation of heart failure related to dilated cardiomyopathy and coronary artery disease using gadolinium-enhanced cardiovascular magnetic resonance. Circulation 2003;108(1):54–9.

42. Ross J Jr. Adaptations of the left ventricle to chronic volume overload. Circ Res 1974;35 (2): suppl II:64-70.

43. Konstam MA. "Systolic and diastolic dysfunction" in heart failure? Time for a new paradigm. J Card Fail 2003;9(1):1–3.

44. Hein S, Arnon E, Kostin S, et al. Progression from compensated hypertrophy to failure in the pressure-overloaded human heart: structural deterioration and compensatory mechanisms. Circulation 2003;107(7):984–91.

45. Messerli FH, Rimoldi SF, Bangalore S. The transition from hypertension to heart failure: contemporary update. JACC Heart Fail 2017;5(8):543–51.

46. Dini FL, Capozza P, Donati F, et al. Patterns of left ventricular remodeling in chronic heart failure: prevalence and prognostic implications. Am Heart J 2011;161(6):1088–95.

47. Marcus ML, Koyanagi S, Harrison DG, et al. Abnormalities in the coronary circulation that occur as a consequence of cardiac hypertrophy. Am J Med 1983;75(3A):62–6.

48. Strauer BE. Myocardial oxygen consumption in chronic heart disease: role of wall stress, hypertrophy and coronary reserve. Am J Cardiol 1979; 44(4):730–40.

49. Dini FL, Ghiadoni L, Conti U, et al. Coronary flow reserve in idiopathic dilated cardiomyopathy: relation with left ventricular wall stress, natriuretic peptides, and endothelial dysfunction. J Am Soc Echocardiogr 2009;22(4):354–60.

50. Nitenberg A, Foult JM, Blanchet F, et al. Multifactorial determinants of reduced coronary flow reserve after dipyridamole in dilated cardiomyopathy. Am J Cardiol 1985;55(6):748–54.

51. Unverferth DV, Magorien RD, Lewis RP, et al. The role of subendocardial ischemia in perpetuating myocardial failure in patients with nonischemic congestive cardiomyopathy. Am Heart J 1983; 105(1):176–9.

52. Vatner SF. Reduced subendocardial myocardial perfusion as one mechanism for congestive heart failure. Am J Cardiol 1988;62(8):94E–8E.

53. Hittinger L, Shannon RP, Bishop SP, et al. Subendomyocardial exhaustion of blood flow reserve and increased fibrosis in conscious dogs with heart failure. Circ Res 1989;65(4):971–80.

54. Lavine SJ, Prcevski P, Held AC, et al. Experimental model of chronic global left ventricular dysfunction secondary to left coronary microembolization. J Am Coll Cardiol 1991;18(7):1794–803.

55. Sabbah HN, Stein PD, Kono T, et al. A canine model of chronic heart failure produced by multiple sequential coronary microembolizations. Am J Physiol 1991;260(4 Pt 2):H1379–84.

56. Beltrami CA, Finato N, Rocco M, et al. Structural basis of end-stage failure in ischemic cardiomyopathy in humans. Circulation 1994;89(1):151–63.

57. Tan LB. Clinical and research implications of new concepts in the assessment of cardiac pumping performance in heart failure. Cardiovasc Res 1987; 21(8):615–22.

58. Dini FL, Mele D, Conti U, et al. Peak power output to left ventricular mass: an index to predict ventricular pumping performance and morbidity in advanced heart failure. J Am Soc Echocardiogr 2010;23(12): 1259–65.

59. Cortigiani L, Sorbo S, Miccoli M, et al. Prognostic value of cardiac power output to left ventricular mass in patients with left ventricular dysfunction and dobutamine stress echo negative by wall motion criteria. Eur Heart J Cardiovasc Imaging 2017;18(2): 153–8.

Myocardial Strain and Dyssynchrony
Incremental Value?

Flemming J. Olsen, MD,
Tor Biering-Sørensen, MD, PhD, MPH*

KEYWORDS

• Heart failure • Speckle tracking • Strain • Dyssynchrony

KEY POINTS

- Global longitudinal strain confers prognostic information independent of conventional echocardiographic measures in systolic heart failure; however, an important interaction for both atrial fibrillation and gender warrants further investigation.
- Longitudinal strain seems to be impaired in heart failure with preserved ejection fraction, suggesting preclinical systolic dysfunction in these patients.
- Spironolactone and sacubitril/valsartan may ameliorate systolic dysfunction by strain measures in heart failure with preserved ejection fraction; however, whether this translates into clinical benefit is unclear.
- Strain imaging can detect left ventricular dyssynchrony in systolic heart failure; however, no measures are currently ready for clinical use. Larger trials are needed to validate the value of strain patterns of left bundle branch block morphology. Whether dyssynchrony is a treatment target in heart failure with preserved ejection fraction is unclear.

IMAGING MYOCARDIAL DEFORMATION USING STRAIN: WHAT, HOW AND WHY
Principles of Myocardial Strain

Cardiac mechanics covers a broad spectrum of cardiac myocardial properties important for both left ventricular systolic and diastolic function. The left ventricular ejection fraction (LVEF) has been the method of choice for estimating cardiac systolic function; however, in recognition of this being a measure of volume expulsion and not a direct measure of myocardial tissue function, increasing focus has been on investigating methods for quantifying specific myocardial tissue function and myocardial viability. Myocardial deformation defines a complex process of myocardial shortening and lengthening in 3 orthogonal axes and covers terms from strain, strain rate, and shear strain, with overall strain being the most extensively investigated deformation parameter in clinical echocardiography and therefore is the focus in this review.[1] Two concepts exist for characterizing myocardial deformation: Lagrangian strain and natural strain. The principle of Lagrangian strain is that the amount of deformation ($\varepsilon(t)$) can be calculated by knowing the initial length of an object at baseline ($L(t_0)$) and the length at the time of interest ($L(t)$): $\varepsilon(t) = [L(t) - L(t_0)]/L(t_0)$. The consensus is that

Disclosures: Dr. Biering-Sørensen has received consultant fees for AmGen and Novartis.
Funding Sources: F.J. Olsen was funded by grants from the Danish Heart Foundation, Herlev & Gentofte Hospital's internal funds and from Herlev & Gentofte Hospital's Cardiologic FUKAP funds. T. Biering-Sørensen was supported by the Fondsbørsvekselerer Henry Hansen og Hustrus Hovedlegat.
Gentofte Hospital, Department of Cardiology, Niels Andersens Vej 65, Hellerup 2900, Denmark
* Corresponding author.
E-mail address: tor.biering@gmail.com

Heart Failure Clin 15 (2019) 167–178
https://doi.org/10.1016/j.hfc.2018.12.002
1551-7136/19/

lengthening is presented as positive strain (percentage in deformation), whereas shortening is negative. The concept of Lagrangian strain builds on defining deformation from a baseline length as reference point. This approach is in contrast to natural strain, where the reference point changes continuously during the cardiac cycle. The methods are comparable with small deformations; however, in myocardial deformation, the difference between the 2 methods becomes too extensive.[2]

Initially, deformation and myocardial strain were derived from tissue Doppler imaging as natural strain, but the high temporal resolution takes its toll on the spatial resolution, the reproducibility is questionable, the images are angle dependent, and extensive segmental analysis is quite time consuming. Focus has therefore shifted toward myocardial speckle tracking, which measures Lagrangian strain and strain rate and remedies these limitations. Speckle tracking represents a more novel technique, in which dedicated software algorithms can identify acoustical markers (or speckles) within the myocardium, which are then followed frame by frame throughout the cardiac cycle (**Fig. 1**). Several guidelines and consensus statements have been published in recent years on how to properly perform speckle tracking in order to standardize the method.[2] Because the method relies on software algorithms, which differs from ultrasound operating systems, there is a significant degree of vendor dependency in measurements, which should be recalled when interpreting speckle tracking results.[3] Depending on operating system, the analysis ranges from manual to semiautomatic and automatic techniques, all of which influence reproducibility and time of analysis.

HEART FAILURE SYNDROMES

Heart failure (HF) has for decades been characterized by clinical hallmarks in conjunction with reduced LVEF. However, the entity of HF has evolved so that these patients now only comprise a subgroup (approximately 50%) of HF patients called heart failure with reduced ejection fraction (HFrEF). Besides this group, the HF syndrome also includes heart failure with preserved ejection fraction (HFpEF), and most recently, heart failure with midrange ejection fraction (HFmrEF). The utility of echocardiographic strain imaging varies widely between these trajectories of EF, and the applications of strain imaging within these subgroups are continuously being expanded and probed in new settings. Because HFmrEF is a fairly new group of unclear phenotypic origin, this review focuses on strain imaging applications in

HFrEF and HFpEF (**Table 1**) because evidence of strain imaging in HFmrEF is sparse but will likely increase in the coming years.

STRAIN IMAGING IN HEART FAILURE WITH REDUCED EJECTION FRACTION

Even though several management strategies are available for patients with HFrEF, the condition is still associated with high mortality and morbidity. Consequently, there is an ongoing need for detecting high-risk patients who require close monitoring and advanced treatments. Although several studies of HF patients revealed global longitudinal strain (GLS) as a promising measure for detecting subclinical left ventricular (LV) dysfunction, the first major study was reported in 2012 by Bertini and colleagues,[4] who investigated the utility of GLS to predict outcome in patients with ischemic cardiomyopathy. In 1060 patients, 309 patients reached a combined end point (HF hospitalization and/or all-cause mortality) within a median follow-up period of 31 months. Even though the investigators found that both LVEF and wall motion score index were independent predictors of outcome when adjusted for clinical confounders, GLS provided the highest C-statistics, suggesting higher predictive value compared with these 2 measures.

The knowledge on prognostic utility of GLS in HF was expanded by Sengeløv and colleagues,[5] who investigated 1065 patients with HFrEF of all causes, and showed prognostic value for predicting all-cause mortality independent and incremental to both echocardiographic and clinical parameters. Importantly, the investigators found that atrial fibrillation (AF) and female sex both modified the relationship between GLS and outcome. The reason for the interaction observed with AF may have related to the variable preload and afterload conditions associated with the cardiac cycle variations, and additionally, due to undersampling owing to the often high heart rate accompanied with AF in relation to the frame rate. Because AF constitutes a major subgroup of HF patients in general, identifying echocardiographic biomarkers in these patients should be a point of focus. Several approaches exist, some being clinically exhaustive, by suggesting measuring over multiple cardiac cycle measurements, and others suggesting indexing to measures to the preceding RR-interval,[6] and most recently, with the RR-interval in question.[7] These approaches, however, need further validation.

The interaction with female sex has since been recognized in the Copenhagen City Heart Study,[8] where GLS was found to be a strong predictor of cardiovascular morbidity and mortality, primarily

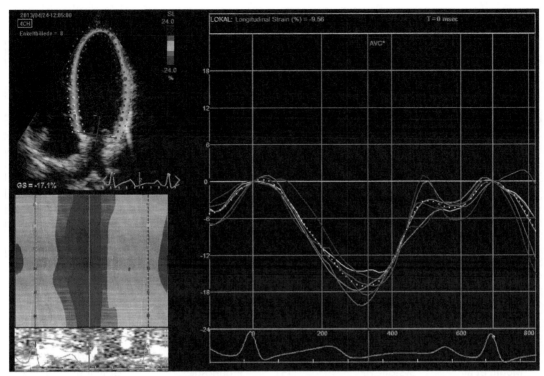

Fig. 1. Myocardial speckle tracking. Left ventricular speckle tracking in the 4-chamber view. The speckle tracking sequence is triggered of the R-wave showing the synchronous contraction of all myocardial segments at the AVC. The global value of LS from all segments is depicted as a white dotted line.

in men. This finding might be explained by smaller hearts observed in women; however, Lumens and colleagues[9] raised an intriguing hypothesis that female hearts may undergo a remodeling process, which is different from men, and this may mediate the gender difference observed between GLS and outcome.

Recently, the prognostic value of GLS in HFrEF was firmly underlined by Park and colleagues,[10] who examined 4172 patients with acute HF of all spectrums and found GLS to be a strong prognosticator of all-cause mortality compared with LVEF with 1740 events. This finding was particularly emphasized among patients with moderately and severely reduced GLS (GLS: 8%–12% and GLS: <8%, respectively).

The reason GLS seems to be an important prognosticator in HFrEF stems from 2 important theories: (1) it is a direct measure of longitudinal myocardial tissue function, (2) it relates closely to amount of fibrosis.[11] The latter is a crucial point, because recognition of impaired systolic function by GLS is one point, but whether medication and other HF-related treatment, that is, CRT, can revert the systolic dysfunction is quite another. This point was recognized in MADIT-CRT, which revealed that the greatest treatment benefit of cardiac resynchronization therapy (CRT) was found in

patients with GLS greater than 8.7%.[12] Similarly, in patients with narrow QRS (<130 ms), the Echo-CRT study found that in patients with GLS less than 6.2% CRT treatment could even have a detrimental effect on outcome.[13] This unfortunate effect likely reflects extensive scar tissue with little chance of myocardial recovery, and not only can CRT treatment not remedy this condition but also it may even have a proarrhythmic effect. In addition, a recent substudy of the MADIT-CRT trial showed that regional strain in the inferior ventricular wall was an independent predictor of outcome.[14] Although cardiac MRI with evaluation of LV fibrosis was not assessed in this study, this may reflect regional fibrosis and thereby an increased risk of arrhythmia. Regional strain may also be important for LV lead placement, in which placement in a fibrotic area is unlikely to improve LV function. Hence, dyssynchrony (as explained in later discussion) only represents one side of the coin in CRT management, with restoration of viable myocardial tissue representing the other side.[15]

MECHANICAL DYSSYNCHRONY IN HEART FAILURE WITH REDUCED EJECTION FRACTION

Treatment effect of CRT for symptomatic (New York Heart Association [NYHA] class III-IV) HFrEF

Table 1
Highlighting selected echocardiographic studies in heart failure

Study	Population	Sample Size (n)	Purpose	Findings
Longitudinal strain in heart failure with reduced ejection fraction				
Bertini et al,[4] 2012	Ischemic cardiomyopathy	1060	Prognostic value of GLS	GLS superior predictor compared with conventional measures
Sengeløv et al,[5] 2015	Systolic HF (all causes)	1065	Prognostic value of GLS	GLS superior predictor compared with conventional measures; significant interaction for AF and female sex
Park et al,[10] 2018	Acute HF, HFrEF, HFmrEF, HFpEF	4172	Prognostic value of GLS	GLS was a superior predictor to LVEF for predicting all-cause mortality across all spectrums of HF
Modin et al,[7] 2018	Systolic HF with AF	151	Prognostic value of GLS/RR	GLS/RR but not GLS or conventional measures predicted outcome
Biering-Sørensen et al,[8] 2017	Community-based cohort (Copenhagen City Heart Study)	1296	Prognostic value of GLS	GLS predictor and improved risk stratification schemes; significant interaction with female sex
Knappe et al,[12] 2011	Systolic HF with CRT treatment (MADIT-CRT substudy)	1077	Dyssynchrony and contraction to identify patients with CRT benefit	Greatest benefit of CRT in patients with GLS >8.7%
Bax et al,[13] 2017	Systolic HF with narrow QRS (Echo-CRT substudy)	755	Prognostic value of GLS in patients with narrow QRS (<130 ms)	GLS significant predictor of outcome, possible detrimental effect of CRT in patients with GLS <6.2%
Biering-Sørensen et al,[14] 2017	Systolic HF with CRT treatment (MADIT-CRT substudy)	1064	Prognostic value of regional strain for ventricular arrhythmias	Inferior wall strain predictor of ventricular arrhythmias; MD was not a significant predictor

(continued on next page)

| Table 1 | | | | |
| (continued) | | | | |

Study	Population	Sample Size (n)	Purpose	Findings
Dyssynchrony in heart failure with reduced ejection fraction				
Beshai et al,[19] 2007	Systolic HF with CRT treatment (RethinQ trial)	172	Effect of CRT on oxygen consumption and outcome	CRT significantly increased oxygen consumption in QRS >120 ms, but not in patients with QRS <120 ms; no significant difference in outcome between study groups
Ruschitzka et al,[20] 2013	Systolic HF and QRS <130 ms with CRT treatment (Echo-CRT trial)	909	Effect of CRT on outcome in patients with systolic HF and narrow QRS	CRT treatment did not show clinical benefit in patients with systolic HF and narrow QRS, was stopped because of potential harm
Chung et al,[21] 2008	Systolic HF with CRT treatment	498	Predictive value of dyssynchrony parameters	Low specificity and high variability in dyssynchrony measures; no parameter recommended for clinical use
Fornwalt et al,[24] 2007	Systolic HF with CRT treatment	23	Test of cross-correlation systolic velocity (XCD) to discriminate dyssynchrony from normal activation	XCD significantly discriminated patients with dyssynchrony from normal activation and showed improvement by CRT
Olsen et al,[25] 2009	Systolic HF with CRT	44	Test of cross-correlation systolic acceleration (XCA) to predict CRT outcome and discriminate from control subjects	XCA significantly discriminated patients with dyssynchrony from normal activation and showed improvement by CRT
Risum et al,[30] 2012	Systolic HF with CRT	n = 67	Regional strain patterns to predict response to CRT	Regional strain pattern was able to predict responders to CRT
Strain imaging in heart failure with preserved ejection fraction				
Shah et al,[32] 2015	HFpEF (TOPCAT substudy)	447	Predictive value of GLS in HFpEF; impact of spironolactone on strain measures	GLS was a significant predictor of outcome, and spironolactone showed trend toward reversing systolic strain in patients from United States

(continued on next page)

Table 1
(continued)

Study	Population	Sample Size (n)	Purpose	Findings
Kraigher-Krainer et al,[33] 2014	HFpEF (PARAMOUNT substudy)	219	Comparison of strain to normal controls and hypertensive subjects; to test the relation to biomarkers and echocardiographic measures	Longitudinal and circumferential strain was significantly lower in HFpEF compared with healthy controls and hypertensive patients; LS was significantly inversely associated with NT-proBNP
Biering-Sørensen et al,[35] 2017	Unexplained dyspnea and normal EF	85	Investigation of longitudinal and circumferential strain to invasive measures during exercise	Ratio of circumferential to LS was the strongest predictor of pulmonary capillary wedge pressure
Biering-Sørensen et al,[38] 2018	HFpEF (PARAMOUNT substudy)	301	Effect of sacubitril/valsartan compared with valsartan on strain measures	Sacubitril/valsartan but not valsartan showed significant improvement in circumferential strain, but showed no effect on LS
Santos et al,[39] 2014	HFpEF (PARAMOUNT substudy)	130	Comparison of dyssynchrony in HFpEF compared with healthy controls	Greater degree of dyssynchrony by MD compared with healthy controls; this related to QRS duration, hypertrophy, and diastolic dysfunction
Menet et al,[40] 2014	HFpEF, HFrEF with narrow QRS, and hypertensive subjects	120	Comparison of dyssynchrony between HFpEF, HFrEF with narrow QRS and hypertensive subjects	No difference in dyssynchrony was found in HFpEF compared with HFrEF with narrow QRS nor with hypertensive subjects
Biering-Sørensen et al,[41] 2017	HFpEF (TOPCAT substudy)	424	Prognostic value of dyssynchrony in HFpEF	Dyssynchrony by MD was not a predictor of outcome in HFpEF

Abbreviations: AF, atrial fibrillation; EF, ejection fraction; NT-proBNP, N-terminal pro–brain natriuretic peptide.

(LVEF <35%) with electrical dyssynchrony (QRS >120 ms) has been established in 2 landmark trials: the COMPANION trial[16] and the CARE-HF trial,[17] and the indication has since been extended to include mildly symptomatic HF (NYHA II) in MADIT-CRT trial.[18] Because CRT is thought to partly exert its effect through resynchronization of LV mechanical activation delay, it has seemed prudent to identify echocardiographic indices of mechanical dyssynchrony (MD). Consequently, there is now a wide armamentarium of dyssynchrony indices, of which time-to-peak measures for long have constituted a cornerstone. Even though electrical dyssynchrony (QRS >120 ms) is an entry criteria for CRT management, patients with narrow and borderline QRS (<130 ms) often exhibit MD as evidenced by different time-to-peak measures. By extension, the RethinQ[19] and the Echo-CRT trials[20] were both conducted with the aim of reversing MD with CRT treatment in such patients; however, none of the studies were able to show clinical benefit. The RethinQ study used septal-to-posterior wall delay by m-mode and peak velocity difference by color tissue Doppler imaging (cTDI) as entry criteria of dyssynchrony.[19] Shortly after the RethinQ study, the PROSPECT trial[21] results were published. The PROSPECT trial sought to investigate the clinical utility of 12 proposed echocardiographic dyssynchrony parameters. Importantly, the trial found poor reproducibility, and despite being predictors of outcome, the sensitivity and specificity were questionable, and the trial concluded that none of the 12 parameters could be recommended for clinical use.[21]

The Echo-CRT study used cTDI opposing wall delay and anteroseptal to posterior wall delay by speckle tracking echocardiography (STE) as entry dyssynchrony criteria, but was stopped early due to futility and potential harm.[20]

In the wake of these trials, several crucial points were made: (1) presence of MD does not necessarily translate into CRT response, (2) specificity of dyssynchrony parameters is crucial, (3) CRT treatment in patients with QRS less than 120 ms does not seem warranted.[22]

Dyssynchrony Without Cardiac Resynchronization Therapy Response

Several hypotheses exist as to why patients with apparent MD should not benefit from CRT treatment. It may relate to extensive scar tissue with reduced myocardial viability, that the measures applied are nonspecific, and that CRT treatment only ameliorates electrical dyssynchrony but not necessarily MD. By extension, the notion that dyssynchrony parameters may predict outcome in

CRT does not necessarily mean that they represent measures of treatment target. In 2009, Fornwalt[23] called for a paradigm shift on dyssynchrony interpretation and outlined a range of important points with regards to dyssynchrony measures and endpoint elucidation. One proposal by Fornwalt and colleagues[24] was to reevaluate the use of time-to-peak analysis, regardless of defined by cTDI or STE, and instead look toward measures that comprise information on myocardial motion throughout the entire cardiac cycle. One proposed method by Fornwalt was by cross-correlation analysis of myocardial velocity (XCD), which showed promise with regards to distinguishing patients with dyssynchrony from normal patients compared with conventional dyssynchrony measures. In 2009, Olsen and colleagues[25] investigated a similar approach with cross-correlation analysis of myocardial acceleration (XCA) compared with conventional measures of dyssynchrony and XCD, which showed clinical value.

A substudy from the EchoCRT revealed that when compared with XCA, entry dyssynchrony criteria were equally distributed among patients with XCA dyssynchrony,[26] once again underlining the nonspecificity of these measures. As outlined by Olsen and colleagues,[25] this method could theoretically be applied in speckle tracking to avoid the limitations of tethering and angle-dependency; however, this has yet to be done. Longitudinal speckle tracking methods for assessment of MD have also been developed, defined as the standard deviation in time-to-peak systolic strain, and have shown promise in various cohorts, including CRT patients.[27] However, recently a substudy of the MADIT-CRT showed no predictive value of MD with regards to ventricular arrhythmias in this large-scale study.[14] Furthermore, MD contemplates the use of time-to-peak analysis, which does not consider whole cardiac cycle myocardial motion as previously mentioned and outlined by Fornwalt and colleagues, and the role of this parameter may therefore be of limited use in these patients.

A substudy of the MADIT-CRT showed increased clinical benefit by CRT in patients with left bundle branch block (LBBB) and with increasing QRS width. In recent years, there has been a continuous search for refining CRT criteria by echocardiography because one-third of patients are nonresponders. Because LBBB is an important target in patients, echocardiographic pattern analysis representing LBBB morphology and activation delay has been extensively studied, because this may help optimize patient selection. Septal flash and apical rocking are 2 well-recognized phenomena with LBBB activation delay,[28] but different contraction patterns of LBBB morphology have been proposed as well.[29] Risum and colleagues[30] investigated a speckle tracking–derived method of regional strain analysis to identify LBBB morphology patterns amenable to CRT treatment (**Fig. 2**). The pattern comprises 3 points: (1) early septal shortening with early lateral wall stretching, (2) septal peak shortening in the early systolic phase (70% of ejection period), and (3) lateral peak shortening after aortic valve closure (AVC). This semiquantitative method seems reliable at identifying LBBB morphology, and thereby, responders to CRT with a high reproducibility, but needs prospective validation in a larger format.

STRAIN IMAGING IN HEART FAILURE WITH PRESERVED EJECTION FRACTION

Even though HFpEF has gained considerable attention, no treatment options currently exist for this syndrome, and treatment largely relies on off-label use or symptomatic treatment with diuretics. Recently, the TOPCAT trial investigated the utility of spironolactone in HFpEF, and even though the study did not show clinical efficacy by the primary endpoint, it did reduce recurrent HF hospitalizations.[31] Furthermore, a geographic regional variation was observed in treatment efficacy based on inclusion from Russia and Georgia compared with the United States, which clouds the clinical efficacy of spironolactone. Recently, an echocardiographic substudy from the TOPCAT trial was published in which Shah and colleagues[32] examined the prognostic value of longitudinal strain (LS) for the prediction of outcome and the effect of spironolactone on echocardiographic measures of cardiac function. The investigators made several important findings: LS was impaired in HFpEF patients compared with matched individuals from a community-based cohort study from the ARIC study, impaired LV strain was associated with an increased risk incremental to clinical risk factors, and measures of LV structure by both c-statistics and net reclassification index, increasing number of echocardiographic abnormalities (E/e′, left ventricular hypertrophy [LVH] and LS) was associated with an increased risk of outcome (regardless of EF), and spironolactone treatment showed a trend toward improvement in LS. Of interest, the investigators did not find a linear relationship between LS and outcome, but rather that an increased risk was mediated by a LS less than 15%.

LVH and diastolic dysfunction have been recognized as key features of HFpEF, and therefore, for long HFpEF was deemed as diastolic HF.

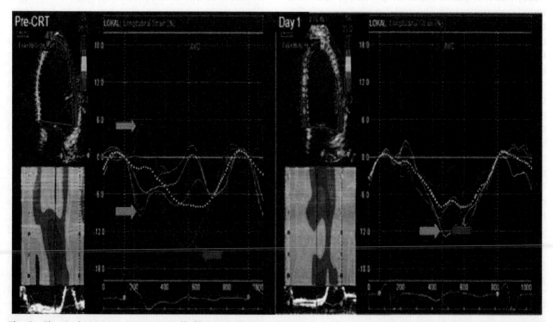

Fig. 2. Classical LBBB strain pattern. (*left*) Pre-CRT classical pattern of LV dyssynchrony, 4-chamber view. The early-activated septal wall shows early peak contraction (*yellow arrow*), whereas the late-activated lateral wall is pre-stretched (*blue arrow*) followed by late peak contraction after AVC (*red arrow*). (*right*) The same patient day 1 after CRT, 4-chamber view. Peak contraction is aligned with improved systolic septal strain (*yellow arrow*), whereas lateral strain is decreased (*red arrow*). (*From* Risum N, Jons C, Olsen NT, et al. Simple regional strain pattern analysis to predict response to cardiac resynchronization therapy: rationale, initial results, and advantages. Am Heart J 2012;163(4):699; with permission.)

However, even though these characteristics are often recognized in HFpEF, findings from the PARAMOUNT trial educated us that LVH and elevated filling pressure (E/e' >15) were only present in approximately half of HFpEF patients,[33] and systolic dysfunction by advanced measures may therefore play an important role in the pathophysiologic development in some HFpEF patients, which was shown in both TOPCAT and PARAMOUNT.[32,33] One theory for why LVEF is preserved in HFpEF has been that impaired longitudinal systolic function was compensated by an increased LV circumferential function, which upholds LVEF.[34] Once circumferential function becomes impaired, LVEF starts to decline (**Fig. 3**).

This notion was substantiated in an invasive study by Biering-Sørensen and colleagues,[35] who investigated patients with preserved EF and unexplained dyspnea, in whom the investigators found that a combination of impaired GLS and increased circumferential strain (CS) was the strongest predictor of elevated pulmonary artery capillary wedge pressure during exercise.

By extension, a substudy from the PARAMOUNT trial revealed that patients with HFpEF exhibit impaired LS, relatively preserved CS, and that CS can discriminate patients with HFpEF symptoms from asymptomatic individuals with similar clinical risk profile.[33] The explanation for why CS is relatively preserved and upholds a normal LVEF in this patient group may be due to subendocardial fiber damage with reduced longitudinal systolic function combined with impaired function of subendocardial helical fibers as well, which results in a relative increase in subepicardial helical fiber function and thus an apparently exaggerated circumferential function[36,37] (**Fig. 4**). Torsional strain imaging by 3-dimensional speckle tracking may play a role in clarifying the theory further, but has yet to be examined for this purpose.

Most recently, preliminary findings from the PARAMOUNT trial suggest that the angiotensin-neprilysin inhibitor (sacubitril/valsartan) attenuates LV CS but not LS in HFpEF patients,[38] suggesting a reversal in one of the important steps in the HFpEF trajectory. The role of sacubitril/valsartan on clinical endpoints remains to be seen in the ongoing PARAGON-HF trial. In summary, both LS and CS play a crucial role in development of HFpEF, and spironolactone and sacubitril/valsartan may improve systolic impairment and thereby potentially improve patient outcomes; however, larger trials are needed to confirm whether the observed improvement in LS and CS also translates into clinical benefit.

DYSSYNCHRONY IN HEART FAILURE WITH PRESERVED EJECTION FRACTION

Contemplating the utility of CRT treatment for systolic HF with electromechanical dyssynchrony, it has been speculated that MD could play a pathophysiological role in the development of HFpEF. A substudy from the PARAMOUNT trial found greater level of MD from enrolled patients compared with healthy control subjects by the standard deviation of time-to-peak method, but also that severity of dyssynchrony is highly related

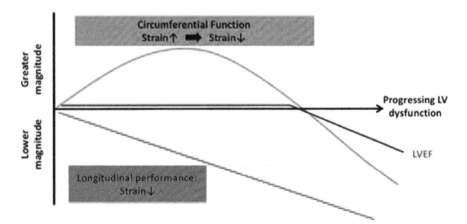

Fig. 3. A model of progressive abnormalities in left ventricular function in HF across LVEF spectrum. Subclinical myocardial dysfunction triggered by cardiovascular risk factors, such as age, hypertension, and diabetes, may present as depressed longitudinal deformation and decreased GLS but increased circumferential deformation and GCS. Progression is characterized by continuous impairment in longitudinal deformation. LVEF decreases at a point when circumferential function also starts to decline. GCS, global circumferential strain. (*From* Modin D, Andersen DM, Biering-Sørensen T. Echo and heart failure: when do people need an echo, and when do they need natriuretic peptides? Echo Res Pract 2018;5(2):R73; with permission.)

A   **Normal Cardiac Function**

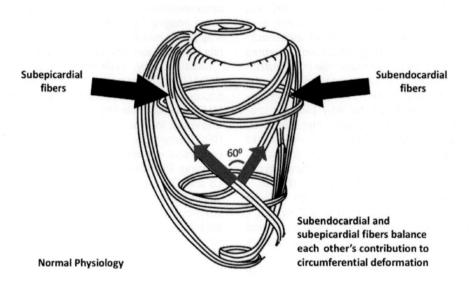

B   **Impaired Longitudinal Function**

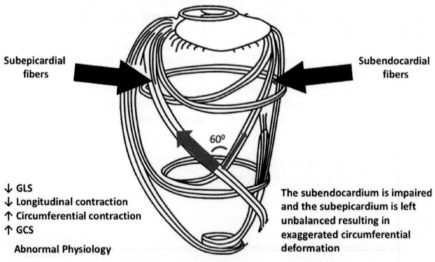

Fig. 4. The myocardial fiber orientation of the left ventricular wall and their directions of contraction. In the subepicardium, myocardial fibers are oriented in a left-handed helix, whereas they run in a right-handed helix in the subendocardium. The cardiac midwall comprises circumferentially oriented fibers. (*A*) In the normal heart, the subepicardial left-handed helical fibers are balanced by the subendocardial right-handed helical fibers, and longitudinal function is normal. (*B*) The subendocardial fibers are most susceptible to dysfunction from hypertension, increasing age, diabetes, and other cardiovascular risk factors. When subendocardial function is lost, longitudinal contraction is impaired, and the subepicardial fibers are left unbalanced. This results in decreased GLS and exaggerated circumferential contraction and GCS. (*Adapted from* Nakatani S. Left ventricular rotation and twist: why should we learn? J Cardiovasc Ultrasound 2011;19(1):2; with permission.)

to QRS width, LVH, and diastolic dysfunction.[39] By extension, Menet and colleagues[40] found no difference in MD in patients with HFpEF compared with HFrEF patients with narrow QRS and compared with controls with hypertension. This similarity across the groups questions the role of dyssynchrony in HFpEF, and whether HFpEF-related dyssynchrony represents a condition that is amenable to treatment with CRT. This notion was substantiated by a substudy of the TOPCAT trial, which found that dyssynchrony by MD did not predict outcome of HF hospitalization or death.[41] Thus, the increased level of MD observed may simply reflect the state of hypertrophy frequently observed in patients with HFpEF and not clinically relevant dyssynchrony. Just as for patients with systolic HF with narrow QRS, LV dyssynchrony may be present without representing an actual treatment target.

SUMMARY

For patients with HFrEF, myocardial strain imaging may provide important prognostic information incremental to echocardiographic and clinical risk factors. Furthermore, echocardiographic substudies suggest that it may help characterize patients who will benefit from CRT management, help guide LV lead placement in CRT, and detect patients in whom treatment could have a detrimental effect.

For HFpEF, myocardial strain imaging has provided important information on the pathophysiologic development of HFpEF and seems to be a potential target in treatment medication, which will help guide clinical trials in the future.

REFERENCES

1. Smiseth OA, Torp H, Opdahl A, et al. Myocardial strain imaging: how useful is it in clinical decision making? Eur Heart J 2016;37(15):1196–207.
2. Voigt J-U, Pedrizzetti G, Lysyansky P, et al. Definitions for a common standard for 2D speckle tracking echocardiography: consensus document of the EACVI/ASE/Industry Task Force to standardize deformation imaging. Eur Heart J Cardiovasc Imaging 2015;16(1):1–11.
3. Risum N, Ali S, Olsen NT, et al. Variability of global left ventricular deformation analysis using vendor dependent and independent two-dimensional speckle-tracking software in adults. J Am Soc Echocardiogr 2012;25(11):1195–203.
4. Bertini M, Ng ACT, Antoni ML, et al. Global longitudinal strain predicts long-term survival in patients with chronic ischemic cardiomyopathy. Circ Cardiovasc Imaging 2012;5(3):383–91.
5. Sengeløv M, Jørgensen PG, Jensen JS, et al. Global longitudinal strain is a superior predictor of all-cause mortality in heart failure with reduced ejection fraction. JACC Cardiovasc Imaging 2015;8(12):1351–9.
6. Lee C-S, Lin T-H, Hsu P-C, et al. Measuring left ventricular peak longitudinal systolic strain from a single beat in atrial fibrillation: validation of the index beat method. J Am Soc Echocardiogr 2012;25(9):945–52.
7. Modin D, Sengeløv M, Jørgensen PG, et al. Global longitudinal strain corrected by RR interval is a superior predictor of all-cause mortality in patients with systolic heart failure and atrial fibrillation. ESC Heart Fail 2018;5(2):311–8.
8. Biering-Sørensen T, Biering-Sørensen SR, Olsen FJ, et al. Global longitudinal strain by echocardiography predicts long-term risk of cardiovascular morbidity and mortality in a low-risk general population: the Copenhagen City Heart Study. Circ Cardiovasc Imaging 2017;10(3) [pii:e005521].
9. Lumens J, Prinzen FW, Delhaas T. Longitudinal strain: "think globally, track locally". JACC Cardiovasc Imaging 2015;8(12):1360–3.
10. Park JJ, Park J-B, Park J-H, et al. Global longitudinal strain to predict mortality in patients with acute heart failure. J Am Coll Cardiol 2018;71(18):1947–57.
11. Roes SD, Mollema SA, Lamb HJ, et al. Validation of echocardiographic two-dimensional speckle tracking longitudinal strain imaging for viability assessment in patients with chronic ischemic left ventricular dysfunction and comparison with contrast-enhanced magnetic resonance imaging. Am J Cardiol 2009;104(3):312–7.
12. Knappe D, Pouleur A-C, Shah AM, et al. Dyssynchrony, contractile function, and response to cardiac resynchronization therapy. Circ Heart Fail 2011;4(4):433–40.
13. Bax JJ, Delgado V, Sogaard P, et al. Prognostic implications of left ventricular global longitudinal strain in heart failure patients with narrow QRS complex treated with cardiac resynchronization therapy: a subanalysis of the randomized EchoCRT trial. Eur Heart J 2017;38(10):720–6.
14. Biering-Sørensen T, Knappe D, Pouleur A-C, et al. Regional longitudinal deformation improves prediction of ventricular tachyarrhythmias in patients with heart failure with reduced ejection fraction: a MADIT-CRT substudy (multicenter automatic defibrillator implantation trial-cardiac resynchronization therapy). Circ Cardiovasc Imaging 2017;10(1) [pii: e005096].
15. Pouleur A-C, Knappe D, Shah AM, et al. Relationship between improvement in left ventricular dyssynchrony and contractile function and clinical outcome with cardiac resynchronization therapy: the MADIT-CRT trial. Eur Heart J 2011;32(14):1720–9.
16. Bristow MR, Saxon LA, Boehmer J, et al. Cardiac-resynchronization therapy with or without an implantable defibrillator in advanced chronic heart failure. N Engl J Med 2004;350(21):2140–50.
17. Cleland JGF, Daubert J-C, Erdmann E, et al. The effect of cardiac resynchronization on morbidity and mortality in heart failure. N Engl J Med 2005;352(15):1539–49.
18. Moss AJ, Hall WJ, Cannom DS, et al. Cardiac-resynchronization therapy for the prevention of heart-failure events. N Engl J Med 2009;361(14):1329–38.

19. Beshai JF, Grimm RA, Nagueh SF, et al. Cardiac-re-synchronization therapy in heart failure with narrow QRS complexes. N Engl J Med 2007;357(24): 2461–71.

20. Ruschitzka F, Abraham WT, Singh JP, et al. Cardiac-resynchronization therapy in heart failure with a nar-row QRS complex. N Engl J Med 2013;369(15): 1395–405.

21. Chung ES, Leon AR, Tavazzi L, et al. Results of the predictors of response to CRT (PROSPECT) trial. Circulation 2008;117(20):2608–16.

22. Yancy CW, McMurray JJV. ECG–still the best for se-lecting patients for CRT. N Engl J Med 2013;369(15): 1463–4.

23. Fornwalt BK. The dyssynchrony in predicting response to cardiac resynchronization therapy: a call for change. J Am Soc Echocardiogr 2011; 24(2):180–4.

24. Fornwalt BK, Arita T, Bhasin M, et al. Cross-correla-tion quantification of dyssynchrony: a new method for quantifying the synchrony of contraction and relaxation in the heart. J Am Soc Echocardiogr 2007;20(12):1330–7.e1.

25. Olsen NT, Mogelvang R, Jons C, et al. Predicting response to cardiac resynchronization therapy with cross-correlation analysis of myocardial systolic ac-celeration: a new approach to echocardiographic dyssynchrony evaluation. J Am Soc Echocardiogr 2009;22(6):657–64.

26. Tayal B, Gorcsan J, Bax JJ, et al. Cardiac resynchro-nization therapy in patients with heart failure and narrow QRS complexes. J Am Coll Cardiol 2018; 71(12):1325–33.

27. Hasselberg NE, Haugaa KH, Bernard A, et al. Left ventricular markers of mortality and ventricular ar-rhythmias in heart failure patients with cardiac re-synchronization therapy. Eur Heart J Cardiovasc Imaging 2016;17(3):343–50.

28. Stankovic I, Belmans A, Prinz C, et al. The associa-tion of volumetric response and long-term survival after cardiac resynchronization therapy. Eur Heart J Cardiovasc Imaging 2017;18(10):1109–17.

29. Leenders GE, Lumens J, Cramer MJ, et al. Septal deformation patterns delineate mechanical dyssyn-chrony and regional differences in contractility: anal-ysis of patient data using a computer model. Circ Heart Fail 2012;5(1):87–96.

30. Risum N, Jons C, Olsen NT, et al. Simple regional strain pattern analysis to predict response to cardiac

resynchronization therapy: rationale, initial results, and advantages. Am Heart J 2012;163(4):697–704.

31. Pitt B, Pfeffer MA, Assmann SF, et al. Spironolactone for heart failure with preserved ejection fraction. N Engl J Med 2014;370(15):1383–92.

32. Shah AM, Claggett B, Sweitzer NK, et al. Prognostic importance of impaired systolic function in heart fail-ure with preserved ejection fraction and the impact of spironolactone. Circulation 2015;132(5):402–14.

33. Kraigher-Krainer E, Shah AM, Gupta DK, et al. Impaired systolic function by strain imaging in heart failure with preserved ejection fraction. J Am Coll Cardiol 2014;63(5):447–56.

34. Shah AM, Solomon SD. Phenotypic and pathophys-iological heterogeneity in heart failure with pre-served ejection fraction. Eur Heart J 2012;33(14): 1716–7.

35. Biering-Sørensen T, Santos M, Rivero J, et al. Left ventricular deformation at rest predicts exercise-induced elevation in pulmonary artery wedge pres-sure in patients with unexplained dyspnoea. Eur J Heart Fail 2017;19(1):101–10.

36. Biering-Sørensen T, Solomon SD. Assessing con-tractile function when ejection fraction is normal: a case for strain imaging. Circ Cardiovasc Imaging 2015;8(11):e004181.

37. Modin D, Andersen DM, Biering-Sørensen T. Echo and heart failure: when do people need an echo, and when do they need natriuretic peptides? Echo Res Pract 2018;5(2):R65–79.

38. Biering-Sorensen T, Shah A, Claggett B, et al. The Angiotensin receptor neprilysin inhibitor (arni), sacu-bitril/valsartan, improves left ventricular myocardial deformation in heart failure with preserved ejection fraction (paramount trial). J Am Coll Cardiol 2018; 71(11 Supplement):A2665.

39. Santos ABS, Kraigher-Krainer E, Bello N, et al. Left ventricular dyssynchrony in patients with heart fail-ure and preserved ejection fraction. Eur Heart J 2014;35(1):42–7.

40. Menet A, Greffe L, Ennezat P-V, et al. Is mechanical dyssynchrony a therapeutic target in heart failure with preserved ejection fraction? Am Heart J 2014; 168(6):909–16.e1.

41. Biering-Sørensen T, Shah SJ, Anand I, et al. Prog-nostic importance of left ventricular mechanical dys-synchrony in heart failure with preserved ejection fraction. Eur J Heart Fail 2017;19(8):1043–52.

Myocardial Scar and Fibrosis
The Ultimate Mediator of Outcomes?

Erik B. Schelbert, MD, MS[a,b,c,d],*

KEYWORDS

- Myocardial fibrosis • Heart failure • Extracellular volume

KEY POINTS

- The key question of "Why does heart muscle fail?" remains unanswered. The lack of agreement on the role of myocardial fibrosis (MF) reflects the cardiology community's lack of a taxonomy to prioritize the origins of the complex myocardial pathology underlying heart failure.
- A large body of literature indicates that myocardial fibrosis may represent a principal pathway mediating the outcomes in heart failure that imparts vulnerability to adverse events.
- Cardiac amyloidosis illustrates how excess protein in the myocardial interstitium culminates in severe heart failure and a dismal prognosis characterized by inexorable clinical decline.
- Given that robust methods now exist to quantify myocardial fibrosis , the cardiology community has the tools to finally establish unequivocally that myocardial fibrosis represents a principal pathway mediating outcomes in heart failure that imparts vulnerability to adverse events.

INTRODUCTION

Myocardial scar and fibrosis may represent one of the principal pathways mediating outcomes in heart failure and thus impart vulnerability to adverse events.[1] Yet, this concept remains controversial. The lack of agreement on the role of myocardial fibrosis (MF) reflects the cardiology community's lack of a taxonomy to prioritize the origins of the complex myocardial pathology underlying heart failure. Specifically, there is no hierarchy that emphasizes the principal causal factors of heart failure. Myriad abnormalities occur in heart failure from the molecular level to the organ level. The key question of "Why does heart muscle fail?" remains unanswered.

The inability to identify causal pathways in heart failure may underlie the series of failed clinical trials over the past 2 decades.[2] Among the pool of variables that associate with outcomes, the cardiology community still struggles to discern primary causal pathology from other secondary pathology that simply represents the secondary downstream effects of other pathology. Therefore, when investigators report variables associated with outcomes, they seldom can resolve whether the variables of interest represent causal pathways that truly mediate disease or whether they simply represent downstream risk markers.

In this review, we compile evidence supporting the concept that MF is causal in heart failure, not simply a downstream marker of risk. We attempt

Disclosure Statement: E.B. Schelbert has served on advisory boards for Bayer and Merck and has received contrast material donated for research purposes from Bracco Diagnostics.
[a] UPMC Cardiovascular Magnetic Resonance Center, Pittsburgh, PA, USA; [b] Heart and Vascular Institute, UPMC, Pittsburgh, PA, USA; [c] Department of Medicine, University of Pittsburgh School of Medicine, 200 Lothrop Street, PUH E E354.2, Pittsburgh, PA 15101, USA; [d] Clinical and Translational Science Institute, University of Pittsburgh, Pittsburgh, PA, USA
* University of Pittsburgh School of Medicine, 200 Lothrop Street, PUH E E354.2, Pittsburgh, PA 15213.
E-mail address: schelberteb@upmc.edu

Heart Failure Clin 15 (2019) 179–189
https://doi.org/10.1016/j.hfc.2018.12.009

to integrate observations from highly controlled experiments, clinical observational data, and clinical trials. Ultimately, the cardiology community requires randomized, controlled trials to demonstrate that reversal of MF represents a legitimate therapeutic target in heart failure. Such trials would illustrate that improvements in MF parallel improved outcomes in heart failure. We hope this work will provide a foundation and further impetus to support such investigations.

DEFINITIONS OF MYOCARDIAL FIBROSIS

Simply defined, MF represents the disproportionate accumulation of fibrillar collagen relative to cardiomyocytes.[1,3] As such, MF refers to increased collagen concentration specifically, not the total content, which obviously represents the product of MF multiplied by left ventricular mass. Therefore, MF designates architectural distortion at the cellular level resulting from excess collagen and interstitial expansion. Type I and to a lesser degree type III collagen predominate in the expanded extracellular matrix, among other components. Interestingly, investigators describe positive correlations between left ventricular mass and MF, observed in both pathology[4–7] studies and cardiovascular magnetic resonance (CMR)[8] studies, suggesting that MF does not occur solely to replace lost cardiomyocytes in otherwise normal myocardium.

Investigators refer to diffuse MF as reactive fibrosis, where fibrillar collagen accumulates in the perivascular space, around cardiomyocyte muscle bundles, and around individual cardiomyocytes,[9] isolating them from capillaries. Reactive fibrosis can lead to cardiomyocyte hypoxia.[10] In contrast, in reparative or replacement fibrosis or simply scar, fibrillar collagen replaces foci of dead cardiomyocytes, forming scars of variable size[9] that may be visible on CMR examinations incorporating late gadolinium enhancement. **Fig. 1** depicts these 2 cellular processes that culminate in MF. Whether these types of MF simply reflect spatial variation of the same process remains uncertain.[9]

Both diffuse MF and replacement fibrosis commonly occur in myocardial disease (**Fig. 2**). Both types of MF are observed in ischemic and nonischemic myocardial injury. Macroscopic scars may result from ischemic[11] or nonischemic[12] injury to the myocardium. Reactive fibrosis may occur in ischemic cardiomyopathy, remote from myocardial infarction.[13] Reactive fibrosis may also occur in various nonischemic cardiomyopathies, including dilated cardiomyopathy,[7] valvular heart disease,[14] and hypertensive heart disease.[6] These types of fibrosis may coexist in the same

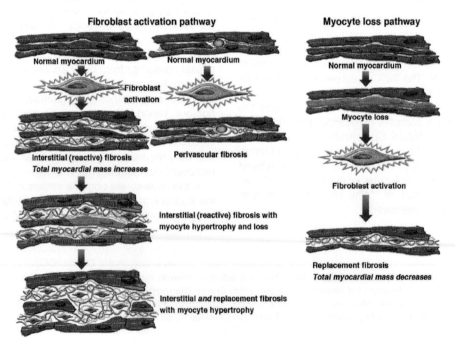

Fig. 1. Myocardial fibrosis may occur through different cellular events. Diffuse reactive myocardial fibrosis follows primary activation of fibroblasts, whereas focal reparative/replacement myocardial fibrosis follows cardiomyocyte loss. (*From* Schelbert EB, Fonarow GC, Bonow RO, et al. Therapeutic targets in heart failure: refocusing on the myocardial interstitium. J Am Coll Cardiol 2014;63(21):2190; with permission.)

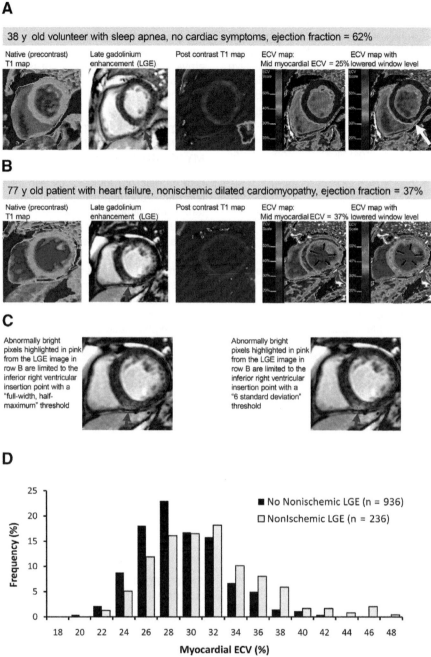

Fig. 2. Myocardial fibrosis (MF) can appear as focal fibrosis (ie, replacement fibrosis, *red* and *white arrows*; A–C) detectable by late gadolinium enhancement (LGE) imaging or diffuse reactive fibrosis (ie, interstitial fibrosis, *panel B*) detectable by extracellular volume mapping. Quantitative extracellular volume fraction (ECV) maps generated from T1 maps can display normal myocardium (A) as well as severe diffuse MF (*black arrows*; B) that is not detectable with LGE imaging (C), and the distributions of ECV in those with and without evident LGE (D) may overlap considerably in large cohorts. Semiautomated quantitative LGE thresholding techniques (C) using 2 common methods fail to identify the severe diffuse MF present in nonenhanced myocardium (*row B*). The upward shift of ECV distributions for those with focal LGE can be small compared with the spectrum of ECV (D). Midmyocardial ECV was measured to avoid contamination from partial volume effects from limited spatial resolution and/or misregistration errors, depicted by the green-colored pixels along the blood pool and myocardium interface. (*From* Schelbert EB, Piehler KM, Zareba KM, et al. Myocardial fibrosis quantified by extracellular volume is associated with subsequent hospitalization for heart failure, death, or both across the spectrum of ejection fraction and heart failure stage. J Am Heart Assoc 2015;4(12):e002613; with permission.)

patients, again raising the issue of whether the they represent truly different entities.[9]

Beyond the excess quantity of MF relative to the mass of cardiomyocytes, MF also implies the potential for changes in its quality. Excessive collagen cross-linking may resist degradation by matrix metalloproteinase and underlie impaired collagen homestasis.[15] The ratio between the C-terminal telopeptide of collagen type I and matrix metalloproteinase-1 in the serum inversely relates to extent of cross-linking. More cross-linking then increases the risk hospitalization for heart failure.[15]

DICHOTOMIZING THE MYOCARDIUM TO EMPHASIZE THE FIBROBLAST AND THE INTERSTITIUM

The concept of MF inherently distinguishes the extracellular compartment containing the fibroblast and the collagen it secretes from the cardiomyocyte compartment containing the sarcomere contractile apparatus.[16,17] As such, it provides an important dimension to characterize cardiac remodeling beyond simply mass, volume, and function. Ultimately, MF implicates disease originating from the fibroblast. Our (Schelbert, unpublished data, 2018) suggest that cardiomyocyte function and fibroblast regulation of the interstitium represent independent and distinct domains of cardiac dysfunction and vulnerability.

DELETERIOUS EFFECTS OF INTERSTITIAL EXPANSION FROM PROTEIN DEPOSITION: AMYLOIDOSIS

Strong evidence exists to demonstrate how excess protein in the interstitium specifically causes cardiac function leading to adverse outcomes. The clinical example of cardiac amyloidosis, a pure interstitial heart disease (where protein depositions occurs independent of cardiomyocyte loss), illustrates how excess interstitial proteins lead to heart failure,[18] microvascular dysfunction,[19] life-threatening ventricular arrhythmia,[20] and death.[18] Such dysfunction and adverse outcomes often occur in the setting of a preserved ejection fraction, emphasizing the inherent importance of the interstitium, irrespective of cardiomyocyte contractility (acknowledging that hypertrophy can mask contractile dysfunction while preserving ejection fraction[21]). Importantly, preventing further amyloid protein deposition, those with transthyretin amyloidosis decreases all-cause mortality and cardiovascular-related

hospitalizations and decreases the decline in functional capacity and quality of life as compared with placebo.[22] This recent trial satisfies a critical condition for causality for amyloidosis: The cessation of the disease process affecting the cardiac interstitium improves patient outcomes.

DELETERIOUS EFFECTS OF INTERSTITIAL EXPANSION FROM PROTEIN DEPOSITION: MYOCARDIAL FIBROSIS

Like cardiac amyloidosis, excess interstitial protein deposition (ie, collagen protein) also characterizes MF, although the extent of excess protein deposition and the occurrence of adverse outcomes are less extreme in MF compared with cardiac amyloidosis. Abundant literature demonstrates the deleterious effects of MF. MF adversely impacts microvascular function,[23] mechanical function,[24–26] and electrical function[27–31] (Fig. 3). Reversing MF in humans with modestly effective pharmacologic therapy targeting the profibrotic renin–angiotensin–aldosterone system (RAAS) improves mechanical function,[24–26] microvascular function,[23] and probably electrical function.[28,32,33] RAAS inhibitors only regress the collagen volume fraction in humans by only an approximate 20% relative change and a 1% absolute change over 6 to 12 months.[23–26,34,35]

We and other investigators have shown that measures of MF associate with outcomes in several selected and unselected patient populations with preserved or reduced ejection fraction.[8,30,36–43] The risk of adverse outcomes in MF parallel the severity of MF (Fig. 4). A dose-response relationship has been demonstrated in large cohorts.[8,38]

ANTIFIBROTIC MEDICATION IMPROVING OUTCOMES IN CLINICAL TRIALS

Unfortunately, the cardiology community lacks a singular trial showing that specific regression of MF improves outcomes. Notably, Zannad and colleagues[44] reported that limitation of the excessive collagen turnover may be one of the various extrarenal mechanisms contributing to the beneficial effect of spironolactone in patients with heart failure with reduced ejection fraction.

Still, compelling circumstantial evidence supports a causal role for MF. Antifibrotic medications that antagonize RAAS improved outcomes in pivotal trials in heart failure with heart failure with reduced ejection fraction that now form the basis of contemporary treatment. Whether their antifibrotic efficacy underlies their beneficial effects

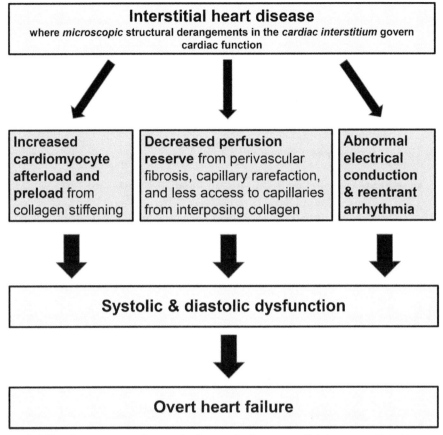

Fig. 3. Myocardial fibrosis represents microscopic changes in the myocardial stroma mediated by excess collagen (mostly type I but also type III) secreted primarily by cardiac fibroblasts in the interstitium, a situation in which synthesis predominates over degradation. (*From* Schelbert EB, Wong TC, Gheorghiade M. Think small and examine the constituents of left ventricular hypertrophy and heart failure: cardiomyocytes vs fibroblasts, collagen, and capillaries in the interstitium. J Am Heart Assoc 2015;4:e002491; with permission.)

remains likely, but consensus does not yet exist for this concept.

Medications that antagonize RAAS may improve outcomes in heart failure with preserved ejection fraction as well,[45–47] but results thus far remain unsatisfying.[48] Several possibilities might explain neutral results of RAAS blockade in heart failure with preserved ejection, including:

1. Limited antifibrotic efficacy of RAAS blockade in humans,[35]
2. Inadvertent inclusion of unsuspected cardiac amyloidosis where (a) events rates are very high in cardiac amyloidosis, (b) the prevalence of cardiac amyloidosis is high in patients with heart failure with preserved ejection[49] (challenging to diagnose without CMR or bone scintigraphy), and (c) RAAS blockade is not effective,
3. Heterogeneous heart failure with preserved ejection populations,[50] without adequate

prevalence of (a) MF or (b) even heart failure with preserved ejection, thereby diluting therapeutic effects in the overall study, and
4. Issues related to suboptimal trial execution related to cross-over, enrollment of patients without heart failure with preserved ejection, poor protocol adherence, and variable rigor of inclusion criteria.[45,47,51]

MYOCARDIAL FIBROSIS PLASTICITY: PREVENTION AND REVERSIBILITY

Several animal studies further support the concept that MF causes adverse outcomes in MF by demonstrating how MF represents a plastic, modifiable substrate amenable to pharmacologic treatment. Among these, Micheletti and colleagues[52] identified Wisper as a cardiac fibroblast–enriched long noncoding RNA that regulates MF, specifically regulating fibroblast proliferation, extracellular matrix deposition, migration, and survival.

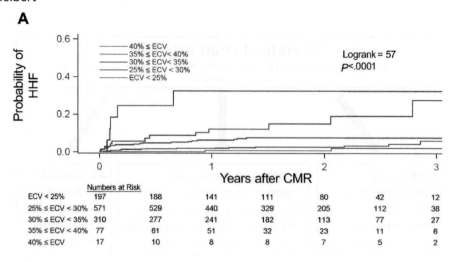

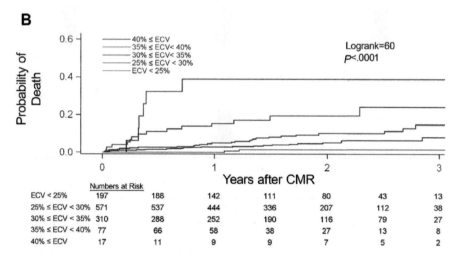

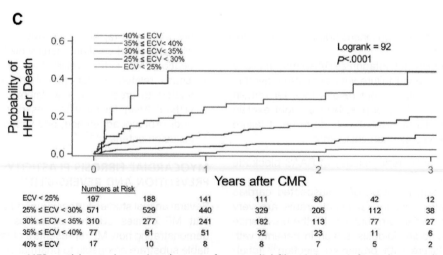

Fig. 4. Among 1172 participants, increasing degrees of myocardial fibrosis in noninfarcted myocardium quantified by the myocardial extracellular volume fraction (ECV) was significantly associated with increased risks of adverse events after cardiovascular magnetic resonance (CMR) scanning: first hospitalization for heart failure (HHF) after CMR (n = 55) (A), all-cause death (n = 74; B), or either HHF or death (n = 111; C). (*From* Schelbert EB, Piehler KM, Zareba KM, et al. Myocardial fibrosis quantified by extracellular volume is associated with subsequent hospitalization for heart failure, death, or both across the spectrum of ejection fraction and heart failure stage. J Am Heart Assoc 2015;4(12):e002613; with permission.)

Wisper as a cardiac fibroblast–enriched superenhancer–associated lncRNA may represent an attractive therapeutic target to reduce the pathologic development of MF and prevent adverse remodeling. Interestingly, Wisper expression was correlated with MF in human patients suffering from aortic stenosis.

Thum and colleagues[53] demonstrated recently that potent modulation of cardiac fibroblast function with miR-21 to mitigate MF improved cardiac function in a rodent model of HF. After integrating their data with prior literature, they further concluded that, "In contrast to the traditional view, in which [myocardial] fibrosis is regarded as a secondary phenomenon, indicative of a primary effect on cardiomyocytes, our results indicate a primary role for cardiac fibroblast activity in myocardial disease."[53]

Yoon and colleagues[54] showed in a rodent model that the matricellular protein CCN5 protects the myocardium through its ability to inhibit MF and preserve cardiac contractility. Even more important, Jeong and colleagues[55] then demonstrated that CCN5 can reverse preexisting established MF by inhibiting the generation of and enhancing apoptosis of myofibroblasts in the myocardium. Collectively, these studies illustrate how MF is preventable and treatable, even after MF occurs, thereby demonstrating reversibility. This plasticity of MF after therapy with improvement of cardiac structure and function further support claims of causality.

NONINVASIVE QUANTIFICATION OF MYOCARDIAL FIBROSIS

To refute or establish that MF causes heart failure and other adverse events, investigators require methods to quantify MF robustly. Extracellular volume (ECV) quantification with CMR offers the most robust estimation of MF.[35] ECV quantifies the expansion of extracellular compartment where collagen resides.[35] ECV does not measure interstitial collagen directly but rather measures the total interstitial space. Still, ECV correlates linearly with the extent of MF, and ECV can be deployed in large-scale studies. ECV measures also include myocardial vasculature, but variation in the microvasculature seems to be small[56] and any capillary rarefaction occurring with MF[57] would only diminish ECV measures. Cardiac computed tomography measures with iodinated contrast agents,[58–63] but few studies have used computed tomography ECV. Native (precontrast) T1[64–70] on CMR scans also increases with MF, whereas post contrast T1[66–68,71–73] decreases, these MF measures remain inferior compared with ECV,

and the latter is not recommended owing to several confounders, which have been discussed elswhere.[17,35,74]

Despite ECV's imperfections, considerable data support ECV as a robust MF measure in noninfarcted myocardium by CMR. First, ECV is well-validated against collagen volume fraction.[66–68,73,75–78] ECV enjoys high reproducibility for repeated CMR scans.[77,79–85] ECV detects clinical reversal of MF.[86] Although other measures may correlate with MF,[65,71,72,87] ECV generally remains superior to native[66–68,76,78] or post contrast T1[66,68,69,73,78] regarding agreement with collagen volume fraction and superior to native T1[88] or post contrast T1[88] for predicting outcomes in large cohorts. Furthermore, inferred functional measures (eg, strain) of MF inherently lack specificity, reflecting either interstitial or cardiomyocyte abnormalities or both, and diastolic Doppler-based parameters remain load dependent.[89–92]

ECV measurement simply uses freely diffusing (ie, non–protein-bound) extracellular molecules as extracellular space markers, a concept published decades ago.[93] ECV is usually expressed a volume percent. Ever since the first CMR ECV publication by Arheden and colleagues,[94] ECV by CMR has generated a significant body of literature. Conceptually, ECV simply reflects the uptake of the extracellular space marker by the myocardium relative to the plasma based on their relative concentrations, assuming equilibration has occurred between plasma and interstitial fluid in the myocardium. Several published reports provide the details, advantages, and potential pitfalls of ECV measurement.[17,35,74,95]

SUMMARY

The cardiology community lacks a taxonomy to prioritize the origins of the complex myocardial pathology underlying heart failure. The key question of "Why does heart muscle fail?" remains unanswered. Nonetheless, a large body of literature indicates that MF represents one of the principal pathways mediating outcomes in heart failure that imparts vulnerability to adverse events. Specifically, MF associates with outcomes in a dose–response fashion, and reversing MF improves several parameters of myocardial dysfunction, leading to improved microvascular function, mechanical function, and electrical function. Modestly effective antifibrotic medications improve outcomes in heart failure with reduced ejection fraction, although for heart failure with preserved ejection the evidence offers no conclusive evidence. Nonetheless, the clinical example of cardiac amyloidosis illustrates how excess protein in the myocardial interstitium culminates in severe HF and dismal prognosis characterized by inexorable clinical decline. Given that robust methods now exist to quantify MF, the cardiology community possess the tools to finally establish unequivocally that MF represents one of the principal pathways mediating outcomes in heart failure that imparts vulnerability to adverse events.

REFERENCES

1. Weber KT, Brilla CG. Pathological hypertrophy and cardiac interstitium. Fibrosis and renin-angiotensin-aldosterone system. Circulation 1991;83:1849–65.
2. Gheorghiade M, Larson CJ, Shah SJ, et al. Developing new treatments for heart failure: focus on the heart. Circ Heart Fail 2016;9:e002727.
3. Swynghedauw B. Molecular mechanisms of myocardial remodeling. Physiol Rev 1999;79:215–62.
4. van Hoeven KH, Factor SM. A comparison of the pathological spectrum of hypertensive, diabetic, and hypertensive-diabetic heart disease. Circulation 1990;82:848–55.
5. Tanaka M, Fujiwara H, Onodera T, et al. Quantitative analysis of myocardial fibrosis in normals, hypertensive hearts, and hypertrophic cardiomyopathy. Br Heart J 1986;55:575–81.
6. Rossi MA. Pathologic fibrosis and connective tissue matrix in left ventricular hypertrophy due to chronic arterial hypertension in humans. J Hypertens 1998;16:1031–41.
7. Beltrami CA, Finato N, Rocco M, et al. The cellular basis of dilated cardiomyopathy in humans. J Mol Cell Cardiol 1995;27:291–305.
8. Schelbert EB, Piehler KM, Zareba KM, et al. Myocardial fibrosis quantified by extracellular volume is associated with subsequent hospitalization for heart failure, death, or both across the spectrum of ejection fraction and heart failure stage. J Am Heart Assoc 2015;4:e002613.
9. González A, Schelbert EB, Diez J, et al. Myocardial interstitial fibrosis in heart failure, biological and translational perspectives. J Am Coll Cardiol 2018;71:1696–706.
10. Sabbah HN, Sharov VG, Lesch M, et al. Progression of heart failure: a role for interstitial fibrosis. Mol Cell Biochem 1995;147:29–34.
11. Kim HW, Farzaneh-Far A, Kim RJ. Cardiovascular magnetic resonance in patients with myocardial infarction: current and emerging applications. J Am Coll Cardiol 2010;55:1–16.
12. Mahrholdt H, Wagner A, Judd RM, et al. Delayed enhancement cardiovascular magnetic resonance assessment of non-ischaemic cardiomyopathies. Eur Heart J 2005;26:1461–74.
13. Beltrami CA, Finato N, Rocco M, et al. Structural basis of end-stage failure in ischemic cardiomyopathy in humans. Circulation 1994;89:151–63.
14. Kanzaki Y, Terasaki F, Okabe M, et al. Images in cardiovascular medicine. Three-dimensional remodeling of cardiomyocytes in a patient with aortic stenosis: scanning electron microscopy. Circulation 2009;119:e10.
15. Lopez B, Ravassa S, Gonzalez A, et al. Myocardial collagen cross-linking is associated with heart failure hospitalization in patients with hypertensive heart failure. J Am Coll Cardiol 2016;67:251–60.
16. Schelbert EB, Wong TC, Gheorghiade M. Think small and examine the constituents of left ventricular hypertrophy and heart failure: cardiomyocytes versus fibroblasts, collagen, and capillaries in the interstitium. J Am Heart Assoc 2015;4:e002491.
17. Moon JC, Messroghli DR, Kellman P, et al. Myocardial T1 mapping and extracellular volume quantification: a Society for Cardiovascular Magnetic Resonance (SCMR) and CMR Working Group of the European Society of Cardiology consensus statement. J Cardiovasc Magn Reson 2013;15:92.
18. Banypersad SM, Moon JC, Whelan C, et al. Updates in cardiac amyloidosis: a review. J Am Heart Assoc 2012;1:e000364.
19. Dorbala S, Vangala D, Bruyere J Jr, et al. Coronary microvascular dysfunction is related to abnormalities in myocardial structure and function in cardiac amyloidosis. JACC Heart Fail 2014;2:358–67.
20. Hamon D, Algalarrondo V, Gandjbakhch E, et al. Outcome and incidence of appropriate implantable cardioverter-defibrillator therapy in patients with cardiac amyloidosis. Int J Cardiol 2016;222:562–8.
21. Stokke TM, Hasselberg NE, Smedsrud MK, et al. Geometry as a confounder when assessing ventricular systolic function: comparison between ejection fraction and strain. J Am Coll Cardiol 2017;70:942–54.
22. Maurer MS, Schwartz JH, Gundapaneni B, et al. Tafamidis treatment for patients with transthyretin amyloid cardiomyopathy. N Engl J Med 2018;379(11):1007–16.
23. Schwartzkopff B, Brehm M, Mundhenke M, et al. Repair of coronary arterioles after treatment with perindopril in hypertensive heart disease. Hypertension 2000;36:220–5.
24. Izawa H, Murohara T, Nagata K, et al. Mineralocorticoid receptor antagonism ameliorates left ventricular diastolic dysfunction and myocardial fibrosis in mildly symptomatic patients with idiopathic dilated cardiomyopathy: a pilot study. Circulation 2005;112:2940–5.
25. Brilla CG, Funck RC, Rupp H. Lisinopril-mediated regression of myocardial fibrosis in patients with hypertensive heart disease. Circulation 2000;102:1388–93.
26. Diez J, Querejeta R, Lopez B, et al. Losartan-dependent regression of myocardial fibrosis is associated with reduction of left ventricular chamber stiffness in hypertensive patients. Circulation 2002;105:2512–7.

27. McLenachan JM, Dargie HJ. Ventricular arrhythmias in hypertensive left ventricular hypertrophy. Relationship to coronary artery disease, left ventricular dysfunction, and myocardial fibrosis. Am J Hypertens 1990;3:735–40.

28. Ramires FJ, Mansur A, Coelho O, et al. Effect of spironolactone on ventricular arrhythmias in congestive heart failure secondary to idiopathic dilated or to ischemic cardiomyopathy. Am J Cardiol 2000;85: 1207–11.

29. Olausson EL, Fröjdh F, Maanja M, et al. Diffuse myocardial fibrosis measured by extracellular volume associates with incident ventricular arrhythmias in implantable cardioverter defibrillator recipients more than focal fibrosis. J Am Coll Cardiol 2018; 71:A1454.

30. Tamarappoo BK, John BT, Reinier K, et al. Vulnerable myocardial interstitium in patients with isolated left ventricular hypertrophy and sudden cardiac death: a postmortem histological evaluation. J Am Heart Assoc 2012;1:e001511.

31. Anderson KP, Walker R, Urie P, et al. Myocardial electrical propagation in patients with idiopathic dilated cardiomyopathy. J Clin Invest 1993;92: 122–40.

32. Pitt B, Zannad F, Remme WJ, et al. The effect of spironolactone on morbidity and mortality in patients with severe heart failure. Randomized Aldactone Evaluation Study Investigators. N Engl J Med 1999;341:709–17.

33. Pitt B, Remme W, Zannad F, et al. Eplerenone, a selective aldosterone blocker, in patients with left ventricular dysfunction after myocardial infarction. N Engl J Med 2003;348:1309–21.

34. Schelbert EB, Fonarow GC, Bonow RO, et al. Therapeutic targets in heart failure: refocusing on the myocardial interstitium. J Am Coll Cardiol 2014;63: 2188–98.

35. Schelbert EB, Sabbah HN, Butler J, et al. Employing extracellular volume cardiovascular magnetic resonance measures of myocardial fibrosis to foster novel therapeutics. Circ Cardiovasc Imaging 2017; 10:e005619.

36. Wong TC, Piehler K, Meier CG, et al. Association between extracellular matrix expansion quantified by cardiovascular magnetic resonance and short-term mortality. Circulation 2012;126:1206–16.

37. Wong TC, Piehler K, Kang IA, et al. Myocardial extracellular volume fraction quantified by cardiovascular magnetic resonance is increased in diabetes and associated with mortality and incident heart failure admission. Eur Heart J 2014;35:657–64.

38. Schelbert EB, Fridman Y, Wong TC, et al. Temporal relation between myocardial fibrosis and heart failure with preserved ejection fraction: association with baseline disease severity and subsequent outcome. JAMA Cardiol 2017;2:1–12.

39. Duca F, Kammerlander AA, Zotter-Tufaro C, et al. Interstitial fibrosis, functional status, and outcomes in heart failure with preserved ejection fraction: insights from a prospective cardiac magnetic resonance imaging study. Circ Cardiovasc Imaging 2016;9:e005277.

40. Duca F, Zotter-Tufaro C, Kammerlander AA, et al. Cardiac extracellular matrix is associated with adverse outcome in patients with chronic heart failure. Eur J Heart Fail 2017;19(4):502–11.

41. Chin CW, Everett RJ, Kwiecinski J, et al. Myocardial fibrosis and cardiac decompensation in aortic stenosis. JACC Cardiovasc Imaging 2017;10(11): 1320–33.

42. Gulati A, Jabbour A, Ismail TF, et al. Association of fibrosis with mortality and sudden cardiac death in patients with nonischemic dilated cardiomyopathy. JAMA 2013;309:896–908.

43. Halliday BP, Gulati A, Ali A, et al. Association between midwall late gadolinium enhancement and sudden cardiac death in patients with dilated cardiomyopathy and mild and moderate left ventricular systolic dysfunction. Circulation 2017;135:2106–15.

44. Zannad F, Alla F, Dousset B, et al. Limitation of excessive extracellular matrix turnover may contribute to survival benefit of spironolactone therapy in patients with congestive heart failure: insights from the randomized aldactone evaluation study (RALES). Rales Investigators. Circulation 2000;102: 2700–6.

45. Pfeffer MA, Claggett B, Assmann SF, et al. Regional variation in patients and outcomes in the treatment of preserved cardiac function heart failure with an aldosterone antagonist (TOPCAT) trial. Circulation 2015;131:34–42.

46. Yusuf S, Pfeffer MA, Swedberg K, et al. Effects of candesartan in patients with chronic heart failure and preserved left-ventricular ejection fraction: the CHARM-preserved trial. Lancet 2003;362: 777–81.

47. Cleland JG, Tendera M, Adamus J, et al. The perindopril in elderly people with chronic heart failure (PEP-CHF) study. Eur Heart J 2006;27:2338–45.

48. Massie BM, Carson PE, McMurray JJ, et al. Irbesartan in patients with heart failure and preserved ejection fraction. N Engl J Med 2008;359:2456–67.

49. Gonzalez-Lopez E, Gallego-Delgado M, Guzzo-Merello G, et al. Wild-type transthyretin amyloidosis as a cause of heart failure with preserved ejection fraction. Eur Heart J 2015;36:2585–94.

50. Lewis GA, Schelbert EB, Williams SG, et al. Biological phenotypes of heart failure with preserved ejection fraction. J Am Coll Cardiol 2017;70:2186–200.

51. Kristensen SL, Kober L, Jhund PS, et al. International geographic variation in event rates in trials of heart failure with preserved and reduced ejection fraction. Circulation 2015;131:43–53.

52. Micheletti R, Plaisance I, Abraham BJ, et al. The long noncoding RNA Wisper controls cardiac fibrosis and remodeling. Sci Transl Med 2017;9 [pii:eaai9118].

53. Thum T, Gross C, Fiedler J, et al. MicroRNA-21 contributes to myocardial disease by stimulating MAP kinase signalling in fibroblasts. Nature 2008;456: 980–4.

54. Yoon PO, Lee MA, Cha H, et al. The opposing effects of CCN2 and CCN5 on the development of cardiac hypertrophy and fibrosis. J Mol Cell Cardiol 2010;49:294–303.

55. Jeong D, Lee M-A, Li Y, et al. Matricellular protein CCN5 reverses established cardiac fibrosis. J Am Coll Cardiol 2016;67:1556–68.

56. Jerosch-Herold M, Sheridan DC, Kushner JD, et al. Cardiac magnetic resonance imaging of myocardial contrast uptake and blood flow in patients affected with idiopathic or familial dilated cardiomyopathy. Am J Physiol Heart Circ Physiol 2008;295: H1234–42.

57. Mohammed SF, Hussain S, Mirzoyev SA, et al. Coronary microvascular rarefaction and myocardial fibrosis in heart failure with preserved ejection fraction. Circulation 2015;131:550–9.

58. Nacif MS, Kawel N, Lee JJ, et al. Interstitial myocardial fibrosis assessed as extracellular volume fraction with low-radiation-dose cardiac CT. Radiology 2012;264:876–83.

59. Bandula S, White SK, Flett AS, et al. Measurement of myocardial extracellular volume fraction by using equilibrium contrast-enhanced CT: validation against histologic findings. Radiology 2013;269: 396–403.

60. Nacif MS, Liu Y, Yao J, et al. 3D left ventricular extracellular volume fraction by low-radiation dose cardiac CT: assessment of interstitial myocardial fibrosis. J Cardiovasc Comput Tomogr 2013;7: 51–7.

61. Kurita Y, Kitagawa K, Kurobe Y, et al. Estimation of myocardial extracellular volume fraction with cardiac CT in subjects without clinical coronary artery disease: a feasibility study. J Cardiovasc Comput Tomogr 2016;10:237–41.

62. Treibel TA, Fontana M, Steeden JA, et al. Automatic quantification of the myocardial extracellular volume by cardiac computed tomography: synthetic ECV by CCT. J Cardiovasc Comput Tomogr 2017;11(3): 221–6.

63. Lee HJ, Im DJ, Youn JC, et al. Myocardial extracellular volume fraction with dual-energy equilibrium contrast-enhanced cardiac CT in nonischemic cardiomyopathy: a prospective comparison with cardiac MR imaging. Radiology 2016;280:49–57.

64. Bull S, White SK, Piechnik SK, et al. Human non-contrast T1 values and correlation with histology in diffuse fibrosis. Heart 2013;99:932–7.

65. Kockova R, Kacer P, Pirk J, et al. Native T1 relaxation time and extracellular volume fraction as accurate markers of diffuse myocardial fibrosis in heart valve disease- comparison with targeted left ventricular myocardial biopsy. Circ J 2016;80:1202–9.

66. Miller CA, Naish J, Bishop P, et al. Comprehensive validation of cardiovascular magnetic resonance techniques for the assessment of myocardial extracellular volume. Circ Cardiovasc Imaging 2013;6: 373–83.

67. de Meester de Ravenstein C, Bouzin C, Lazam S, et al. Histological Validation of measurement of diffuse interstitial myocardial fibrosis by myocardial extravascular volume fraction from Modified Look-Locker imaging (MOLLI) T1 mapping at 3 T. J Cardiovasc Magn Reson 2015;17:48.

68. Inui K, Tachi M, Saito T, et al. Superiority of the extracellular volume fraction over the myocardial T1 value for the assessment of myocardial fibrosis in patients with non-ischemic cardiomyopathy. Magn Reson Imaging 2016;34:1141–5.

69. Ide S, Riesenkampff E, Chiasson DA, et al. Histological validation of cardiovascular magnetic resonance T1 mapping markers of myocardial fibrosis in paediatric heart transplant recipients. J Cardiovasc Magn Reson 2017;19:10.

70. Puntmann VO, Peker E, Chandrashekhar Y, et al. T1 mapping in characterizing myocardial disease: a comprehensive review. Circ Res 2016;119:277–99.

71. Iles L, Pfluger H, Phrommintikul A, et al. Evaluation of diffuse myocardial fibrosis in heart failure with cardiac magnetic resonance contrast-enhanced T1 mapping. J Am Coll Cardiol 2008;52:1574–80.

72. Sibley CT, Noureldin RA, Gai N, et al. T1 Mapping in cardiomyopathy at cardiac MR: comparison with endomyocardial biopsy. Radiology 2012;265:724–32.

73. White SK, Sado DM, Fontana M, et al. T1 mapping for myocardial extracellular volume measurement by CMR: bolus only versus primed infusion technique. JACC Cardiovasc Imaging 2013;6:955–62.

74. Messroghli DR, Moon JC, Ferreira VM, et al. Clinical recommendations for cardiovascular magnetic resonance mapping of T1, T2, T2* and extracellular volume: a consensus statement by the Society for Cardiovascular Magnetic Resonance (SCMR) endorsed by the European Association for Cardiovascular Imaging (EACVI). J Cardiovasc Magn Reson 2017;19:75.

75. Flett AS, Hayward MP, Ashworth MT, et al. Equilibrium contrast cardiovascular magnetic resonance for the measurement of diffuse myocardial fibrosis: preliminary validation in humans. Circulation 2010; 122:138–44.

76. Aus dem Siepen F, Buss SJ, Messroghli D, et al. T1 mapping in dilated cardiomyopathy with cardiac magnetic resonance: quantification of diffuse myocardial fibrosis and comparison with

endomyocardial biopsy. Eur Heart J Cardiovasc Imaging 2014;16:210–6.

77. Fontana M, White SK, Banypersad SM, et al. Comparison of T1 mapping techniques for ECV quantification. Histological validation and reproducibility of ShMOLLI versus multibreath-hold T1 quantification equilibrium contrast CMR. J Cardiovasc Magn Reson 2012;14:88.

78. Zeng M, Zhang N, He Y, et al. Histological validation of cardiac magnetic resonance T mapping for detecting diffuse myocardial fibrosis in diabetic rabbits. J Magn Reson Imaging 2016;44:1179–85.

79. McDiarmid AK, Swoboda PP, Erhayiem B, et al. Single bolus versus split dose gadolinium administration in extra-cellular volume calculation at 3 Tesla. J Cardiovasc Magn Reson 2015;17:6.

80. Schelbert EB, Testa SM, Meier CG, et al. Myocardial extravascular extracellular volume fraction measurement by gadolinium cardiovascular magnetic resonance in humans: slow infusion versus bolus. J Cardiovasc Magn Reson 2011;13:16.

81. Kawel N, Nacif M, Zavodni A, et al. T1 mapping of the myocardium: intra-individual assessment of post-contrast T1 time evolution and extracellular volume fraction at 3T for Gd-DTPA and Gd-BOPTA. J Cardiovasc Magn Reson 2012;14:26.

82. Chin CW, Semple S, Malley T, et al. Optimization and comparison of myocardial T1 techniques at 3T in patients with aortic stenosis. Eur Heart J Cardiovasc Imaging 2014;15:556–65.

83. Singh A, Horsfield MA, Bekele S, et al. Myocardial T1 and extracellular volume fraction measurement in asymptomatic patients with aortic stenosis: reproducibility and comparison with age-matched controls. Eur Heart J Cardiovasc Imaging 2015;16:763–70.

84. Liu S, Han J, Nacif MS, et al. Diffuse myocardial fibrosis evaluation using cardiac magnetic resonance T1 mapping: sample size considerations for clinical trials. J Cardiovasc Magn Reson 2012;14:90.

85. McDiarmid AK, Broadbent DA, Higgins DM, et al. The effect of changes to MOLLI scheme on T1 mapping and extra cellular volume calculation in healthy volunteers with 3 tesla cardiovascular magnetic resonance imaging. Quant Imaging Med Surg 2015;5:503–10.

86. Heydari B, Abdullah S, Pottala JV, et al. Effect of Omega-3 acid ethyl esters on left ventricular remodeling after acute myocardial infarction: the OMEGA-REMODEL randomized clinical trial. Circulation 2016;134:378–91.

87. Child N, Suna G, Dabir D, et al. Comparison of MOLLI, shMOLLLI, and SASHA in discrimination between health and disease and relationship with histologically derived collagen volume fraction. Eur Heart J Cardiovasc Imaging 2018;19(7):768–76.

88. Treibel TA, Fridman Y, Hackman B, et al. Extracellular volume associates with outcomes more strongly than native or post-contrast myocardial T1. Eur Heart J Cardiovasc Imaging 2016;17:i1–80.

89. Rommel KP, von Roeder M, Latuscynski K, et al. Extracellular volume fraction for characterization of patients with heart failure and preserved ejection fraction. J Am Coll Cardiol 2016;67:1815–25.

90. Obokata M, Kane GC, Reddy YN, et al. Role of diastolic stress testing in the evaluation for heart failure with preserved ejection fraction: a simultaneous invasive-echocardiographic study. Circulation 2017;135:825–38.

91. Sharifov OF, Schiros CG, Aban I, et al. Diagnostic accuracy of tissue Doppler index E/e' for evaluating left ventricular filling pressure and diastolic dysfunction/heart failure with preserved ejection fraction: a systematic review and meta-analysis. J Am Heart Assoc 2016;5:e002530.

92. Santos M, Rivero J, McCullough SD, et al. E/e' ratio in patients with unexplained dyspnea: lack of accuracy in estimating left ventricular filling pressure. Circ Heart Fail 2015;8:749–56.

93. Brading AF, Jones AW. Distribution and kinetics of CoEDTA in smooth muscle, and its use as an extracellular marker. J Physiol 1969;200:387–401.

94. Arheden H, Saeed M, Higgins CB, et al. Measurement of the distribution volume of gadopentetate dimeglumine at echo-planar MR imaging to quantify myocardial infarction: comparison with 99mTc-DTPA autoradiography in rats. Radiology 1999;211:698–708.

95. Kellman P, Arai AE, Xue H. T1 and extracellular volume mapping in the heart: estimation of error maps and the influence of noise on precision. J Cardiovasc Magn Reson 2013;15:56.

Importance of the Left Atrium: More Than a Bystander?

Kalie Y. Kebed, MD[a], Karima Addetia, MD, FASE[b], Roberto M. Lang, MD, FESC, FRCP[c],*

KEYWORDS

- Left atrium • Left atrial appendage • Three-dimensional echocardiography • Strain
- Diastolic dysfunction

KEY POINTS

- The cause of left atrial enlargement is multifactorial and associated with adverse outcomes in multiple disease states.
- Growing evidence supports the clinical importance of left atrial size and function for risk-stratification of patients with heart failure.
- The left atrium modulates left ventricular filling via its reservoir, conduit, and booster functions. These can be measured volumetrically and with speckle tracking strain, are altered in response to age and diastolic function, and are correlated with outcomes.
- Increasing accessibility and automation of 3-dimensional echocardiography and longitudinal strain analyses allow the application of left atrial size and function in routine clinical practice.

INTRODUCTION

Emerging data suggest that the left atrium (LA) is much more than simply a conduit for left ventricular (LV) filling, and its size and remodeling are recognized as a predictor of poor outcomes in multiple disease states. LA dilation has been associated with increased risk of atrial fibrillation (AF), ischemic stroke, mortality after acute myocardial infarction, and heart failure with both reduced and preserved LV systolic function.[1–4] In patients with heart failure, LA size provides incremental prognostic information over LV systolic and diastolic function.[5]

The causal pathway linking LA size with adverse outcomes is not entirely clear, which highlights the fact that LA dilation can be multifactorial, resulting from valvular disease, systemic hypertension, and any condition causing elevated LV filling pressures (**Box 1**). Furthermore, dilation itself predisposes to adverse outcomes, such as the development of AF and ischemic stroke.[1,6] Hence, LA size may be considered a barometer for the combined effect of these conditions longitudinally.

LEFT ATRIAL ANATOMY

Embryologically, most of the LA is derived from the primitive pulmonary vein and is characterized by smooth endocardium, whereas the left atrial appendage (LAA) is the only part from the primitive LA and has pectinate muscle and trabeculations. The LA is the most posterior of all the cardiac chambers, resting adjacent to the esophagus. In addition to the LAA, the LA is composed of a body, which receives passive pulmonary venous

Disclosure: K.Y. Kebed and K. Addetia have nothing to disclose. RML received a research grant from Philips Healthcare.
[a] Section of Cardiology, University of Chicago Medicine, The University of Chicago Medical Center, 5758 South Maryland Avenue, MC 9067, DCAM 5502, Chicago, IL 60637, USA; [b] Section of Cardiology, University of Chicago Medicine, The University of Chicago Medical Center, 5758 South Maryland Avenue, MC 9067, DCAM 5504, Chicago, IL 60637, USA; [c] Noninvasive Cardiac Imaging Laboratories, Section of Cardiology, Heart & Vascular Center, University of Chicago Medicine, The University of Chicago Medical Center, 5758 South Maryland Avenue, MC 9067, DCAM 5509, Chicago, IL 60637, USA
* Corresponding author.
E-mail address: rlang@medicine.bsd.uchicago.edu

Heart Failure Clin 15 (2019) 191–204
https://doi.org/10.1016/j.hfc.2018.12.001

flow, a vestibule surrounding the mitral orifice, and a shared interatrial septum with the right atrium. The pulmonary veins drain into the posterior LA body, with the ostia of the left pulmonary veins higher than the right. The left circumflex artery and great cardiac vein run together in the left atrioventricular groove. The coronary sinus travels along the epicardial aspect of the posteroinferior wall.[7]

In utero, the interatrial septum is formed by the septum primum growing from the roof of the atria toward the endocardial cushion. Fenestrations then form within the septum primum. The septum secundum then forms by an in-folding of the atrial walls and through the overlap of the septum primum to the left acts as a conduit for right-to-left shunting of oxygenated blood in fetal circulation. After birth, if the primum and secundum septum fail to fuse, this results in a patent foramen ovale at the anterosuperior edge of the fossa ovalis.[8]

When viewed from the right atrium on transesophageal echocardiography (TEE), the atrial septum can appear falsely larger. The true septum is the fossa ovalis, and the muscular rim that surrounds it. The aortic mound is the anterior portion of the septum, which lies immediately behind the aortic root. Understanding LA anatomy and its relationship to other adjacent structures is very important, especially with the increase in percutaneous therapies requiring transseptal puncture.[7]

LEFT ATRIAL APPENDAGE ANATOMY

TEE been extensively used to characterize LAA structure and function and is the gold standard for assessing for the presence of LAA thrombus with a sensitivity of 92% to 100% and specificity of 98% to 99%.[9] Although the LAA is sometimes visualized on transthoracic echocardiographic (TTE) imaging in the parasternal short axis through the cardiac base and the apical 2-chamber view, TEE is far superior to TTE in LAA assessment. In most patients, the LAA lies on the anterolateral aspect of the LA with an oval-shaped orifice separated from the left upper pulmonary vein by the left lateral ridge.[7,10] There are significant variations in the size, shape, and relation to adjacent structures, and with the expanding use of the Watchman LAA occluder device for stroke prevention, it is important to clearly define the LAA anatomy. **Fig. 1** shows a comprehensive assessment of the LAA before WATCHMAN implantation. The LAA can be single- or multilobed and morphologically has been classified having 4 broad categories. In one multimodality imaging study, the most common morphologies of the LAA were chicken wing (48%), cactus (30%), windsock (19%), and cauliflower (3%), as seen in **Fig. 2** A–D. The chicken wing morphology, after adjusting for other comorbidities, has been associated with higher thromboembolic risk.[11] The inner surface of the LAA has pectinate muscle bundles that can mimic thrombi or other intracardiac masses.

If the images of the LAA are suboptimal, microbubble contrast agents can be used to help eliminate artifacts, enhance visualization of the cavity, and assess for filling defects that can represent thrombus. Three-dimensional echocardiography (3DE) is a helpful adjunct in assessing the LAA by differentiating thrombus from pectinate muscle and defining the LAA's relationship to surrounding structures. In a TEE and computed tomography (CT) study, LAA orifice area on CT correlated well with area on 3D TEE ($r = 0.98$) but not with area on 2-dimensional (2D) TEE calculated assuming an ellipsoid shape using diameters obtained from the orthogonal plane ($r = 0.13$). Bland-Altman analysis demonstrated that 2D TEE systematically underestimated LAA orifice area compared with 3D TEE.[12]

3DE is also superior in planning for and real-time imaging guidance during percutaneous device therapy for LAA occlusion. Several catheter-based LAA closure devices have been developed over the years, and currently, the Watchman Left Atrial Appendage Closure Implant (Boston Scientific, Massachusetts, USA) is commercially available in the United States. The Amplatzer Cardiac Plug (Abbott, Illinois, USA) is available in select international markets. In the PROTECT Atrial Fibrillation, a prospective, randomized trial, LAA closure with the Watchman was noninferior to warfarin therapy in preventing cardiovascular death, stroke, or systemic embolization in patients with nonvalvular AF after 3.8 years of follow-up and was superior for cardiovascular and all-cause mortality.[13] Five-year follow-up data show that LAA closure with the Watchman device provides

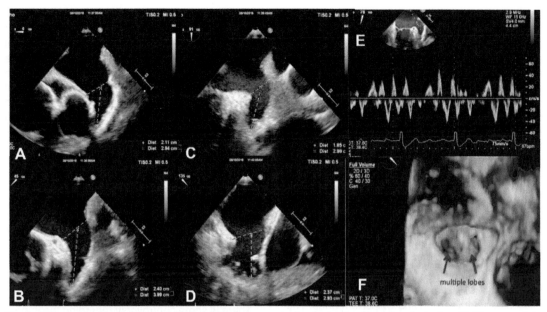

Fig. 1. TEE examination of the LAA before Watchman occluder device implantation, including 2DE images of the LAA at 0°, 45°, 90°, and 135° (*A–D*), pulsed Doppler LAA velocities (*E*), and 3DE enface of the LAA ostium (*F*).

stroke prevention in nonvalvular AF comparable to warfarin, with additional reductions in major bleeding and mortality.[14]

In sinus rhythm, the LAA is highly contractile with cavity obliteration at its apex, which prevents thrombus formation. LAA contraction can be assessed by pulsed-wave Doppler in the proximal third of the LAA and in normal subjects is biphasic with velocities ranging from 50 ± 6 cm/s to 83 ± 25 cm/s with filling velocities

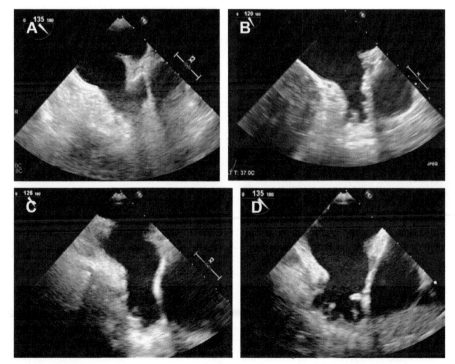

Fig. 2. TTE examinations of LAA morphologies: chicken wing (*A*), cactus (*B*), windsock (*C*), and cauliflower (*D*).

ranging from 46 ± 12 cm/s to 60 ± 19 cm/s. AF causes LAA remodeling with sac dilation and reduction in pectinate muscles. Doppler examination in AF shows loss of the normal pattern and lower velocities (see **Fig. 1**E). Velocities less than 40 cm/s are associated with higher risk of stroke and spontaneous echo contrast and less than 20 cm/s with identification of LAA thrombus.[9,15,16] After cardioversion, albeit spontaneous, chemical, or electrical, there is temporary stunning with a paradoxic worsening of LA and LAA mechanical function and reduction in LAA flow velocities that typically resolve after a few days, underscoring the importance of adequate anticoagulation.[17]

LEFT ATRIAL PHYSIOLOGY

The LA is a complex chamber with multiple functions, and it is important to recognize the dynamic relationship between LA and LV performance. The principal role of the LA is to modulate LV filling via its reservoir, conduit, and booster functions. During the reservoir phase, which is governed by LA compliance, the LA stores pulmonary venous return during LV contraction and isovolumic relaxation. In the conduit phase, the LA passively transfers blood to the LV. Last, LA contraction during the booster phase in late diastole contributes about a quarter of LV stroke volume[18,19] (**Fig. 3**, top row).

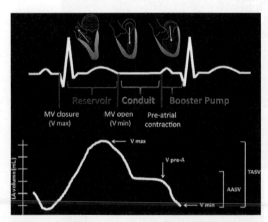

Fig. 3. Left atrial reservoir, conduit, and booster LA function in relation to the cardiac cycle (*top*) with the corresponding LA volume curves during these phases (*bottom*). The maximal volume (V_{max}) at end-systole just before the opening of the mitral valve, minimal volume (V_{min}) at end-diastole before mitral valve closure, and the volume before atrial contraction (V_{preA}) before mitral valve reopening at the time of the P wave on ECG. TASV is $V_{max} - V_{min}$ and the AASV is the $V_{preA} - V_{min}$, which represents the LA booster phase.

The volumes of the LA during these phases can be defined as maximal volume (V_{max}) at end-systole just before the opening of the mitral valve, minimal volume (V_{min}) at end-diastole before mitral valve closure, and the volume before atrial contraction (V_{preA}) before mitral valve reopening at the time of the P wave on electrocardiogram (ECG) (see **Fig. 3**, bottom row). From these 3 volumes, the following parameters can be obtained:

1. Total atrial stroke volume (TASV): $V_{max} - V_{min}$.
2. Total atrial emptying fraction: TASV/$V_{max} \times 100$.
3. Active atrial stroke volume (AASV): $V_{preA} - V_{min}$.
4. Active atrial emptying fraction: AASV/$V_{preA} \times 100$.
5. Atrial expansion index: TASV/$V_{min} \times 100$.
6. Passive atrial emptying fraction: ($V_{max} - V_{preA}$)/$V_{max} \times 100$.[20]

There is some controversy regarding the impact of aging on total LA volume, by both 2-dimensional echocardiography (2DE) and 3DE, but there are data to suggest that phasic -contributions to LA volume change with age. As patients age, there is a decrease in conduit phase (passive emptying) and an increase in booster (active emptying) contribution representing impaired LV diastolic relaxation.[21–23] In a study of 276 healthy volunteers, 3DE LA volumes indexed to body surface area increased with age,[24] whereas another multicenter of the Normal Reference Ranges for Echocardiography in 371 healthy individuals found a trend toward increased LA volume with age that did not reach statistical significance.[23] LA volume is greater in men compared with women, but this difference is attributable to differences in body surface area; therefore, indexed volumes are similar.[24]

CLINICAL IMPLICATIONS OF LEFT ATRIAL ABNORMALITIES

LA preload is largely volume dependent. The LA manifests adaptive changes in its structure and mechanics in response to changes in compliance of the LV, the primary determinant of LA afterload. These changes are well described in the setting of abnormal patterns of LV filling. Previous studies have shown that increasing LA volume and pressure leads to LA dilation with an initial increase in contractile function followed by worsening LA function with further dilation, similar to the Frank-Starling pressure volume relationship in the LV.[18] In the absence of mitral valve disease and AF, an increase in LA size most commonly reflects increased wall tension as a result of chronic elevation of LA pressure.[25–27] This increase in LA size also results in impaired LA function due to atrial myopathy.[28] LA size has been found to be an important marker for the chronicity of elevated LV filling pressures and a powerful predictor of adverse cardiovascular outcomes, including stroke, development of AF, congestive heart failure, and death.[1,2,5,6,29–32] There are also data to suggest using LA size is a therapeutic target. Medical therapy with angiotensin-converting enzyme inhibitor and angiotensin-receptor blockers resulted in reverse remodeling and decrease in LA size.[33,34] Therefore, accurate and reproducible measurement of atrial volumes is important in clinical practice.

MEASUREMENT OF LEFT ATRIAL SIZE

The LA can be imaged with cardiac CT, cardiac MRI, and with the echocardiography being best suited in most situations with the ability to image in real time with good spatial and temporal resolution to assess not only size but also function with Doppler and strain imaging.[35–42] TTE is the most frequently used imaging modality for measuring atrial size. TTE is superior to TEE in evaluating LA size. Because of the close proximity of the LA to the esophagus, it is difficult to view the entire endocardial boundary in the TEE sector. In addition, because patients referred for TEE usually have underlying cardiac pathologic condition, reference values for LA size by TEE have not been established.

Among the different echocardiographic parameters available for assessing LA size, including diameter, area, and the LA volumes has been identified as the most accurate and robust predictor of cardiovascular outcomes.[43] Attention has turned toward establishing the most accurate echocardiographic method to measure LA volumes and identifying normal values and partitions for severity of atrial enlargement, given its clinical implications.

Historically, LA size was assessed using M-mode echocardiography acquired from the parasternal long-axis view. In this transducer position, the anteroposterior dimension of the LA was recorded. Because this measurement is highly reproducible, it was widely adopted by echocardiography laboratories worldwide. It soon became obvious, however, that the LA does not dilate symmetrically in all directions when it enlarges. In fact, there are data to suggest that left atrial enlargement in the anteroposterior direction is constricted by the presence of the spine and sternum, and accordingly, most LA enlargement tends to occur in the superior-

inferior direction.[38] Because of this, the use of M-mode echocardiography (which measures LA size in the anteroposterior direction) was strongly discouraged by the American Society of Echocardiography (ASE) 2005 chamber quantification guidelines, and measurement of LA volumes was recommended for clinical practice.[44]

2DE measurements of atrial volumes assume a certain atrial shape and as a result depend on the specific imaging plane used. For standardization purposes, current 2015 ASE guidelines recommend that the atria be measured in apical 4- and 2-chamber views while excluding the LAA and pulmonary ostia at ventricular end systole.[45] However, these views maximize often the long axis of the left ventricle, rather than the dimensions of the atria, resulting in foreshortening of the atria. Both the 2005 and the current 2015 chamber quantification guidelines recommend the use of the biplane method of disks or alternatively the area-length method for the measurement of LA volumes. The LA endocardial border is traced and volume computed by adding the volume of a stack of 20 cylinders of length (L) and area calculated by orthogonal minor and major transverse axes (a_i and b_i) assuming an oval shape.

$$LA\ volume = \left(\frac{\pi}{4}\right)\sum_{i=1}^{20} a_i \times b_i \times \frac{L}{20}$$

The LA endocardial borders should be traced in both the apical 4- and the 2-chamber views. Alternatively, a biplane calculation could also be performed using the LA areas and length measured from both the apical 4- (A1) and 2-chamber (B1) views. The LA volume is calculated as using the area-length method:

$$LA\ volume = \frac{\left(\frac{8}{3\pi}\right) \times A1 \times B1}{L} = \frac{0.85 \times A1 \times B1}{L}$$

where L is the shortest distance between the midline of the plane of mitral annulus to the opposite superior side (roof) of the LA measured in either the 4- or 2-chamber views. As well, it is assumed that the difference between L measured in the 2- and 4-chambers views is no more than 5 mm (**Fig. 4**). Although the area-length method still assumes an ellipsoidal LA shape, it has the advantage of reducing linear dimensions to a single measurement. The area-length method has been shown to result in atrial volumes that are slightly larger than those obtained using the biplane method of disks.[41]

There was a major increase in the published values for normal LA volumes between the 2005 and 2015 chamber quantification guidelines. The

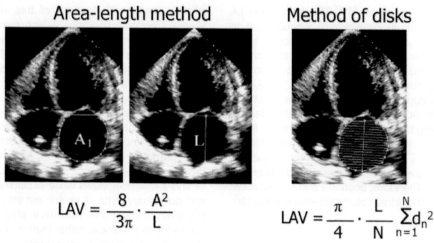

Area-length method

$$LAV = \frac{8}{3\pi} \cdot \frac{A^2}{L}$$

Method of disks

$$LAV = \frac{\pi}{4} \cdot \frac{L}{N} \sum_{n=1}^{N} d_n^2$$

Fig. 4. Apical 4-chamber images of the LA depicting both the area-length and biplane method of disks equations for calculation of LA volumes.

upper normal reference value increased from 28 mL/m^2 for both men and women in 2005 to 34 mL/m^2 in 2015[44,45] (**Table 1**). The main reason for this change is that the 2015 document had access to normative LA volume data obtained from a large number of studies conducted after the 2005 guidelines had been published. Just as it is important not to foreshorten the left ventricle when obtaining measurements of LV volumes and ejection fraction, it is just as crucial to not foreshorten the LA. The need for such "atrial-focused views" has been recognized for over a decade. The long axes of the left ventricle and LA almost always lie in different planes, which explains why dedicated acquisitions of the LA must be obtained to optimize volume measurements (**Fig. 5**). In these LA-focused views, care must be taken to maximize the long-axis length and the base of the LA in both the apical 4- and the apical 2-chamber views in order to avoid foreshortening. If acquired adequately, the length of the LA in the 2 apical views should be nearly identical. As outlined in **Table 2**, 6 of the 13 studies with a total of 3066 subjects out of the total 4701 normal subjects (65%) used to define normative values specifically stated that non-foreshortened atrial-focused views were used.[2,4,19,29–31,35,37,40,42,46–48] This large percentage of the data can probably explain

Table 1
Normative left atrial values

Left Atrial Parameter	Reference	Value
LA volume (2DE)	Lang et al,[45] 2015	LAVi upper limit 34 mL/m^2
LA volume (3DE)	Wu et al,[51] 2013, n = 124 Badano et al,[24] 2016, n = 276 Sugimoto et al,[23] 2018, n = 371	LAVi upper limit 33 mL/m^2 LAVi upper limit 43 mL/m^2 LAVi upper limit 41 mL/m^2
LA volume (CMR)	Maceira et al,[39] 2010, n = 120 Hudsmith et al,[65] 2005, n = 108	LAVi mean 40 ± 7 mL/m^2 LAV mean 103 ± 30 mL (men), 89 ± 21 mL (women)
LA strain	Miglioranza et al,[56] 2016, P-wave reference, n = 171	LA LS pos 19.7% ± 5.6%, LA LS neg −14.5% ± 2.4%, and LA LS total 33.3% ± 5.7%
	Saraiva et al,[55] 2010, P-wave reference, n = 64	LA LS pos 23.2% ± 6.7%, LA LS neg −14.6% ± 3.5%, and LA LS total 37.6% ± 7.6%
	Sun et al,[61] 2013, R-wave reference, n = 121	LA LS pos 46.8% ± 7.7%

Abbreviations: LAVi, left atrial volume index; LA LS, left atrial longitudinal strain positive, negative, total.

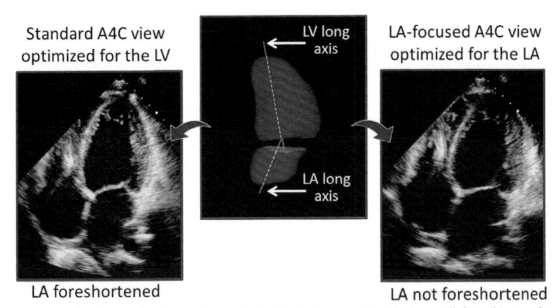

Standard A4C view optimized for the LV

LV long axis ←

LA long axis ←

LA-focused A4C view optimized for the LA

LA foreshortened

LA not foreshortened

Fig. 5. Example of an apical 4-chamber view, optimized to depict maximal length of the LV (*left*). In this view, the LA is foreshortened, in contrast with an LA-focused view specifically optimized to visualize the atrium at its maximal length (*right*). Atrial foreshortening occurs because the long axes of the ventricle are not the same, as depicted in this 3D reconstruction of both left heart chambers (*center*).

Table 2
Studies cited by the recent chamber quantification guidelines update as a basis for an increase in normal values for left atrial volumes

Source	Total Patients	Normal Subjects	Method	View	Indexed Mean LA Volume (mL/m^2)
Tsang et al,[29] 2002	140	44	Biplane A-L	Standard apical	22 ± 5 (no diastolic dysfunction)
Barnes et al,[4] 2004	1554	1462	Biplane A-L	Standard apical	34 ± 14 (no history of stroke)
Takemoto et al,[31] 2005	1375	1237	Biplane A-L	Standard apical	32 ± 12 (non-HF)
Orban et al,[46] 2008	24	24	Biplane A-L	Standard apical	17 ± 3
Yoshida et al,[2] 2009	111	20	Biplane MOD	Standard apical	14 ± 4
Whitlock et al,[35] 2010	103	18	Biplane A-L	Standard apical	23 ± 6
Cacciapuoti et al,[47] 2012	77	15	Biplane MOD	Standard apical	23 ± 4
Thomas et al,[19] 2002	92	92	Biplane MOD	Zoomed apical	23 ± 7
Tsang et al,[33] 2006	423	255	Biplane A-L	Non-forshortened atrial apical	36 ± 10 (sinus rhythm, no CV events)
Yamaguchi et al,[48] 2006	105	105	Biplane MOD	Non-forshortened atrial apical	22 ± 4
Nistri et al,[37] 2011	418	418	Biplane A-L	Dedicated LA	32.2 ± 9
Iwataki et al,[42] 2012	200	77	Biplane MOD	Non-forshortened atrial apical	27 ± 5
Kou et al,[40] 2014	734	734	Both	Atrial focused	29 ± 7 (A-L) and 26 ± 6 (MOD)

Abbreviations: A-L, area-length; CV, cardiovascular; HF, heart failure; MOD, method of disks.

the increase in the recommended normal values in the revised 2015 guidelines.[49]

3-DIMENSIONAL ASSESSMENT OF THE LEFT ATRIUM

Previous studies have shown that 3DE minimizes the inaccuracies associated with geometric assumptions and mostly eliminates the errors associated with foreshortening by allowing the operator to manually select orthogonal planes that maximize the long axis of the chamber being quantified.[50] In order to obtain good-quality 3D images, first, the 2DE image should be optimized in an apical LA focused view as described above by modifying the gain, compress, and time gain compensation controls. For best temporal resolution, a multibeat, wide-angle full-volume acquisition, including the entire LA cavity in the pyramidal scan, should be obtained. This acquisition should be done during a breath-hold to minimize stitch artifact from respiratory motion. Simultaneous real-time multiplanar mode should be used to minimize any dropout, especially of the posterior LA wall.

To perform 3DE analysis, depending on the software used, a combination of 2-, 3-, and 4-chamber views is selected from 3DE pyramidal data set. In these views, the LA boundaries can be manually initialized on 2 frames depicting minimal and maximal left atrial volumes (LAVs). These initialized LA boundaries are then used to reconstruct the LA endocardial surface throughout the cardiac cycle. This reconstruction can be repeated for each frame of the cardiac cycle, resulting in a dynamic cast of LA cavity, and for each consecutive frame, the voxel count inside the 3D surface is used to measure the LA volume. This analysis results in a smooth interpolated LA volume time curve with effective temporal resolutions of 150 to 200 samples per second (**Fig. 6**, left).[50] It has been suggested that because the LA wall lacks the trabeculations found in the LV wall, 3D LA volumes more closely approximate those obtained with cardiac magnetic resonance imaging (CMR).[36] **Fig. 6** (right) highlights the results of the comparisons between the 2DE and 3DE measurements of the maximal LA volumes, respectively, against the corresponding CMR values in a study of 92 patients.[50] 2DE-derived values of the LA volume correlated well with CMR reference values ($r = 0.74$). However, Bland-Altman analysis revealed negative biases of 31 mL ($P<.001$), reflecting a systematic underestimation of the LA volume by the 2DE technique. There was a trend toward increased bias in patients with enlarged atria compared with those with normal atrial sizes. The corresponding 3DE measurements resulted in even better correlations with CMR ($r = 0.93$) with only minimal bias of 1 mL (not significant) for maximal LA volume. The

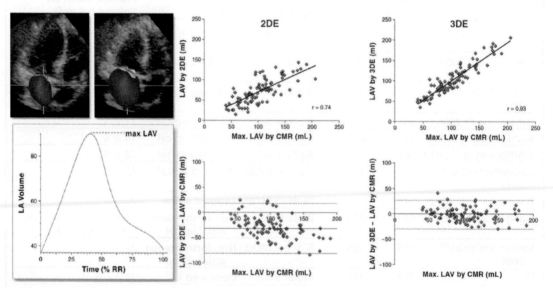

Fig. 6. Example of the LA cavity cast shown at 2 different phases of the cardiac cycle depicting the minimal and maximal LAV and the corresponding time curve depicting the LAV throughout the cardiac cycle from 0% to 100% of the R-R interval (*left*). Linear regression and Bland-Altman analyses of 2DE and 3DE measurements of maximal LAV. Correlation coefficients (*r* values) are shown; solid horizontal lines depict the bias of each technique (mean difference from the CMR reference, whereas dashed lines indicate the limits of agreement; 2 standard deviations around the mean difference) (*right*).

limits of agreement for the 3DE measurements were considerably tighter than those of the 2DE data.

There are conflicting data on the relationship between 3DE- and 2DE-derived LA volumes with some studies finding significantly larger normal reference values for maximum LA volumes obtained by 3D echocardiography (20%–30% larger) versus those obtained using the 2D biplane Simpson method performed on atrial-focused views, where others have found similar values between the 2 methods.[24,49,51] In those with differences in 2DE and 3DE LA volume, the 3DE-derived LA volume had a stronger and additive prognostic value with higher risk ratios compared with 2DE-derived volume.[51] 2DE, 3DE, and CMR normative LA volumes are summarized in **Table 1**.

Despite the well-known advantages of 3DE, this modality is not routinely used in clinical practice for a variety of reasons, including the need for 3DE-specific expertise and the additional time needed for 3DE imaging. Philips HeartModel A.I. is a fully automated program, validated and found to be reasonably accurate when compared with CMR measurements in a group of more than 150 patients, which simultaneously detects LA and LV endocardial surfaces using an adaptive analytics algorithm that consists of knowledge-based identification of initial global shape and orientation followed by patient-specific adaptation. In a study of 30 patients, the average acquisition time for a 3DE full-volume data set of the LA and LV was 20 seconds, and analysis time was 17 seconds, providing 3D volumes throughout the cardiac cycle (**Fig. 7**). By automating some of the manual steps required for 3D analysis, integration of 3D analysis into the workflow of a busy echocardiography laboratory[52] may become possible in the future.

3DE also allows for the assessment of LA shape, which may help to risk-stratify increases in LA volume. Study of LA shape has provided insight into the potential mechanism that determines blood stasis, which predisposes to embolic events in patients with mitral stenosis. It has been reported that patients in whom the LA remodels from an ellipsoidal to a more spherical shape are at greater risk of embolic events.[53] Spherical remodeling is thought to result in an increase in atrial wall tension that predisposes patients to AF and is less effective for atrial contraction. Although these findings are physiologically important, at this time the clinical utility of LA shape remains uncertain.

DIASTOLIC FUNCTION AND THE LEFT ATRIUM

In addition to volumetric data throughout the cardiac cycle as described above, LA and diastolic function can be assessed with spectral Doppler of transmitral, pulmonary venous and LAA flow, tissue Doppler, and LA strain.[18,54–57] Dysfunction in LA phases leads to impaired LV filling and the development of heart failure with preserved ejection fraction (HFpEF). In the absence of atrial arrhythmias and significant mitral valve disease, LA size and function can act as a surrogate for LV diastolic disease, thus assessing that the LA is vital in diagnosing these patients.[2,32] According to the 2016 ASE Diastolic Function guidelines, LA volume index greater than 34 mL/m² along with abnormal mitral annular tissue velocities (septal <7 cm/s, lateral <10 m/s), average E/e' ratio >14, and peak tricuspid regurgitation velocity greater than 2.8 m/s are the 4 parameters used to assess for diastolic dysfunction (**Table 3**). LV diastolic function is normal if more than half of the available

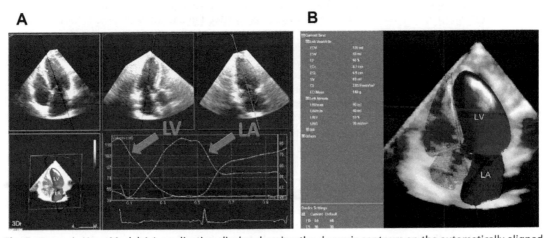

Fig. 7. Dynamic HeartModel A.I. application display showing the dynamic contours on the automatically aligned AP4, AP3, and AP2 views along with the volume waveform and the 3D shell of the left atrial and ventricular cavity.

Table 3
2016 diastolic function guidelines

LA volume index >34 mL/m^2 Abnormal mitral annular tissue velocities (septal <7 cm/s, lateral <10 m/s) Peak TR velocity >2.8 m/s Average E/e' ratio >14	LV diastolic function is normal if more than half of the available variables do not meet the cutoff values for identifying abnormal function. LV diastolic dysfunction is present if more than half of the available parameters meet these cutoff values.

variables do not meet the cutoff values for identifying abnormal function. LV diastolic dysfunction is present if more than half of the available parameters meet these cutoff values. The study is inconclusive if half of the parameters do not meet the cutoff values.[58] The mitral E velocity reflects the LA-LV pressure gradient in early diastole and is affected by LV relaxation and LA pressure. The mitral A velocity is the LA-LV pressure gradient in late diastole affected by LV compliance and LA contractile function. The mitral inflow velocities are used to identify LV filling patterns. Along with tissue Doppler, these can be used to estimate filling pressures. Mean LA pressure can also be assessed with pulmonary venous S/D ratio, isovolumic relation time, Ar-A duration, and in the absence of pulmonary disease, diastolic PA pressure from a pulmonic regurgitation jet. These updated and simplified guidelines for the estimation of filling pressures are more user-friendly and efficient than the 2009 guidelines and provide accurate estimates of LV filling pressure in most patients when compared with invasive measurements.[59] The simplicity of the new algorithm did not compromise its accuracy and is likely to encourage its incorporation into clinical decision making.

LEFT ATRIAL STRAIN

Strain imaging using 2D speckle tracking of the LA has been used for the assessment of left atrial

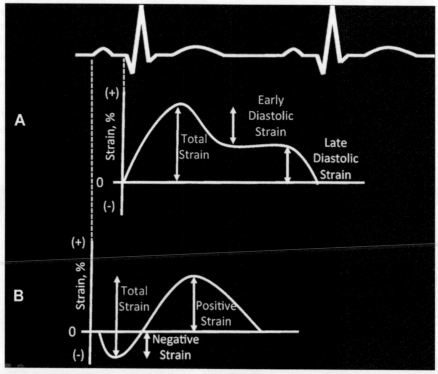

Fig. 8. LA strain time curves and an electrocardiogram using an R-wave zero reference (*A*) and P-wave zero reference point (*B*). Using the R-wave reference point, the total LA strain is positive and the sum of the early and late diastolic strain. Using the P-wave reference point, the total LA strain is the sum of the negative and positive strain.

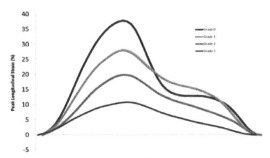

Fig. 9. Peak longitudinal strain curves are depicted as the mean of each subgroup of diastolic dysfunction from grade 0 to grade 4. Diastolic dysfunction grade based on the 2009 ASE guidelines.

function. LA strain is angle independent, and thus less susceptible to the limitations of Doppler echocardiographic assessment of strain. Alterations in LA strain have been described in patients with hypertension, AF, and diastolic heart failure.[56,57] Reduction in LA strain was found to be an important predictor in separating patients with clinical HFpEF and asymptomatic diastolic dysfunction.[60] To obtain LA strain, using 2D speckle tracking software, the LA endocardial border is traced in the apical 4-chamber view, taking care to exclude the appendage and pulmonary veins from the LA cavity, generating an LA longitudinal strain curve throughout the cardiac cycle. The peak negative strain corresponds to the LA contractile function and the peak positive strain corresponds to the LA conduit function. The sum of the peak positive and negative strains is considered to be total LA strain, corresponding to LA reservoir function. Studies using either the R wave (**Fig. 8**A) or the P wave (see **Fig. 8**B) as the zero-reference point have generated completely different normative values.[55,56,61] The single additional measurement of LA strain using 2D speckle tracking may be a valuable diagnostic tool in the evaluation of diastolic dysfunction (**Fig. 9**).[62] In addition, changes in LA strain have been shown to be independent of LA volume in patients with HFpEF[63] and correlated well with filling pressures in patients with systolic heart failure.[64] However, peak LA strain is susceptible to the effects of age, obesity, valvular disease, such as mitral regurgitation, and AF.[54]

SUMMARY

Alterations in LA size and function have been associated with adverse cardiovascular outcomes. LA enlargement is both a marker of severity and chronicity of diastolic dysfunction and magnitude of LA pressure elevation. LA size assessment is important in routine clinical practice because it holds

clinical and prognostic significance. LA volumes should be measured using dedicated, focused views and reported indexed to body surface area. Although 2DE methods for measuring LA volumes are recommended, 3DE methods are likely more accurate and are a stronger predictor of mortality. However, routine use of 3DE to obtain LA volumes is limited by the time required to analyze the data set to obtain this measurement and the lack of large population-based normal values. These issues are being addressed by the development of automated chamber quantification programs for 3DE data, and large 3DE studies on LA size in normal and abnormal patients. In addition, changes in LA strain are associated with clinical HFpEF and elevated filling pressures in patients with LV systolic dysfunction. Last, it has been demonstrated that medical therapy can result in reverse remodeling of the LA with improvement in size and function,[33,34] suggesting the possibility of using LA as a future therapeutic target.

REFERENCES

1. Tsang TS, Barnes ME, Bailey KR, et al. Left atrial volume: important risk marker of incident atrial fibrillation in 1655 older men and women. Mayo Clin Proc 2001;76(5):467–75.
2. Yoshida C, Nakao S, Goda A, et al. Value of assessment of left atrial volume and diameter in patients with heart failure but with normal left ventricular ejection fraction and mitral flow velocity pattern. Eur J Echocardiogr 2009;10(2):278–81.
3. Moller JE, Hillis GS, Oh JK, et al. Left atrial volume: a powerful predictor of survival after acute myocardial infarction. Circulation 2003;107(17):2207–12.
4. Barnes ME, Miyasaka Y, Seward JB, et al. Left atrial volume in the prediction of first ischemic stroke in an elderly cohort without atrial fibrillation. Mayo Clin Proc 2004;79(8):1008–14.
5. Rossi A, Temporelli PL, Quintana M, et al. Independent relationship of left atrial size and mortality in patients with heart failure: an individual patient meta-analysis of longitudinal data (MeRGE Heart Failure). Eur J Heart Fail 2009;11(10):929–36.
6. Tsang TS, Barnes ME, Gersh BJ, et al. Risks for atrial fibrillation and congestive heart failure in patients ≥65 years of age with abnormal left ventricular diastolic relaxation. Am J Cardiol 2004;93(1):54–8.
7. Ho SY, McCarthy KP, Faletra FF. Anatomy of the left atrium for interventional echocardiography. Eur J Echocardiogr 2011;12(10):i11–5.
8. Calvert PA, Rana BS, Kydd AC, et al. Patent foramen ovale: anatomy, outcomes, and closure. Nat Rev Cardiol 2011;8(3):148–60.
9. Beigel R, Wunderlich NC, Ho SY, et al. The left atrial appendage: anatomy, function, and noninvasive

evaluation. JACC Cardiovasc Imaging 2014;7(12): 1251–65.

10. Agmon Y, Khandheria BK, Gentile F, et al. Echocardiographic assessment of the left atrial appendage. J Am Coll Cardiol 1999;34(7):1867–77.

11. Di Biase L, Santangeli P, Anselmino M, et al. Does the left atrial appendage morphology correlate with the risk of stroke in patients with atrial fibrillation? Results from a multicenter study. J Am Coll Cardiol 2012;60(6):531–8.

12. Shah SJ, Bardo DM, Sugeng L, et al. Real-time three-dimensional transesophageal echocardiography of the left atrial appendage: initial experience in the clinical setting. J Am Soc Echocardiogr 2008;21(12):1362–8.

13. Reddy VY, Sievert H, Halperin J, et al. Percutaneous left atrial appendage closure vs warfarin for atrial fibrillation: a randomized clinical trial. JAMA 2014; 312(19):1988–98.

14. Reddy VY, Doshi SK, Kar S, et al. 5-Year outcomes after left atrial appendage closure: from the PREVAIL and PROTECT AF trials. J Am Coll Cardiol 2017;70(24):2964–75.

15. Transesophageal echocardiographic correlates of thromboembolism in high-risk patients with non-valvular atrial fibrillation. The Stroke Prevention in Atrial Fibrillation Investigators Committee on Echocardiography. Ann Intern Med 1998;128(8): 639–47.

16. Garcia-Fernandez MA, Torrecilla EG, San Roman D, et al. Left atrial appendage Doppler flow patterns: implications on thrombus formation. Am Heart J 1992;124(4):955–61.

17. Ito T, Suwa M, Otake Y, et al. Assessment of left atrial appendage function after cardioversion of atrial fibrillation: relation to left atrial mechanical function. Am Heart J 1998;135(6 Pt 1):1020–6.

18. Hoit BD. Left atrial size and function: role in prognosis. J Am Coll Cardiol 2014;63(6):493–505.

19. Thomas L, Levett K, Boyd A, et al. Compensatory changes in atrial volumes with normal aging: is atrial enlargement inevitable? J Am Coll Cardiol 2002; 40(9):1630–5.

20. Anwar AM, Soliman OI, Geleijnse ML, et al. Assessment of left atrial volume and function by real-time three-dimensional echocardiography. Int J Cardiol 2008;123(2):155–61.

21. Boyd AC, Schiller NB, Leung D, et al. Atrial dilation and altered function are mediated by age and diastolic function but not before the eighth decade. JACC Cardiovasc Imaging 2011;4(3):234–42.

22. Nikitin NP, Witte KK, Thackray SD, et al. Effect of age and sex on left atrial morphology and function. Eur J Echocardiogr 2003;4(1):36–42.

23. Sugimoto T, Robinet S, Dulgheru R, et al. Echocardiographic reference ranges for normal left atrial function parameters: results from the EACVI NORRE

study. Eur Heart J Cardiovasc Imaging 2018;19(6): 630–8.

24. Badano LP, Miglioranza MH, Mihaila S, et al. Left atrial volumes and function by three-dimensional echocardiography: reference values, accuracy, reproducibility, and comparison with two-dimensional echocardiographic measurements. Circ Cardiovasc Imaging 2016;9(7) [pii:e004229].

25. Appleton CP, Galloway JM, Gonzalez MS, et al. Estimation of left ventricular filling pressures using two-dimensional and Doppler echocardiography in adult patients with cardiac disease. Additional value of analyzing left atrial size, left atrial ejection fraction and the difference in duration of pulmonary venous and mitral flow velocity at atrial contraction. J Am Coll Cardiol 1993;22(7):1972–82.

26. Geske JB, Sorajja P, Nishimura RA, et al. The relationship of left atrial volume and left atrial pressure in patients with hypertrophic cardiomyopathy: an echocardiographic and cardiac catheterization study. J Am Soc Echocardiogr 2009;22(8):961–6.

27. Guron CW, Hartford M, Rosengren A, et al. Usefulness of atrial size inequality as an indicator of abnormal left ventricular filling. Am J Cardiol 2005; 95(12):1448–52.

28. Ersboll M, Andersen MJ, Valeur N, et al. The prognostic value of left atrial peak reservoir strain in acute myocardial infarction is dependent on left ventricular longitudinal function and left atrial size. Circ Cardiovasc Imaging 2013;6(1):26–33.

29. Tsang TS, Barnes ME, Gersh BJ, et al. Left atrial volume as a morphophysiologic expression of left ventricular diastolic dysfunction and relation to cardiovascular risk burden. Am J Cardiol 2002; 90(12):1284–9.

30. Tsang TS, Abhayaratna WP, Barnes ME, et al. Prediction of cardiovascular outcomes with left atrial size: is volume superior to area or diameter? J Am Coll Cardiol 2006;47(5):1018–23.

31. Takemoto Y, Barnes ME, Seward JB, et al. Usefulness of left atrial volume in predicting first congestive heart failure in patients > or = 65 years of age with well-preserved left ventricular systolic function. Am J Cardiol 2005;96(6):832–6.

32. Gottdiener JS, Kitzman DW, Aurigemma GP, et al. Left atrial volume, geometry, and function in systolic and diastolic heart failure of persons > or =65 years of age (the cardiovascular health study). Am J Cardiol 2006;97(1):83–9.

33. Tsang TS, Barnes ME, Abhayaratna WP, et al. Effects of quinapril on left atrial structural remodeling and arterial stiffness. Am J Cardiol 2006;97(6):916–20.

34. Gerdts E, Wachtell K, Omvik P, et al. Left atrial size and risk of major cardiovascular events during antihypertensive treatment: losartan intervention for endpoint reduction in hypertension trial. Hypertension 2007;49(2):311–6.

35. Whitlock M, Garg A, Gelow J, et al. Comparison of left and right atrial volume by echocardiography versus cardiac magnetic resonance imaging using the area-length method. Am J Cardiol 2010;106(9): 1345–50.

36. Rodevan O, Bjornerheim R, Ljosland M, et al. Left atrial volumes assessed by three- and two-dimensional echocardiography compared to MRI estimates. Int J Card Imaging 1999;15(5):397–410.

37. Nistri S, Galderisi M, Ballo P, et al. Determinants of echocardiographic left atrial volume: implications for normalcy. Eur J Echocardiogr 2011;12(11): 826–33.

38. Maddukuri PV, Vieira ML, DeCastro S, et al. What is the best approach for the assessment of left atrial size? Comparison of various unidimensional and two-dimensional parameters with three-dimensional echocardiographically determined left atrial volume. J Am Soc Echocardiogr 2006;19(8):1026–32.

39. Maceira AM, Cosin-Sales J, Roughton M, et al. Reference left atrial dimensions and volumes by steady state free precession cardiovascular magnetic resonance. J Cardiovasc Magn Reson 2010; 12:65.

40. Kou S, Caballero L, Dulgheru R, et al. Echocardiographic reference ranges for normal cardiac chamber size: results from the NORRE study. Eur Heart J Cardiovasc Imaging 2014;15(6):680–90.

41. Jiamsripong P, Honda T, Reuss CS, et al. Three methods for evaluation of left atrial volume. Eur J Echocardiogr 2008;9(3):351–5.

42. Iwataki M, Takeuchi M, Otani K, et al. Measurement of left atrial volume from transthoracic three-dimensional echocardiographic datasets using the biplane Simpson's technique. J Am Soc Echocardiogr 2012;25(12):1319–26.

43. Pritchett AM, Jacobsen SJ, Mahoney DW, et al. Left atrial volume as an index of left atrial size: a population-based study. J Am Coll Cardiol 2003; 41(6):1036–43.

44. Lang RM, Bierig M, Devereux RB, et al. Recommendations for chamber quantification: a report from the American Society of Echocardiography's Guidelines and Standards Committee and the Chamber Quantification Writing Group, developed in conjunction with the European Association of Echocardiography, a branch of the European Society of Cardiology. J Am Soc Echocardiogr 2005;18(12):1440–63.

45. Lang RM, Badano LP, Mor-Avi V, et al. Recommendations for cardiac chamber quantification by echocardiography in adults: an update from the American Society of Echocardiography and the European Association of Cardiovascular Imaging. Eur Heart J Cardiovasc Imaging 2015;16(3):233–70.

46. Orban M, Bruce CJ, Pressman GS, et al. Dynamic changes of left ventricular performance and left atrial volume induced by the mueller maneuver in healthy young adults and implications for obstructive sleep apnea, atrial fibrillation, and heart failure. Am J Cardiol 2008;102(11):1557–61.

47. Cacciapuoti F, Scognamiglio A, Paoli VD, et al. Left atrial volume index as indicator of left ventricular diastolic dysfunction: comparation between left atrial volume index and tissue myocardial performance index. J Cardiovasc Ultrasound 2012; 20(1):25–9.

48. Yamaguchi K, Tanabe K, Tani T, et al. Left atrial volume in normal Japanese adults. Circ J 2006;70(3): 285–8.

49. Kebed K, Kruse E, Addetia K, et al. Atrial-focused views improve the accuracy of two-dimensional echocardiographic measurements of the left and right atrial volumes: a contribution to the increase in normal values in the guidelines update. Int J Cardiovasc Imaging 2017;33(2):209–18.

50. Mor-Avi V, Yodwut C, Jenkins C, et al. Real-time 3D echocardiographic quantification of left atrial volume: multicenter study for validation with CMR. JACC Cardiovasc Imaging 2012;5(8): 769–77.

51. Wu VC, Takeuchi M, Kuwaki H, et al. Prognostic value of LA volumes assessed by transthoracic 3D echocardiography: comparison with 2D echocardiography. JACC Cardiovasc Imaging 2013;6(10): 1025–35.

52. Narang A, VV, Tamborini G, et al. 3D echocardiographic automated quantification of left ventricular and left atrial time-volume curves: comparison with MRI. Nashville (TN): American Society of Echocardiography; 2018.

53. Nunes MC, Handschumacher MD, Levine RA, et al. Role of LA shape in predicting embolic cerebrovascular events in mitral stenosis: mechanistic insights from 3D echocardiography. JACC Cardiovasc Imaging 2014;7(5):453–61.

54. Singh A, Medvedofsky D, Mediratta A, et al. Peak left atrial strain as a single measure for the non-invasive assessment of left ventricular filling pressures. Int J Cardiovasc Imaging 2018. [Epub ahead of print].

55. Saraiva RM, Demirkol S, Buakhamsri A, et al. Left atrial strain measured by two-dimensional speckle tracking represents a new tool to evaluate left atrial function. J Am Soc Echocardiogr 2010;23(2): 172–80.

56. Miglioranza MH, Badano LP, Mihaila S, et al. Physiologic determinants of left atrial longitudinal strain: a two-dimensional speckle-tracking and three-dimensional echocardiographic study in healthy volunteers. J Am Soc Echocardiogr 2016;29(11): 1023–34.e3.

57. Buggey J, Hoit BD. Left atrial strain: measurement and clinical application. Curr Opin Cardiol 2018; 33(5):479–85.

58. Nagueh SF, Smiseth OA, Appleton CP, et al. Recommendations for the evaluation of left ventricular diastolic function by echocardiography: an update from the American Society of Echocardiography and the European Association of Cardiovascular Imaging. Eur Heart J Cardiovasc Imaging 2016;17(12): 1321–60.

59. Balaney B, Medvedofsky D, Mediratta A, et al. Invasive validation of the echocardiographic assessment of left ventricular filling pressures using the 2016 diastolic guidelines: head-to-head comparison with the 2009 guidelines. J Am Soc Echocardiogr 2018;31(1):79–88.

60. Kurt M, Wang J, Torre-Amione G, et al. Left atrial function in diastolic heart failure. Circ Cardiovasc Imaging 2009;2(1):10–5.

61. Sun JP, Yang Y, Guo R, et al. Left atrial regional phasic strain, strain rate and velocity by speckle-tracking echocardiography: normal values and effects of aging in a large group of normal subjects. Int J Cardiol 2013;168(4):3473–9.

62. Singh A, Addetia K, Maffessanti F, et al. LA strain for categorization of LV diastolic dysfunction. JACC Cardiovasc Imaging 2017;10(7):735–43.

63. Santos AB, Kraigher-Krainer E, Gupta DK, et al. Impaired left atrial function in heart failure with preserved ejection fraction. Eur J Heart Fail 2014; 16(10):1096–103.

64. Cameli M, Lisi M, Mondillo S, et al. Left atrial longitudinal strain by speckle tracking echocardiography correlates well with left ventricular filling pressures in patients with heart failure. Cardiovasc Ultrasound 2010;8:14.

65. Hudsmith LE, Petersen SE, Francis JM, et al. Normal human left and right ventricular and left atrial dimensions using steady state free precession magnetic resonance imaging. J Cardiovasc Magn Reson 2005;7(5):775–82.

Right Ventricular Size and Function in Chronic Heart Failure: Not to Be Forgotten

Xiao Zhou, MD, PhD[a], Francesco Ferrara, MD, PhD[b],
Carla Contaldi, MD[b], Eduardo Bossone, MD, PhD, FESC[c],*

KEYWORDS

- Right heart • Pulmonary circulation • Pulmonary hypertension • Chronic heart failure
- Echocardiography • Cardiac magnetic resonance • Exercise Doppler echocardiography
- Nuclear imaging

KEY POINTS

- Chronic heart failure (CHF) is a growing public health problem impacting heavily on patient survival, quality of life, and health care costs.
- Contemporary studies have demonstrated the strong prognostic value of right ventricular (RV) dysfunction and related pulmonary hypertension in CHF.
- A multimodality imaging approach is essential to detect early-stage RV and pulmonary vascular remodeling and dysfunction.

INTRODUCTION

Chronic heart failure (CHF) is a growing public health problem impacting heavily on patient survival, quality of life, and health care costs. The main causes include coronary artery disease (CAD), hypertension, valve disease, and cardiomyopathies.[1,2] CHF is classified in 3 distinct phenotypes: heart failure with preserved ejection fraction ≥50% (HFpEF), heart failure with mid-range ejection fraction 40% to 49% (HFmrEF), and heart failure with reduced ejection fraction <40% (HFrEF). Generally, the diagnosis of CHF requires 3 conditions to be simultaneously satisfied: (a) signs or symptoms of CHF; (b) reduced, normal, or only mildly abnormal left ventricular (LV) systolic function; (c) evidence of diastolic LV dysfunction and relevant structural heart disease and elevated brain natriuretic peptide levels.[1,2] Herein, the authors focus on the role of right ventricular (RV) structure and function in heart failure (HF) as

assessed by multimodality imaging approach, namely, echocardiography, chest computed tomography (CT), cardiovascular magnetic resonance (CMR), and nuclear imaging, and discuss its diagnostic and prognostic implications, highlighting recent advances.

RIGHT VENTRICULAR STRUCTURE AND FUNCTION IN HEART FAILURE

Contemporary studies have demonstrated the strong prognostic value of right ventricular (RV) dysfunction and related pulmonary hypertension (PH) in CHF.[3–6] In left heart disease, the passive backward transmission of the pressure elevation contributes to higher postcapillary pulmonary artery pressure (PAP). During the initial stage, the RV can adapt to increased afterload (better to volume overload) by hypertrophy and increased contractility by way of LaPlace's law. However, these mechanisms are often insufficient, and

Disclosure: The authors have nothing to disclose.
[a] PLA Chinese Hospital, Beijing, China; [b] Cardiology Division, Cava de' Tirreni Hospital, University of Salerno, Via Enrico de Marinis, 84013 Cava de' Tirreni SA, Italy; [c] Cardiology Division, A. Cardarelli Hospital, Naples, Italy
* Corresponding author. Hospital Antonio Cardarelli, Via Antonio Cardarelli, 9, 80131 Napoli, Italy.
E-mail address: ebossone@hotmail.com

maladaptive changes can subsequently lead to right heart dilatation up to RV failure.[7,8] An intricate molecular model of cardiopulmonary interaction (metabolic shifts, altered gene expression, neurohormonal signal alterations, hypoxic environment, oxidative stress, and inflammation), the occurrence of ischemia, and unfavorable ventricular interdependence concomitant with overload pressure may contribute to the progression from adaptive to maladaptive RV hypertrophy and dysfunction.[7,8] In this regard, a multimodality imaging approach is essential to detect early-stage RV and pulmonary vascular remodeling and dysfunction.

STANDARD ECHOCARDIOGRAPHY

Transthoracic Doppler echocardiography (TTE) represents a key imaging test of diagnostic-prognostic CHF algorithm.[1,2] In addition to a comprehensive evaluation of the left heart, it allows assessment of the right heart structure, function, and pressures in virtually any clinical setting.[9–11]

Right Heart Structure and Function

In CHF patients, enlarged right heart dimensions along with dysfunction and PH represent an important predictor of morbidity and mortality.[1,2]

The right atrium can be measured as the right atrial volume in a single-plane 4-chamber view.[12,13] RV size can be estimated as RV end-diastolic and end-systolic areas, and RV basal, midcavity, and longitudinal diameters preferably indexed to body surface area. RV outflow tract (RVOT) and pulmonary artery diameters may also be obtained[11,12] (Table 1).

Furthermore, standard TTE indices may be applied to explore the longitudinal shortening (tricuspid annular plane systolic excursion [TAPSE] and RV tissue Doppler imaging [TDI] and Systolic Velocity of Lateral Tricuspid Annulus Displacement [peak s1]) and transverse motion of the RV (RV functional area change [FAC]).[12–15] In particular, TAPSE, being simple and reproducible, represents one of the most widely used indices of RV systolic performance.[11,12,14,15] However, it is based on a one-dimensional measurement, and it is therefore only partially representative of global RV function, especially in PH patients with dilated RV cavity and volume overload, where it can overestimate RV function.[11,12] Guazzi and colleagues[16] have proposed the benefit of the relationship between TAPSE and systolic pulmonary artery pressure (sPAP) as a useful clinical index of the length/force ratio for a better RV function evaluation, predicting outcome in patients with HF. However, it

should be highlighted that 3-dimensional echocardiography (3DE) and CMR are more accurate and precise in assessing dimensions and function of right heart (Table 2).

Right Heart Pressures

sPAP is usually estimated by a simplified Bernoulli equation, applied to the peak tricuspid regurgitation velocity (TRV), then adding right atrial pressure (RAP) (estimated by collapsibility index of the inferior vena cava) ($4 \times TRV^2 + RAP$). Furthermore, shorter acceleration time (<100 milliseconds) and notched (mid or late) pattern of the pulsed-wave (PW) Doppler of the RVOT reflect an increase of mean pulmonary artery pressure (mPAP) and pulmonary vascular resistance (PVR), respectively.[11,12,17] An elevated ratio of peak mitral inflow to early diastolic annular velocity (E/e') along with an increase of left atrial (LA) volume indicates an elevated LA pressure, suggesting a left heart cause of PH[18] (see Table 1).

STRESS ECHOCARDIOGRAPHY

Stress echocardiography (exercise or pharmacologic) is an established tool for the detection of inducible ischemia/myocardium viability and the noninvasive hemodynamic assessment of heart valve diseases (dynamic mitral regurgitation, low-flow–low-gradient aortic stenosis).[19,20] Furthermore, exercise Doppler echocardiography (EDE) may unmask LV diastolic dysfunction. In this regard, an exercise-induced increase in E/e' greater than 13 may be useful to confirm the diagnosis of HFpEF in patients with exertional dyspnea, preserved left ventricular ejection fraction (LVEF), and normal diastolic parameters at rest.[1] EDE has recently been implemented in the evaluation of the right heart pulmonary circulation unit (RH-PCU) of patients affected by CHF, allowing the documentation of substantial and variable changes in functional mitral regurgitation and sPAP.[19] In this regard, depressed RV systolic function at rest along with the lack of increase in sPAP during exercise is related to impaired RV contractile reserve, a marker of adverse prognosis.[21–23] Guazzi and colleagues[24] in 97 patients with advanced stages of CHF (mean age 64 years, 70% men, mean LVEF 33% ± 10%) demonstrated that group C patients (TAPSE at peak exercise <15.5 mm as a measure of reduced RV contractile reserve) showed more severe degree of dyspnea, reduced exercise tolerance, worse LV/LA remodeling, and higher mortality. In the multiple regression analysis, ΔsPAP (Δ = peak minus rest) and severe MR at rest emerged as the strongest cardiac correlates of RV contractile reserve in the

Table 1
Key multi-imaging indices for evaluation of the right heart structure, function, and pressures in chronic heart failure

Key Multimaging Indices	Cut-Off Values	Pitfalls and Remarks
Right heart structure		
Echocardiography		
2D RV diameters	2D RV dimensions: >42 mm at the base, >35 mm at the midlevel	These 2D indices may be late signs of RV remodeling to PH
RV D-shape	LV eccentricity index >1 in systole ± diastole	May differentiate right heart pressure vs volume overload
2D RV wall thickness	2D RV wall thickness >5 mm from the subcostal view	
2D RA volume	2D RA volume/BSA (A-L) >36 mL/m^2 in men >31 mL/m^2 in women	Should be preferred single-plane A-L at end-systole in apical 4-chamber view; 2D RA volume may be underestimated compared with 3DE and CMR imaging reference values
3D RA volume	3D RA volume	No geometric assumption; 3DE tends to less underestimate RA volume than 2D measures compared with gold-standard CMR; dependent on image quality; requires patient's cooperation, offline analysis, and experience
2D RVOT dilatation	PSAX distal diameter >27 mm at end-diastole	
3D RV volume	3D RV EDV/BSA >87 mL/m^2 in men >74 mL/m^2 in women 3D RV ESV >44 mL/m^2 in men >36 mL/m^2 in women	Independent of geometric assumptions but dependent on image quality and regular rhythm; 3DE tends to less underestimate RV volumes than 2D measures compared with gold-standard CMR; lack of data in wide population, requires patient's cooperation, offline analysis, and experience
CMR		
RV volume	RV EDV/BSA >121 mL/m^2 in men >112 mL/m^2 in women RV ESV >59 mL/m^2 in men >52 mL/m^2 in women	Independent of geometric assumptions; may be considered the gold standard
RV mass	RV mass/BSA >29 g/m^2 in men >28 g/m^2 in women	Independent of geometric assumptions; may be considered the gold standard
RA volume	RA volume/BSA (MOD) >47 mL/m^2	Independent of geometric assumptions; may be considered the gold standard

(continued on next page)

Table 1
(continued)

Key Multimaging Indices	Cut-Off Values	Pitfalls and Remarks
Right heart function		
Echocardiography		
TAPSE	<16 mm	Angle and load dependent; may be not fully representative of RV global function. There are no well-defined reference values to assess RV contractile reserve with exercise. TAPSE is generally reduced in patients after cardiac surgery. Prognostic value in CHF
RV FAC $100 \times (EDA - ESA)/EDA$	<35%	Poorly reproducible in case of suboptimal image quality especially during exercise
S′ TDI	10 cm/s	Angle-dependent; not fully representative of RV global function; S′ is generally reduced in patients after cardiac surgery
RV LPSS	$\geq -19\%$	Vendor dependent; prognostic value; good sensitivity for estimate of RV function
3D RV EF $100 \times (EDV - ESV)/EDV$	<50%	RV EF is a global measure of RV systolic performance; independent of geometric assumptions but dependent on image quality; good correlation with RV EF by CMR; lack of data in wide population and requires offline analysis and experience
CMR		
RV EF	<50%	May be considered the gold standard
Right heart pressures		
Echocardiography		
sPAP (mm Hg) $4 \times TRV^2 + RAP$	TRV >2.8–2.9 m/s or not measurable sPAP >34–36 mm Hg	Signal acquisition may be difficult because of respiratory excursion; sweep velocity should be at least 100 mm/s measuring only the well-defined dense spectral profile. If there is a weak TR jet, the intravenous use of agitated saline may provide a more complete TR envelope with attention to avoiding artifacts (fringes) and overestimation
RAP (mm Hg) IVC size and collapsibility	<2.1 cm, collapse >50%: RAP = 3–5 mm Hg	
mPAP (mm Hg) $(0.6 \times PASP + 2) + RAP$	$\geq$25 mm Hg	

(continued on next page)

Table 1
(continued)

Key Multimaging Indices	Cut-Off Values	Pitfalls and Remarks
PVR TRV/VTI_{RVOT} (cm) × 10 + 0.16	<1.5 WU normal PVR >0.2 = PVR >2 WU	Methods for estimating PVR are less well validated; should not be used as a substitute for the invasive evaluation of PVR
AT_{RVOT}	<100 m/s	Heart rate should be in the normal range of 60 to <100 beats/min
FVE_{RVOT}	Midsystolic notching	It is indicative of high pulmonary vascular resistances; lack of data in wide population of PH patients
E/e' LAP = 1.9 + 1.24 E/e'	Average E/e' ratio <10 LAP >15 mm Hg	Angle dependent; proper attention to the location of the sample size

Abbreviations: 2D, 2-dimensional; 3- A-L, area-length; AT, acceleration time by PW Doppler; BSA, body surface area; ED, end diastole; EDA, end-diastolic area; EDV, end-diastolic volume; EF, ejection fraction; ESV, end-systolic volume; FAC, fractional area change; FVE, flow velocity envelope; IVC, inferior vena cava; LAP, left atrial pressure; MOD, method of disks summation; PVD, pulmonary vascular disease; PVR, pulmonary vascular resistance; RA, right atrium; S', peak velocity of the lateral tricuspid annulus as measured by tissue Doppler imaging; TR, tricuspid regurgitation; TRV, tricuspid regurgitation peak velocity; VTI, velocity-time integral; WU, woods unit.

overall HFrEF population. Although the above reports are very promising, challenges remain on proving the feasibility, reproducibility, and the standardization of EDE in exploring the full physiopathologic response of the RH-PCU and related prognostic impact among different clinical conditions.[25]

NONCONVENTIONAL ECHOCARDIOGRAPHY

Major recent advances in echocardiography, including RV strain imaging and 3DE, allow better assessment of RV volume and function and provide additional diagnostic and prognostic information (see **Table 2**).

Strain

RV free-wall longitudinal strain (RVLS) measures longitudinal shortening of the RV wall during systole (good correlation with gold-standard CMR-derived RV ejection fraction[26]) (see **Table 1**). Interestingly, it may detect silent RV dysfunction in the early disease course when all conventional indices appear within normal limits, and it may provide incremental prognostic information and improved risk stratification in PH, congenital heart disease, and HF.[5,27–29]

Three-Dimensional Echocardiography

Three-dimensional (3D) right heart modeling reconstruction has emerged as a useful tool for overcoming intrinsic limitations of standard TTE. Although CMR is the gold standard for RV volumetric measurements, 3DE should be considered a valid alternative, being cost-effective and feasible in every clinical scenario.[30] The right ventricular ejection fraction (RVEF) derived by 3DE proved to be highly accurate, using CMR as a reference, and to be an independent predictor of poor cardiovascular outcomes in patients with different cardiovascular diseases[31] (see **Table 1**). In the Atherosclerosis Risk in Communities study, including more than 1000 elderly participants, lower RVEF assessed by 3DE and worse RV-PA coupling (ie, lower RVEF/sPAP ratio) were both associated with incident HF or death independent of LVEF and N-terminal pro b–type natriuretic peptide (hazard ratio [HR], 1.20; 95% confidence interval [CI], 1.02–1.42 per 5% decrease in RVEF; $P = .03$; HR, 1.65, 95% CI, 1.15–2.37 per 0.5 unit decrease in RVEF/sPAP ratio; $P = .007$).[32] However, it should be highlighted that 3DE requires higher costs than standard TTE for dedicated transducers, hardware, and software, and it needs expertise, good-qualityimages, and additional time to perform measurements.[33]

COMPUTED TOMOGRAPHY

CT imaging is a widely available tool that can provide important and accurate information on intrathoracic organs[3] (see **Table 2**). In patients

Table 2
Relative strengths and weaknesses of different multimodality imaging techniques in assessment of right heart structure, function, and pressures in patients with chronic heart failure

	Echocardiography	CT	CMR	Nuclear Imaging
Availability	++++	+++	++	++
Portability	++++	-	-	-
Cost	Low	Medium	High	Medium
Speed of acquisition	++++	++++	+	+
Radiation risk	-	+++[c]	-	++++
Suitability for sick or claustrophobic patients	++++	++++	+/-	+/-
Contrast agents	+/-	++++	+[a]	-
Temporal resolution	++++	++	+++	-[b]
Spatial resolution	++	++++	+++	+
Right heart structure	+++	++	++++	-
RV function	+++	-	++++	++
Tissue characterization	+	+	++++	+
Myocardial viability	+	+	++++	++++
First-pass perfusion	++	-	++++	++++
Coronary artery imaging	+	+++	++	-
Assessment of pressure gradients	++++	-	+	-
Clinical application	• Allows to assess right heart structure, function, and pressures at rest and during exercise in virtually any clinical setting • 3DE and strain permit better assess to right heart structure and function	• Ruling out underlying CAD and lung disease (interstitial, COPD, CTEPH, cancer)	• May be useful to specify the cause of CHF (differential diagnosis between ischemic vs nonischemic cardiomyopathy) • Higher accuracy to evaluate right heart structure and function	• Assess myocardial ischemia and viability in underlying suspected CAD

Abbreviations: COPD, chronic obstructive pulmonary disease; CTEPH, chronic thromboembolic pulmonary hypertension.
[a] Renal insufficiency (GFR <30 mL/min) contraindicates the use of gadolinium contrast agents.
[b] Temporal resolution for nuclear techniques is variable and depends on the radiotracer and counts.
[c] Radiation risk is significantly higher when the cine ventricular function and first-pass perfusion are performed.

affected by long-standing dyspnea, chest CT rules out underlying lung disease (chronic obstructive pulmonary disease, chronic thromboembolic PH, interstitial lung disease, and pulmonary diseases with mixed restrictive and obstructive pattern, lung cancer).[3] It also permits detection of rare cases of pulmonary veno-occlusive disease (septal thickening, centrilobular ground-glass opacities, and lymph node enlargement) and pulmonary capillary hemangiomatosis.[17] Furthermore, cardiac CT may be considered to noninvasively assess coronary artery stenosis as a cause of LV dysfunction in patients with CHF and low to intermediate pretest probability of CAD or those with equivocal noninvasive stress tests.[1,2,34]

On the other hand, in the acute clinical setting of patients presenting to the emergency room with chest pain and/or dyspnea, CT has been proposed as "triple out strategy" differentiating acute coronary syndrome versus acute aortic syndrome versus acute pulmonary embolism. It should be noted that acquiring information throughout the cardiac cycle (spiral or helical acquisition mode), cardiac CT may also be able to assess RV volume and RVEF with good levels of correlation with CMR (gold standard), but at an unacceptable price of high radiation exposure[3] (see **Table 2**).

NUCLEAR IMAGING

Single-photon emission computed tomography (SPECT) is usually implemented to assess LV ischemia and myocardial viability. In this regard, among patients with known or suspected CAD, regional LV ischemia involving the inferior and lateral walls, assessed by SPECT, confers increased likelihood of RV dysfunction, which is related to exercise tolerance, independently by LV dysfunction.[35] Advanced nuclear imaging techniques have also been applied to acquire information on RV myocardial perfusion, volume, and function in CHF.[1,2] In symptomatic patients without overt CAD, a recent study highlights the role of impaired coronary flow reserve, assessed with stress myocardial perfusion PET, as an independent predictor of diastolic dysfunction and cardiovascular outcomes, including HFpEF hospitalization.[36] Furthermore, several studies have explored the potential utility of [18F]fluorodeoxyglucose PET uptake in the RV metabolism to improve diagnosis, management, and prognostication of the patient with PH. In particular, myocardial standardized uptake value (SUV) measurements (RV/LV SUV ratio) strongly correlated with PH severity.[37,38]

However, nuclear assessment of the RV still suffers several technical limitations and exposes the patient to substantial ionizing radiation burden, which restricts its potential use as an alternative to TTE or CMR in daily clinical practice (see **Table 2**).

CARDIOVASCULAR MAGNETIC RESONANCE

CMR is considered the gold standard for noninvasive quantification of heart volumes, mass, and ejection fraction (see **Table 1**).

In CHF patients, CMR may be useful to specify the cause (ie, early diagnosis of arrhythmogenic RV cardiomyopathy), estimate the survival, and guide treatment decisions, allowing for noninvasive morphologic and functional evaluation, as well as tissue characterization and blood flow. In women with suspected CAD as a cause of CHF and PH, the CE-MARC trial demonstrated higher diagnostic accuracy on the use of CMR compared with SPECT during stress test with adenosine for identification of significant coronary artery stenosis, including perfusion, cine imaging, and scar in a single scan session.[39] Furthermore, late gadolinium enhancement (LGE) is useful to differentiate between ischemic and nonischemic cardiomyopathy. The typical nonischemic patterns are diffuse subendocardial, mesocardiac, and subepicardic, never correspond to a coronary vascular distribution, and independently predict major adverse cardiovascular events, including hospitalization for decompensated HF, sudden and noncardiac sudden death, malignant ventricular arrhythmias, and all-cause mortality.[40,41]

In the presence of PH, LGE is frequently localized in the RV insertion points of the interventricular septum (RVIP), corresponding to higher-fiber stress zones. RVIP LGE extension should be considered a noninvasive marker of advanced PH.[42] Furthermore, the RV myocardial extracellular contrast volume of distribution by T1-mapping is increased, and it is indicative of higher RV myocardial fibrosis.[43] Interestingly, in the case of PH, 4-dimensional (4D) flow-CMR shows flow turbulence and characteristic vortices of blood flow in the main pulmonary artery, and the pulmonary artery vortex duration is related to elevated mPAP.[44] RV volume, function, and mass can be quantified by 4D flow CMR with precision and interobserver agreement comparable to cine steady-state free precession CMR.[45] However, CMR have some nonnegligible clinical limitations compared with echocardiography, including local expertise, lower availability, higher costs, claustrophobia, safety in patients with metallic implants (including cardiac devices), and chronic renal failure (glomerular filtration rate <30 mL/min) with the use of gadolinium contrast agents[3] (see **Table 2**).

Finally, the multi-imaging flow chart of the RH-PCU in CHF along with the specific role of each imaging modality is depicted in **Fig. 1**.

PROGNOSTIC IMPLICATIONS

Although in recent decades pharmacologic and device therapeutic interventions have substantially improved outcomes, the CHF prognosis is still poor, implying an increasing economic and social burden.[1,2]

Numerous multiparametric prognostic markers of death and/or HF hospitalization have been identified in patients with CHF, including comorbidities, functional capacity, biomarkers, multimodality imaging indices, and hemodynamics.[1,2] However, precise risk stratification in CHF and its clinical applications remain challenging. In this regard, a prognostic pivotal role is played by right heart–pulmonary circulation structural and functional abnormalities.[6] In 658 patients with HFrEF, Ghio and colleagues[46] demonstrated that sPAP ≥40 mm Hg and TAPSE ≤14 mm were associated with worst outcome (death, urgent heart transplant,

ventricular fibrillation), and their combination improved risk stratification. Guazzi and colleagues,[47] using the EDE as a tool for CHF risk stratification, demonstrated that the lowest tertile of the TAPSE/sPAP ratio (<0.35 mm/mm Hg) was a marker of significant intrinsic RV dysfunction and independently predictive of adverse outcomes in HFpEF (death and hospitalization). In CHF patients with nonischemic cardiomyopathy, CMR assessment of RVEF provides important prognostic information independent of established risk factors, such as LVEF. RVEF is also strongly associated with indices reflecting intrinsic myocardial contractility and increased afterload from pulmonary vascular dysfunction.[48] Furthermore, in PH patients, CMR evidence of RVIP-LGE is a marker of poorer prognosis, predicting clinical worsening.[42] In the future, CMR could potentially help in risk stratification so that appropriate therapy can be given in a timely manner.

Finally, in **Table 3**, the authors report the major prognostic studies of multi-imaging parameters of right heart structure, function, and pressures in patients with CHF.[49–53]

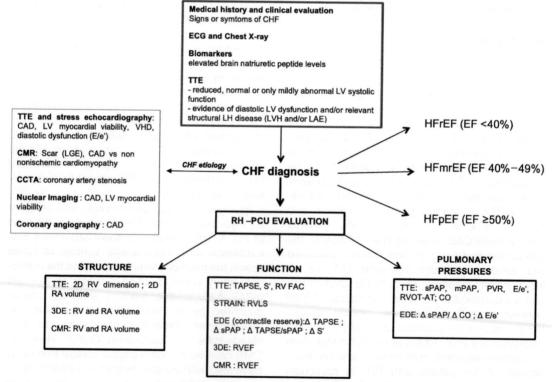

Fig. 1. Multi-imaging evaluation of the RH-PCU in CHF. CCTA, coronary computed tomography angiography; CO, cardiac output; ECG, electrocardiogram; LAE, left atrium enlargement; LH, left heart; LVH, left heart hypertrophy; PCU, pulmonary circulation unit; RV-FAC, right ventricular fractional area change; RVOT-AT, right ventricular outflow tract acceleration time; S', peak systolic tissue velocity at the tricuspid annulus; VHD, valvular heart disease.

Table 3
Major prognostic studies of multi-imaging parameters of right heart structure, function, and pressures in patients with chronic heart failure

Author, y	Patients (M/F) Age (Mean ± SD)	CHF Phenotype	Parameters	Follow-Up	Remarks
Resting echocardiography					
Lam et al,[49] 2009	244 (109 M) 76 ± 13	HFpEF LVEF ≥50% Framingham criteria	sPAP >35 mm Hg	2.4 ± 1.2 y	sPAP >48 mm Hg had worse all-cause mortality than sPAP <48 mm Hg (P<.01)
Ghio et al,[46] 2013	658 (563 M) 63 ± 12	LVEF <45%	TAPSE sPAP	38 mo	sPAP ≥40 mm Hg and TAPSE ≤14 mm were associated with worst outcome (death, urgent heart transplant, ventricular fibrillation) Their combination improved risk stratification
Guazzi et al,[16] 2015	459 Survivors (389; 84% M) 62.2 ± 10.1 Nonsurvivors (70; 86% M) 64.2 ± 8.1	HFrEF HFpEF	TAPSE sPAP Group D (TAPSE/sPAP <0.35 mm/mm Hg)	4 y	Group D had the highest risk (HR 5.6; 3.5–8.9, P<.001), the worst RV-pulmonary pressure coupling (TAPSE <16 and sPAP >40 mm Hg), the lowest peak O₂, and the highest EOV rate
Carluccio et al,[29] 2018	200 (151 M) 66 ± 11	HFrEF with TAPSE >16 mm	RVLS	28 mo	RVLS > −15.3% was associated with outcomes and reclassified patients with TAPSE >16 mm
EDE					
Bandera et al,[50] 2014	136/86 M Group A[a] 36/20 F 67 ± 10 Group B[a] 100/30 F 61 ± 12	HFrEF HFpEF	Peak sPAP Peak TAPSE	—	Peak SPAP (odds ratio, 1.06; CI 1.01–1.11; P = .01) and ex. TAPSE (odds ratio, 0.88; CI 0.80–0.97; P = .01) as main cardiac determinants of ΔVO₂/ΔWR flattening

(continued on next page)

Table 3
(continued)

Author, y	Patients (M/F) Age (Mean ± SD)	CHF Phenotype	Parameters	Follow-Up	Remarks
Guazzi et al,[24] 2016	97 (30 F) 64 ± 11	HFrEF	RVECR (median exercise-induced TAPSE increase; group C <15.5 mm at peak exercise)	16 mo	Group C showed more severe degree of dyspnea, reduced exercise tolerance, worse LV/LA remodeling, and higher mortality rate
Cardiovascular magnetic resonance					
Aschauer et al,[51] 2016	171 (61 M) 70.0 ± 8.6	HFpEF LVEF >50%	RVEF RVFAC TAPSE	573 ± 387 d	RVEF <45% was independently associated with event-free survival (HR: 4.90 [95% CI: 2.46–9.75]). RVEF was superior to RVFAC and TAPSE for prediction of cardiac events
Freed et al,[52] 2016	308	HFpEF LVEF ≥50% Framingham criteria	RV FAC <35% TAPSE <16 mm RVLS > −20%	—	RV strain was associated with outcome (univariate HR: 1.30 [95% CI: 1.07–1.58]). Using multivariate analysis, RV strain was not retained, whereas LA strain and LA stiffness were
Pueschner et al,[48] 2017	M/F: 222/201 54.4 (45.8–65.8)	RV HF in nonischemic cardiomyopathy	RVEF	6.2 y (2.9–7.6 y)	Cardiac mortality
Tampakakis,[53] 2018	1036	HFrEF or HFpEF with PH	Pulmonary arterial compliance, elastance, resistance	—	Pulmonary arterial compliance and elastance were more strongly associated with outcome than resistance or transpulmonary gradient

Abbreviations: —, not reported; EOV, exercise oscillatory ventilation; ex., exercise; F, female; FAC, fractional area change; M, male; RVECR, right ventricular exercise contractile reserve; ΔVO_2, delta oxygen consumption; ΔWR, delta work rate.
[a] ΔVO_2/ΔWR flattening (group A), not flattening (group B).

SUMMARY AND FUTURE DIRECTIONS

CHF represents a worrisome syndrome needing a multidisciplinary approach. In this scenario, a comprehensive assessment of the RH-PCU should not be forgotten in order to unmask early dysfunction signs and to undertake optimal individualized therapeutic interventions.

REFERENCES

1. Ponikowski P, Voors AA, Anker SD, et al, ESC Scientific Document Group. 2016 ESC guidelines for the diagnosis and treatment of acute and chronic heart failure: the task force for the diagnosis and treatment of acute and chronic heart failure of the European Society of Cardiology (ESC)Developed with the special contribution of the Heart Failure Association (HFA) of the ESC. Eur Heart J 2016;37(27):2129–200.
2. Yancy CW, Jessup M, Bozkurt B, et al. 2017 ACC/AHA/HFSA focused update of the 2013 ACCF/AHA guideline for the management of heart failure: a report of the American College of Cardiology/American Heart Association Task Force on Clinical Practice Guidelines and the Heart Failure Society of America. Circulation 2017;136(6):e137–61.
3. Bossone E, Dellegrottaglie S, Patel S, et al. Multimodality imaging in pulmonary hypertension. Can J Cardiol 2015;31(4):440–59.
4. Mehta SR, Eikelboom JW, Natarajan MK, et al. Impact of right ventricular involvement on mortality and morbidity in patients with inferior myocardial infarction. J Am Coll Cardiol 2001;37:37–43.
5. Fine NM, Chen L, Bastiansen PM, et al. Outcome prediction by quantitative right ventricular function assessment in 575 subjects evaluated for pulmonary hypertension. Circ Cardiovasc Imaging 2013;6:711–21.
6. Ghio S, Gavazzi A, Campana C, et al. Independent and additive prognostic value of right ventricular systolic function and pulmonary artery pressure in patients with chronic heart failure. J Am Coll Cardiol 2001;37(1):183–8.
7. Harrison A, Hatton N, Ryan JJ. The right ventricle under pressure: evaluating the adaptive and maladaptive changes in the right ventricle in pulmonary arterial hypertension using echocardiography (2013 Grover Conference series). Pulm Circ 2015;5(1):29–47.
8. Vonk-Noordegraaf A, Haddad FF, Chin KM, et al. Right heart adaptation to pulmonary arterial hypertension: physiology and pathobiology. J Am Coll Cardiol 2013;62(25 Suppl):D22–33.
9. Bossone E, Ferrara F, Grünig E. Echocardiography in pulmonary hypertension. Curr Opin Cardiol 2015;30(6):574–86.
10. Bossone E, D'Andrea A, D'Alto M, et al. Echocardiography in pulmonary arterial hypertension: from diagnosis to prognosis. J Am Soc Echocardiogr 2013;26(1):1–14.
11. Rudski LG, Lai WW, Afilalo J, et al. Guidelines for the echocardiographic assessment of the right heart in adults: a report from the American Society of Echocardiography endorsed by the European Association of Echocardiography, a registered branch of the European Society of Cardiology, and the Canadian Society of Echocardiography. J Am Soc Echocardiogr 2010;23:685–713.
12. Lang RM, Badano LP, Mor-Avi V, et al. Recommendations for cardiac chamber quantification by echocardiography in adults: an update from the American Society of Echocardiography and the European Association of Cardiovascular Imaging. J Am Soc Echocardiogr 2015;28:1–39.
13. Ferrara F, Gargani L, Ruohonen S, et al. Reference values and correlates of right atrial volume in healthy adults by two-dimensional echocardiography. Echocardiography 2018;5(8):1097–107.
14. Ghio S, Recusani F, Klersy C, et al. Prognostic usefulness of the tricuspid annular plane systolic excursion in patients with congestive heart failure secondary to idiopathic or ischemic dilated cardiomyopathy. Am J Cardiol 2000;85:837–42.
15. Ferrara F, Rudski LG, Vriz O, et al. Physiologic correlates of tricuspid annular plane systolic excursion in 1168 healthy subjects. Int J Cardiol 2017;223:736–43.
16. Guazzi M, Naeije R, Arena R, et al. Echocardiography of right ventriculoarterial coupling combined with cardiopulmonary exercise testing to predict outcome in heart failure. Chest 2015;148(1):226–34.
17. Galiè N, Humbert M, Vachiery JL, et al. 2015 ESC/ERS guidelines for the diagnosis and treatment of pulmonary hypertension: The Joint Task Force for the Diagnosis and Treatment of Pulmonary Hypertension of the European Society of Cardiology (ESC) and the European Respiratory Society (ERS): Endorsed by: Association for European Paediatric and Congenital Cardiology (AEPC), International Society for Heart and Lung Transplantation (ISHLT). Eur Heart J 2016;37(1):67–119.
18. Nagueh SF, Smiseth OA, Appleton CP, et al. Recommendations for the evaluation of left ventricular diastolic function by echocardiography: an update from the American Society of Echocardiography and the European Association of Cardiovascular Imaging. J Am Soc Echocardiogr 2016;29(4):277–314.
19. Rudski LG, Gargani L, Armstrong WF, et al. Stressing the cardiopulmonary vascular system: the role of echocardiography. J Am Soc Echocardiogr 2018;31(5):527–50.

20. Lancellotti P, Pellikka PA, Budts W, et al. The clinical use of stress echocardiography in non-ischaemic heart disease: recommendations from the European Association of Cardiovascular Imaging and the American Society of Echocardiography. Eur Heart J Cardiovasc Imaging 2016; 17(11):1191–229.

21. Lewis GD, Bossone E, Naeije R, et al. Pulmonary vascular hemodynamic response to exercise in cardiopulmonary diseases. Circulation 2013;128: 1470–9.

22. Grünig E, Tiede H, Enyimayew EO, et al. Assessment and prognostic relevance of right ventricular contractile reserve in patients with severe pulmonary hypertension. Circulation 2013;128:2005–15.

23. Naeije R, Saggar R, Badesch D, et al. Exercise-induced pulmonary hypertension. Translating patho-physiological concepts into clinical practice. Chest 2018;154(1):10–5.

24. Guazzi M, Villani S, Generati G, et al. Right ventricular contractile reserve and pulmonary circulation uncoupling during exercise challenge in heart failure: pathophysiology and clinical phenotypes. JACC Heart Fail 2016;4(8):625–35.

25. Ferrara F, Gargani L, Armstrong WF, et al. The right heart international network (RIGHT-NET): rationale, objectives, methodology, and clinical implications. Heart Fail Clin 2018;14(3):443–65.

26. Freed BH, Tsang W, Bhave NM, et al. Right ventricular strain in pulmonary arterial hypertension: a 2D echocardiography and cardiac magnetic resonance study. Echocardiography 2015;32(2):257–63.

27. Puwanant S, Park M, Popović ZB, et al. Ventricular geometry, strain, and rotational mechanics in pulmonary hypertension. Circulation 2010;121(2):259–66.

28. Utsunomiya H, Nakatani S, Okada T, et al. A simple method to predict impaired right ventricular performance and disease severity in chronic pulmonary hypertension using strain rate imaging. Int J Cardiol 2011;147(1):88–94.

29. Carluccio E, Biagioli P, Alunni G, et al. Prognostic value of right ventricular dysfunction in heart failure with reduced ejection fraction: superiority of longitudinal strain over tricuspid annular plane systolic excursion. Circ Cardiovasc Imaging 2018;11(1): e006894.

30. Addetia K, Maffessanti F, Yamat M, et al. Three-dimensional echocardiography-based analysis of right ventricular shape in pulmonary arterial hypertension. Eur Heart J Cardiovasc Imaging 2016; 17(5):564–75.

31. Nagata Y, Wu VC, Kado Y, et al. Prognostic value of right ventricular ejection fraction assessed by transthoracic 3D echocardiography. Circ Cardiovasc Imaging 2017;10(2):e5384.

32. Nochioka K, Querejeta Roca G, Claggett B, et al. Right ventricular function, right ventricular-pulmonary artery coupling, and heart failure risk in 4 US communities: the atherosclerosis risk in communities (ARIC) study. JAMA Cardiol 2018;3(10): 939–48.

33. Ferrara F, Gargani L, Ostenfeld E, et al. Imaging the right heart pulmonary circulation unit: Insights from advanced ultrasound techniques. Echocardiography 2017;34(8):1216–31.

34. Goldstein JA, Chinnaiyan KM, Abidov A, et al. The CT-STAT (coronary computed tomographic angiography for systematic triage of acute chest pain patients to treatment) trial. J Am Coll Cardiol 2011;58: 1414–22.

35. Kim J, Di Franco A, Seoane T, et al. Right ventricular dysfunction impairs effort tolerance independent of left ventricular function among patients undergoing exercise stress myocardial perfusion imaging. Circ Cardiovasc Imaging 2016;9(11) [pii:e005115].

36. Taqueti VR, Solomon SD, Shah AM, et al. Coronary microvascular dysfunction and future risk of heart failure with preserved ejection fraction. Eur Heart J 2017;39:840–9.

37. Saygin D, Highland KB, Farha S, et al. Metabolic and functional evaluation of the heart and lungs in pulmonary hypertension by gated 2-[18F]-Fluoro-2-deoxy-D-glucose positron emission tomography. Pulm Circ 2017;7(2):428–38.

38. Graham BB, Kumar R, Mickael C, et al. Severe pulmonary hypertension is associated with altered right ventricle metabolic substrate uptake. Am J Physiol Lung Cell Mol Physiol 2015;309:L435–40.

39. Greenwood JP, Motwani M, Maredia N, et al. Comparison of cardiovascular magnetic resonance and single-photon emission computed tomography in women with suspected coronary artery disease from the Clinical Evaluation of Magnetic Resonance Imaging in Coronary Heart Disease (CE-MARC) Trial. Circulation 2014;129(10):1129–38.

40. Halliday BP, Cleland JGF, Goldberger JJ, et al. Personalizing risk stratification for sudden death in dilated cardiomyopathy: the past, present, and future. Circulation 2017;136:215–31.

41. Pi SH, Kim SM, Choi JO, et al. Prognostic value of myocardial strain and late gadolinium enhancement on cardiovascular magnetic resonance imaging in patients with idiopathic dilated cardiomyopathy with moderate to severely reduced ejection fraction. J Cardiovasc Magn Reson 2018;20(1):36.

42. Freed BH, Gomberg-Maitland M, Chandra S, et al. Late gadolinium enhancement cardiovascular magnetic resonance predicts clinical worsening in patients with pulmonary hypertension. J Cardiovasc Magn Reson 2012;14:11.

43. Mehta BB, Auger DA, Gonzalez JA, et al. Detection of elevated right ventricular extracellular volume in pulmonary hypertension using Accelerated and Navigator-Gated Look-Locker Imaging for Cardiac

T1 Estimation (ANGIE) cardiovascular magnetic resonance. J Cardiovasc Magn Reson 2015;17:110.

44. Reiter G, Reiter U, Kovacs G, et al. Magnetic resonance-derived 3-dimensional blood flow patterns in the main pulmonary artery as a marker of pulmonary hypertension and a measure of elevated mean pulmonary arterial pressure. Circ Cardiovasc Imaging 2008;1(1):23–30.

45. Hanneman K, Kino A, Cheng JY, et al. Assessment of the precision and reproducibility of ventricular volume, function, and mass measurements with ferumoxytol-enhanced 4D flow MRI. J Magn Reson Imaging 2016;44(2):383–92.

46. Ghio S, Temporelli PL, Klersy C, et al. Prognostic relevance of a non-invasive evaluation of right ventricular function and pulmonary artery pressure in patients with chronic heart failure. Eur J Heart Fail 2013;15(4):408–14.

47. Guazzi M, Dixon D, Labate V, et al. RV contractile function and its coupling to pulmonary circulation in heart failure with preserved ejection fraction: stratification of clinical phenotypes and outcomes. JACC Cardiovasc Imaging 2017;10(10 Pt B):1211–21.

48. Pueschner A, Chattranukulchai P, Heitner JF, et al. The prevalence, correlates, and impact on cardiac mortality of right ventricular dysfunction in nonischemic cardiomyopathy. JACC Cardiovasc Imaging 2017;10(10 Pt B):1225–36.

49. Lam CS, Roger VL, Rodeheffer RJ, et al. Pulmonary hypertension in heart failure with preserved ejection fraction: a community-based study. J Am Coll Cardiol 2009;53(13):1119–26.

50. Bandera F, Generati G, Pellegrino M, et al. Role of right ventricle and dynamic pulmonary hypertension on determining ΔVO2/ΔWork Rate flattening: insights from cardiopulmonary exercise test combined with exercise echocardiography. Circ Heart Fail 2014;7(5):782–90.

51. Aschauer S, Kammerlander AA, Zotter-Tufaro C, et al. The right heart in heart failure with preserved ejection fraction: insights from cardiac magnetic resonance imaging and invasive haemodynamics. Eur J Heart Fail 2016;18(1):71–80.

52. Freed BH, Daruwalla V, Cheng JY, et al. Prognostic utility and clinical significance of cardiac mechanics in heart failure with preserved ejection fraction: importance of left atrial strain. Circ Cardiovasc Imaging 2016;9(3) [pii:e003754].

53. Tampakakis E, Shah SJ, Borlaug BA, et al. Pulmonary effective arterial elastance as a measure of right ventricular afterload and its prognostic value in pulmonary hypertension due to left heart disease. Circ Heart Fail 2018;11(4):e004436.

Valve Disease in Heart Failure
Secondary but Not Irrelevant

Patrizio Lancellotti, MD, PhD[a,b,]*, Raluca Dulgheru, MD[a],
Stella Marchetta, MD[a], Cécile Oury, PhD[a],
Madalina Garbi, MD, PhD[c]

KEYWORDS

- Secondary mitral regurgitation • Secondary tricuspid regurgitation • Valvular heart failure
- Mechanism • Treatment

KEY POINTS

- Secondary (functional) mitral regurgitation is a common and insidious complication of heart failure patients with ischemic or idiopathic systolic left ventricular dysfunction.
- Secondary (functional) tricuspid regurgitation has long been neglected and regarded as a surrogate of a more fundamental condition (left-sided valvular lesions, pulmonary hypertension, or atrial fibrillation).
- When present, secondary mitral or tricuspid regurgitation may exhibit a broad range of severity. Any degree of secondary mitral or tricuspid regurgitation conveys an adverse prognosis, with a graded relationship between severity of regurgitation and reduced survival.
- Imaging and more specifically echocardiography plays a central role in diagnosis and serial assessment of secondary regurgitation as well as for timing the intervention and guiding the procedure.
- By convention, secondary mitral or tricuspid regurgitation is graded into mild, moderate, and severe. For tricuspid regurgitation, massive and torrential regurgitation are to be considered.

INTRODUCTION

Valve disease caused by the remodeling of cardiac chambers may complicate heart failure, worsening both symptoms and prognosis. This type of valve disease involves the atrioventricular valves because of their intricate structure and function with the adjacent cardiac chambers, and it is the result of dilatation of the annulus of the valve and of distortion of the subvalvular apparatus. Affecting the valves indirectly, because of changes in size, shape, and function of the ventricles and/or of the atria, it is named secondary or functional valve disease. By comparison, primary valve disease affects the valves directly, causing changes of the leaflets or cusps.

Secondary valve disease may complicate both heart failure with reduced ejection fraction (HFrEF) and heart failure with preserved ejection fraction (HFpEF).[1] In HFrEF, the secondary mitral regurgitation (MR) is predominantly ventricular-secondary, due to remodeling (increased tethering force) and dysfunction (reduced closing force) of the left ventricle as a result of ischemic or nonischemic myocardial disease.[2] In HFpEF, the secondary MR is predominantly atrial-secondary, due to

Disclosure Statement: The authors have nothing to disclose.
[a] Department of Cardiology, Heart Valve Clinic, University of Liege Hospital, GIGA Cardiovascular Sciences, CHU Sart Tilman, Domaine Universitaire du Sart Tilman, Batiment B35, Liege, Belgium; [b] Gruppo Villa Maria Care and Research, Anthea Hospital, Bari, Italy; [c] King's Health Partners, King's College London NHS Foundation Trust, King's College Hospital, Denmark Hill, London SE5 9RS, UK
* Corresponding author. Department of Cardiology, University Hospital, Université de Liège, CHU du Sart Tilman, Domaine Universitaire du Sart Tilman, Batiment B35, Liège 4000, Belgium.
E-mail address: plancellotti@chu.ulg.ac.be

Heart Failure Clin 15 (2019) 219–227
https://doi.org/10.1016/j.hfc.2018.12.014

dilatation of the left atrium as a result of diastolic dysfunction with increased left atrial pressure (increased pushing force) and/or atrial fibrillation. Similarly, secondary tricuspid regurgitation (TR) can be ventricular-secondary or atrial-secondary.

Ventricular-secondary valve disease evolves with the progression of heart failure and varies in severity with the response of heart failure to medical treatment[3] (**Fig. 1**). Ventricular-secondary MR may worsen as a result of systolic dyssynchrony due to left bundle branch block, improving with cardiac resynchronization therapy.[4] There seems to be a certain threshold, a stage of no return, when secondary valve disease stops responding to heart failure treatment and drives the worsening of heart failure.[5,6] This threshold signals development of valvular heart failure.[6] It also signals the need for valve-specific management, valve repair; however, further evidence is needed regarding timing of valve repair before or after reaching this threshold.

Atrial-secondary valve disease responds to diuretics and, in the case of atrial fibrillation, it responds to the specific treatment[7]: rate control, cardioversion, or ablation.

HEMODYNAMICS OF MITRAL REGURGITATION

MR creates a volume overload state. The duration and severity of MR are the main determinants of the adaptive cardiac changes in response to volume overload. The regurgitant volume reflects the sum of regurgitant flow throughout systole and is determined by the MR orifice area, the left ventricle/left atrial pressure gradient, and the duration of the systole. It is typically lower in secondary than in primary MR. Secondary MR has a different physiology as compared with primary MR, because it is the consequence of an initial ventricular disease. The left ventricle and left atrial dilatation are in excess to the degree of MR. The left atrial pressure is often elevated despite lower regurgitant volume than in primary MR. Furthermore, the consequences of regurgitation on the left ventricular and left atrial volumes and function provide indirect signs on the chronicity and severity of the regurgitation. The excess regurgitant blood entering in the left atrium may induce a progressive increase in pulmonary arterial pressure and a significant right atrial and tricuspid annulus dilatation, contributing to TR development.

Imaging Assessment of Secondary Mitral Regurgitation

The role of echocardiography
Echocardiography plays a central role in diagnosis and serial assessment of secondary MR as well as for timing the intervention and guiding the procedure.[2,8–12] The assessment begins with the left

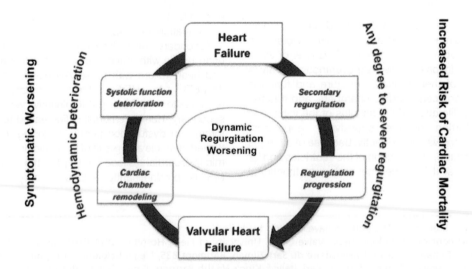

Fig. 1. Vicious cycle associated with secondary regurgitation in heart failure (HF). Secondary regurgitation progression contributes to a cascade of events progressing to poor prognosis. At each point of this cycle, imaging, and, in particular, echocardiography, plays a major role.

ventricle (**Fig. 2**) and the left atrium, to define the specific secondary MR mechanism.

In nonischemic cardiomyopathy, dilatation of the left ventricle with spherical remodeling and displacement of the papillary muscles away from the mitral valve annulus results in symmetric tethering of the mitral valve leaflets (**Fig. 3**), restricting their descent toward the closure plane. Consequently, the coaptation point is displaced toward the apex of the left ventricle, and the coaptation length is reduced or the leaflets fail to coapt. Concomitantly, the mitral valve annulus may be dilated as a result of dilatation of the left ventricle, with or without dilatation of the left atrium as well. The mitral valve leaflets' failure to coapt all throughout systole causes an anatomic regurgitation orifice parallel with the coaptation line, semilunar in shape, having a large dimension in the bicommissural view and small dimensions in all other views (**Fig. 4**). Therefore, the vena contracta of the regurgitant jet in color-flow Doppler imaging is larger in a bicommissural 2-chamber view, and smaller in the other views (**Fig. 5**). The proximal isovelocity surface area (PISA) method of MR quantification assumes a circular regurgitant orifice, thus being likely invalid in ventricular-secondary MR. However, the effective regurgitant orifice area (EROA) can be directly measured using 3-dimensional echocardiography-guided planimetry.

In ischemic cardiomyopathy, the mechanism of ventricular-secondary MR may be similar with the mechanism in nonischemic cardiomyopathy, in case scar involves the distal myocardial segments and in the absence of scar. Myocardial scar involving basal and midmyocardial segments, causing eccentric expansion of the left ventricular wall, results in asymmetric tethering of one of the mitral valve leaflets. The MR orifice shape depends on the extent of the scar circularly, on the perimeter of the mitral valve annulus, to involve a small segment, a scallop or a larger proportion of the leaflet of the mitral valve. The jet resembles that of MR due to mitral valve prolapse of the opposite leaflet. This is because asymmetric tethering and restriction of one of the mitral valve leaflets results in relative prolapse of the opposite leaflet that has free excursion toward the mitral valve annulus in systole; however, this relative prolapse does not result in mitral valve leaflet systolic excursion beyond the mitral valve annulus, within the left atrium.

In atrial-secondary MR,[13] the systolic excursion of the mitral valve leaflets toward the closure plane is not restricted. The leaflets are fully unfolded and stretched, attempting but failing to cover the systolic valve area, enlarged because of annular dilatation with or without loss of posterior annulus systolic sphincter mechanism.[14]

The role of stress echocardiography

Exercise echocardiography with supine bicycle exercise can be used for the assessment of secondary MR to explain symptoms or to establish prognosis.[15–17]

In nonischemic cardiomyopathy, exertion-induced increase in myocardial contractility with consequent decrease in left ventricular cavity size may result in MR severity decrease, predictive of response to medical treatment and good prognosis. The severity of MR can increase on exertion, particularly in the case of exertion-induced systolic dyssynchrony.[15,16]

In ischemic cardiomyopathy, the severity of MR can increase on exertion because of induced ischemia or simply because of change in balance of tethering forces of the valve as a result of an

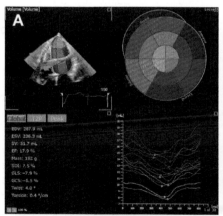
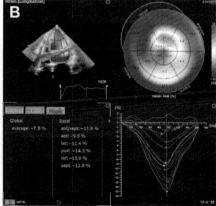

Fig. 2. Assessment of the left ventricle: (*A*) 3-dimensional echo-based assessment of volumes, ejection fraction, systolic dyssynchrony; (*B*) 3-dimensional echo-based assessment of Global Longitudinal Strain and systolic dyssynchrony based on peak strain.

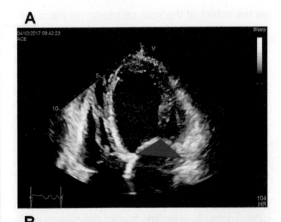

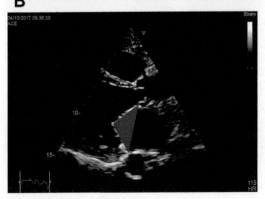

Fig. 3. Symmetric tenting (enclosed red area *arrow head*) of the mitral valve leaflets in dilated cardiomyopathy: (*A*) 4-chamber view; (*B*) parasternal long-axis view.

increase in contractility in areas with no scar, whereas areas with scar remain akinetic or become dyskinetic.[18]

Exertion-induced dynamic MR was also associated with HFpEF, related to increase in left ventricular filling pressures.[19]

The role of cardiac magnetic resonance
The role of cardiac magnetic resonance in the assessment of secondary MR is still to be defined based on evidence.[8] There are limited outcome data and also limited data on regurgitant volume and regurgitant fraction thresholds for severity grading. However, cardiac magnetic resonance provides gold-standard assessment of volumes and ejection fraction of the left ventricle, assessment of the myocardial scar, and assessment of the left atrial volume. Furthermore, the quantification of MR severity based on regurgitant volume and regurgitant fraction does not depend on the shape of the regurgitant orifice or on existence of multiple jets.[8]

Grading mitral regurgitation severity
By convention, MR is graded into mild, moderate, and severe. When present, secondary MR may exhibit a broad range of severity. Any degree of secondary MR conveys an adverse prognosis, with a graded relationship between severity of regurgitation and reduced survival. In the American guidelines, on the basis of the criteria used for determination of severe MR in randomized controlled trials of surgical intervention, both primary and secondary MR are considered severe if EROA is ≥ 40 mm^2, regurgitant volume is ≥ 60 mL, and regurgitant fraction is $\geq 50\%$.[8] In the european society of cardiology guidelines, the corresponding thresholds of severity for secondary MR, which are of prognostic value, are 20 mm^2 and 30 mL, respectively (**Table 1**).[9] These differences in the definition of severe secondary MR are generating considerable controversy within the cardiology community. Noteworthy, in secondary MR, a concomitant increase in MR severity (EROA ≥ 13 mm^2) and in pulmonary arterial pressure (>60 mm Hg of systolic arterial pressure) identifies a subset of patients with moderate MR at high risk of cardiac-related death.[17]

HEMODYNAMICS OF TRICUSPID REGURGITATION

As for secondary MR, secondary TR begets TR. Indeed, TR itself leads to further RV dilation and dysfunction, right atrial enlargement, more tricuspid annular dilatation and tethering, and worsening TR. With increasing TR, the right ventricle dilates and eventually fails, causing increased right ventricular diastolic pressure and, in advanced situation, a shift of the interventricular septum toward the left ventricle. Such ventricular interdependence might reduce the left ventricular cavity size (pure compression), causing restricted left ventricular filling and increased left ventricular diastolic and pulmonary artery pressure. The resulting increase in left and right atrial pressures may promote atrial fibrillation and precipitate symptom onset.

Imaging Assessment of Secondary Tricuspid Regurgitation

The role of echocardiography
As for MR, echocardiography plays a central role in the assessment of secondary TR for diagnosis, follow-up, timing of intervention, and procedure guiding.[8–11,20,21] The morphology of the tricuspid valve is more complex, and the diagnosis of secondary TR is more difficult to make. Three-dimensional echocardiography is essential, because 2-dimensional echocardiography is a poor assessment tool for identification of the 3 valve leaflets and detection of the regurgitation

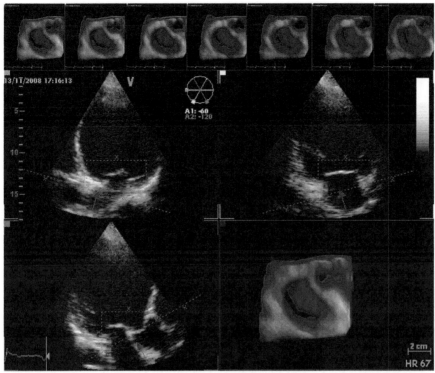

Fig. 4. Failure of mitral valve leaflets to coapt all throughout systole (illustrated with the help of 3-dimensional echo surgical view, in all the systolic frames) causing an anatomic regurgitant orifice parallel with the coaptation line.

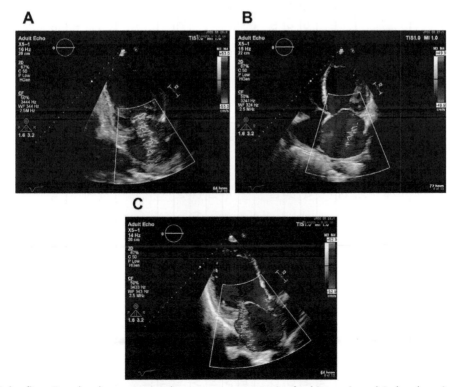

Fig. 5. Color-flow Doppler demonstrating large vena contracta in the bicommissural 2-chamber view (*A*) and smaller vena contracta in 4-chamber (*B*) and 3-chamber (apical long-axis) view (*C*) in ventricular-secondary MR.

Table 1
Mitral and tricuspid regurgitation grading

	MR	TR		
	Severe	Severe	Massive	Torrential
Qualitative				
Morphology	Abnormal/flail/large coaptation defect			
Color Doppler of regurgitant jet	Very large central jet or eccentric wall impinging jet			
Continuous wave signal of regurgitant jet	Dense/triangular with early peaking	Dense/triangular with early peaking	Peak TR velocity <2 m/s	—
Semiquantitative				
Vena contracta width (mm)	>7 (>8 for biplane)	7–13.9	14–20	>21
PISA radius (mm)	Large flow convergence zone	>9	—	—
Venous flow (pulmonary/hepatic)	Systolic vein flow reversal			
Inflow	Mitral E-wave dominant (>1.2–1.5)	Tricuspid E-wave dominant (≥1 cm/s)		
Quantitative				
EROA (mm²) by PISA	≥20 (EACVI) ≥40 (ASE) (may be lower in secondary MR with elliptical EROA)	40–59	60–79	≥80
EROA (mm²) by 3-dimensional	≥41	75–94	95–114	≥115
R Vol (mL) by PISA	≥30 (EACVI) ≥60 (ASE) (may be lower in low flow conditions)	45–59	60–74	≥75

Abbreviations: ASE, American Society of Echocardiography; EACVI, European Association of Echocardiography; R Vol, regurgitant volume.

mechanism. Furthermore, primary TR is often complicated by a secondary mechanism, because of the susceptibility of the right ventricle to dilatation, as a result of volume overload.

The assessment should begin with the right ventricle (**Fig. 6**) and the right atrium. Dilatation of the right ventricle may occur as a result of systolic dysfunction due to myocardial disease or pressure overload; it may also occur as a result of volume overload due to a pathologic intercavitary communication (usually atrial septal defect) or as a result of primary TR or primary pulmonary valve regurgitation. The dilatation of the right ventricle causes dilatation of the tricuspid valve annulus and distortion of the subvalvular apparatus restricting the systolic excursion of the leaflets. As for secondary MR, the annulus can be dilated purely because of dilatation of the right atrium, usually due to chronic atrial fibrillation. In the process of dilatation, the annulus takes a more circular shape (**Fig. 7**), because the increase in dimensions occurs mainly in the direction less supported by the atrioventricular junction fibrous skeleton (**Fig. 8**).

The same quantification methods as for MR can be applied; however, it is supported by less evidence.[8] Systolic flow reversal in the hepatic veins is present with severe TR. Lack of coaptation of the tricuspid valve leaflets creating an anatomic regurgitant orifice defines free (massive) TR; in this case, the right atrial pressure is very high and the TR jet velocity is very low, regardless of the pulmonary artery pressure, being no longer useful for the estimation of systolic pulmonary artery pressure.

The role of stress echocardiography
The role of stress echocardiography in the assessment of TR, particularly secondary TR, is less well defined. However, increased contractility of the right ventricle may result in reduction in TR severity in the case of ventricular-secondary TR due to right ventricle myocardial disease. In the case of TR secondary to pulmonary hypertension and consequent right ventricular pressure overload, further increase in systolic pulmonary artery pressure on exertion may result in an increase in TR severity.

The role of cardiac magnetic resonance
Cardiac magnetic resonance is less established for the assessment of TR severity; however, it is

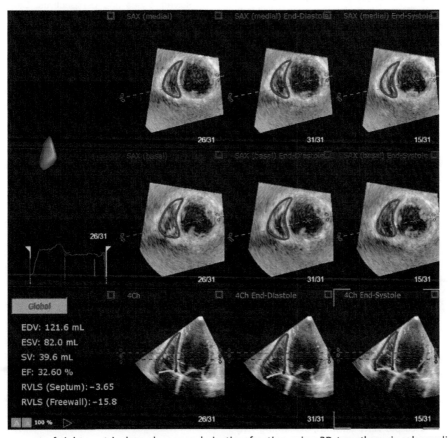

Fig. 6. Assessment of right ventricular volumes and ejection fraction using 3D transthoracic echocardiography.

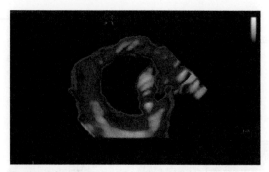

Fig. 7. Dilated tricuspid valve annulus, circular in shape.

the gold standard for the assessment of the right ventricular volumes and ejection fraction, and derived quantification techniques can be used.[8]

Grading tricuspid regurgitation severity

Traditionally, TR is graded into mild, moderate, and severe, following the severity grading conventions that also apply to mitral, aortic, and pulmonary valves. Severe TR is defined quantitatively as an EROA of ≥ 40 mm^2 and a regurgitant volume of ≥ 45 mL according to both the European and the American recommendations.[8,22] Massive TR is referred to as TR that is beyond severe, and it is associated with a low TR jet velocity of less than 2 m/s because there is near equalization of right ventricular and right atrial pressures. Expansion of TR severity grading to include massive (EROA 60–79 mm^2) and torrential (EROA ≥ 80 mm^2) TR, based on quantitative assessment, has been recently proposed.[23] Natural history studies have

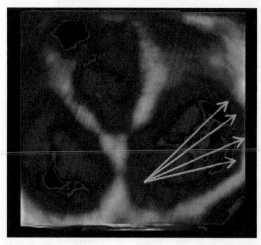

Fig. 8. Three-dimensional echocardiography image obtained with oblique rendering of the base of the heart to visualize the annuli of both atrioventricular valves. The arrows show the direction of maximal dilatation of the tricuspid valve annulus, explaining why the annulus acquires a more circular shape.

shown that patients' prognosis worsened as the severity of TR increases, supporting the case for grading TR beyond severe to reflect the differential outcomes.[24]

SUMMARY

Secondary regurgitation caused by the remodeling and dysfunction of left or right heart chamber may complicate heart failure, worsening both symptoms and prognosis. Outcome studies have shown that patients' prognosis worsened as the severity of secondary regurgitation increases. Imaging and more specifically echocardiography plays a central role for diagnosis and serial assessment of secondary regurgitation as well as for timing the intervention and guiding the procedure.

REFERENCES

1. Ennezat PV, Sylvestre Maréchaux S, Pibarot P, et al. Secondary mitral regurgitation in heart failure with reduced or preserved left ventricular ejection fraction. Cardiology 2013;125:110–7.
2. Lancellotti P, Zamorano JL, Vannan MA. Imaging challenges in secondary mitral regurgitation: unsolved issues and perspectives. Circ Cardiovasc Imaging 2014;7:735–46.
3. Asgar AW, Mack MJ, Stone GW. Secondary mitral regurgitation in heart failure. pathophysiology, prognosis, and therapeutic considerations. J Am Coll Cardiol 2015;65:1231–48.
4. Breithardt OA, Sinha AM, Schwammenthal E, et al. Acute effects of cardiac resynchronization therapy on functional mitral regurgitation in advanced systolic heart failure. J Am Coll Cardiol 2003;41:765–70.
5. Bartko PE, Pavo N, Pérez-Serradilla A, et al. Evolution of secondary mitral regurgitation. Eur Heart J Cardiovasc Imaging 2018;19:622–9.
6. Lancellotti P, Garbi M. Progression of secondary mitral regurgitation: from heart failure to valvular heart failure. Eur Heart J Cardiovasc Imaging 2018;19:613–4.
7. Gertz ZM, Raina A, Saghy L, et al. Evidence of atrial functional mitral regurgitation due to atrial fibrillation. Reversal with arrhythmia control. J Am Coll Cardiol 2011;58:1474–81.
8. Zoghbi WA, Adams D, Bonow RO, et al. Recommendations for noninvasive evaluation of native valvular regurgitation: a report from the American Society of Echocardiography developed in collaboration with the society for cardiovascular magnetic resonance. J Am Soc Echocardiogr 2017;30:303–71.
9. Baumgartner H, Falk V, Bax JJ, et al, ESC Scientific Document Group. 2017 ESC/EACTS Guidelines for the management of valvular heart disease. Eur Heart J 2017;38:2739–91.

10. Nishimura RA, Otto CM, Bonow RO, et al. 2014 AHA/ACC guidelines for the management of patients with valvular heart disease. J Am Coll Cardiol 2014;63: e57–185.

11. Nishimura RA, Otto CM, Bonow RO, et al. 2017 AHA/ACC focused update of the 2014 AHA/ACC guideline for the management of patients with valvular heart disease: a report of the American College of Cardiology/American Heart Association task force on clinical practice guidelines. Circulation 2017; 135(25):e1159–95.

12. Rossi A, Dini FL, Faggiano P, et al. Independent prognostic value of functional mitral regurgitation in patients with heart failure. A quantitative analysis of 1256 patients with ischaemic and non-ischaemic dilated cardiomyopathy. Heart 2011;97:1675–80.

13. Ring L, Dutka DP, Wells FC, et al. Mechanisms of atrial mitral regurgitation: insights using 3D transoesophageal echo. Eur Heart J Cardiovasc Imaging 2014;15:500–8.

14. Silbiger JJ. Mechanistic insights into ischemic mitral regurgitation: echocardiographic and surgical implications. J Am Soc Echocardiogr 2011;24:707–19.

15. Pierard LA, Lancellotti P. Stress testing in valve disease. Heart 2007;93:766–72.

16. Lancellotti P, Magne J. Stress echocardiography in regurgitant valve disease. Circ Cardiovasc Imaging 2013;6:840–9.

17. Lancellotti P, Gérard PL, Piérard LA. Long-term outcome of patients with heart failure and dynamic functional mitral regurgitation. Eur Heart J 2005;26: 1528–32.

18. Lancellotti P, Lebrun F, Piérard LA. Determinants of exercise-induced changes in mitral regurgitation in patients with coronary artery disease and left ventricular dysfunction. J Am Coll Cardiol 2003;42: 1921–8.

19. Maréchaux S, Terrade J, Biausque F, et al. Exercise-induced functional mitral regurgitation in heart failure and preserved ejection fraction: a new entity. Eur J Echocardiogr 2010;11:E14.

20. Dreyfus GD, Martin RP, Chan KMJ, et al. Functional tricuspid regurgitation. A need to revise our understanding. J Am Coll Cardiol 2015;65:2331–6.

21. Muraru D, Surkova E, Badano LP. Revisit of functional tricuspid regurgitation; current trends in the diagnosis and management. Korean Circ J 2016; 46:443–55.

22. Lancellotti P, Tribouilloy C, Hagendorff A, et al. Scientific Document Committee of the European Association of Cardiovascular Imaging. Recommendations for the echocardiographic assessment of native valvular regurgitation: an executive summary from the European Association of Cardiovascular Imaging. Eur Heart J Cardiovasc Imaging 2013;14: 611–44.

23. Lancellotti P, Fattouch K, Yun Go Y. Secondary tricuspid regurgitation in patients with left ventricular systolic dysfunction: cause for concern or innocent bystander? Eur Heart J 2018. https://doi.org/10.1093/eurheartj/ehy522.

24. Topilsky Y, Inojosa JL, Benfari G, et al. Clinical presentation and outcome of tricuspid regurgitation in patients with systolic dysfunction. Eur Heart J 2018. https://doi.org/10.1093/eurheartj/ehy434.

Resting and Exercise Doppler Hemodynamics
How and Why?

Shane Nanayakkara, MBBS[a,b,c,*],
David M. Kaye, MBBS, PhD[a,d],
Thomas H. Marwick, MBBS, MPH, PhD[a,b]

KEYWORDS

- Diastole • Heart failure • Exercise • Invasive • Pressure • Pulmonary hypertension
- Valvular heart disease • Stress test

KEY POINTS

- Rest and exercise hemodynamics are useful in prognostic and therapeutic decision making across the spectrum of heart failure.
- Several hemodynamic measures may appear normal at rest and require dynamic challenge, such as exercise, to provoke symptoms and reveal abnormal physiology.
- Invasive cardiac catheterization remains the gold standard but may be limited by practicality; consequently, several echocardiographic and MRI parameters are becoming of increasing interest, particularly in regard to quantifying the ventriculo-vascular interaction for both the pulmonary and systemic circulation.
- Consensus around appropriate exercise protocols and invasive validation of noninvasive parameters are required.

INTRODUCTION

Exercise intolerance is the clinical hallmark of the failing heart. Evidence of hemodynamic derangement is often not always present at rest, necessitating dynamic challenges to accentuate abnormalities. Although cardiac catheterization remains the gold standard method for hemodynamic assessment, it is limited by practicality, access, risk, and its invasive nature; consequently, there is a need to better understand noninvasive measures.

The etiology of exercise intolerance can be divided into 3 key physiologic components, as seen in **Fig. 1**. These components can coexist in the same patient and can vary within the same underlying condition due to the interaction with the duration of disease and comorbid

Disclosure Statement: The authors have nothing to disclose.
Funding: S. Nanayakkara is supported by a scholarship from the National Heart Foundation of Australia and the Baker Bright Sparks program. D.M. Kaye is supported by a Fellowship from the National Health and Medical Research Council of Australia. The Baker Heart and Diabetes Institute is supported in part by the Victorian Government's Operational Infrastructure Support Program.
[a] Department of Cardiology, The Alfred, 55 Commercial Road, Melbourne, Victoria 3004, Australia; [b] Baker Heart and Diabetes Institute, 75 Commercial Road, Melbourne, Victoria 3004, Australia; [c] Department of Medicine, Nursing and Health Sciences, Monash University, Melbourne, Australia; [d] Heart Failure Research Laboratory, Baker Heart and Diabetes Institute, 75 Commercial Road, Melbourne, Victoria 3004, Australia
* Corresponding author. Department of Cardiology, Alfred Hospital, Commercial Road, Melbourne, Victoria 3004, Australia.
E-mail address: shane.nanayakkara@baker.edu.au

Heart Failure Clin 15 (2019) 229–239
https://doi.org/10.1016/j.hfc.2018.12.003

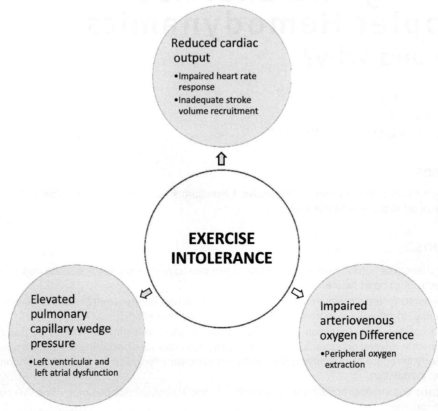

Fig. 1. Physiologic determinants of exercise intolerance in heart failure.

conditions. Analyzing these mechanisms, in particular the interactions, may be challenging. Pseudodeficiency can inhibit interpretation, whereby 1 factor limits exercise capacity sufficiently to prevent another factor from reaching its physiologic potential.[1] As such, accurate quantification of peak exercise capacity is important, such as through the use of cardiopulmonary exercise testing[2] (**Fig. 2**).

This review discusses the how and the why of rest and exercise hemodynamics in the failing heart, in regard to both noninvasive and invasive methods.

METHODS TO CHALLENGE THE LEFT VENTRICLE
Exercise Testing

Conventional exercise testing, performed on a treadmill or upright cycle, has the disadvantage of limiting access to peak imaging, so most studies are performed immediately postexercise. This has the disadvantage of potentially missing signals that rapidly dissipate. Supine exercise is more amenable to imaging, but the position changes preload, and therefore subjects begin at different points on the diastolic pressure-volume curve. Left ventricular (LV) volumes and stroke volume are larger when supine at rest, and with exercise.[3] Maeder and colleagues[4] demonstrated a steeper response in the heart rate (HR)/peak oxygen consumption (Vo_2) relationship in patients with heart failure with preserved ejection fraction (HFpEF) compared with controls. Peak HR is higher[5,6] and mean arterial pressure is lower during upright exercise.[6] Peak LV filling pressure (FP) is slightly lower when upright, although there is controversy as to whether exercise capacity is changed by position. The absolute changes in key parameters are similar between both positions.[7]

Few studies have directly compared the impact of exercise modalities in patients with heart failure. Kim and colleagues performed cardiopulmonary exercise testing in 18 patients with heart failure with reduced ejection fraction (HFrEF), comparing upright ergometry with treadmill testing, demonstrating that VO_2 was greater in those on the treadmill due to both a higher peak arteriovenous oxygen difference and cardiac output, the latter predominantly due to stroke volume rather than HR. Further studies are required to elucidate the mechanisms for this difference.

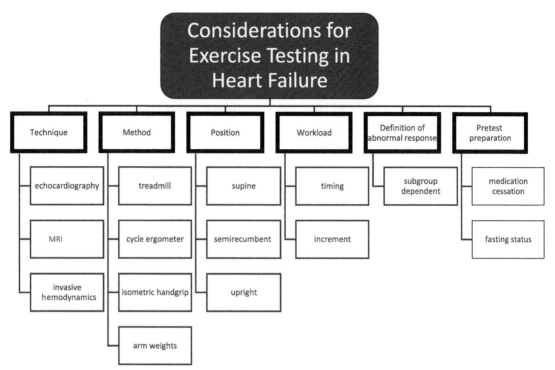

Fig. 2. Considerations for exercise testing in heart failure.

A large systematic review of diastolic stress testing suggested a specific protocol using a semisupine bicycle to facilitate both imaging and hemodynamic measures, with a gradual ramped resistance targeting HR initially and then symptom exhaustion.[8]

Preload Alteration

Although fluid challenge can be used as an alternative hemodynamic challenge,[9] this does not simulate the complex hemodynamics of exertion and has been demonstrated to be inferior to exercise.[10] Passive leg elevation does increase FP through increased venous return; however, the magnitude is small compared with exercise,[11] and the response is heterogeneous.[12] Alternatively, preload can be reduced through negative pressure of the lower body, induced either via nitroprusside or via suction from a vacuum pump using a tank sealed around the legs.

PARAMETERS

Several hemodynamic parameters are relevant to the failing heart (**Table 1**). Fundamentally, dyspnea occurs most commonly due to an elevation of LVFP, and accurate noninvasive estimation at rest and at peak exercise has remained the holy grail. Elevation of LVFP is primarily a compensatory response to preserve cardiac output in heart failure, with the magnitude of elevation indexed to workload proving highly prognostic.[13] Beyond accurate LVFP measurement, invasive catheterization allows for robust measures of contractility and diastolic function that are independent of external factors, such as preload-recruitable stroke work, LV end-systolic elastance, tau (time constant of pressure decay), and the maximal rate of pressure decay ($dPdt_{min}$).

The downstream consequences of elevated LVFP, such as left atrial dysfunction, pulmonary hypertension, right ventricular (RV) impairment, and elevated venous pressures, are all readily measured with noninvasive tests. Increasingly, there has been interest in capturing more complex hemodynamic relationships, such as the ventriculovascular interaction,[14] rather than these parameters in isolation. Such measures are well served by the information provided on imaging studies, with increasing capacity to define anatomy, estimate velocity, and characterize tissue all with a single test.

DISEASES

Patients with heart failure, regardless of ejection fraction (EF), display varying levels of pulmonary vascular remodeling, left atrial dysfunction, dynamic mitral regurgitation, and peripheral oxygen extraction abnormalities. Consequently, the physiologic response to exercise is variable, and accurate and deep phenotypic identification allows for precise targeted therapy.

Table 1
Key indices measuring hemodynamics of the failing heart

	Right Atrial	Right Ventricular	Pulmonary Arterial	Left Atrial	Left Ventricular	Aortic
Clinical	Jugular venous pressure	RV heave	Loud pulmonary component of the second heart sound		Third or fourth heart sounds	Sphygmomanometry
Blood		BNP		ANP	BNP	
Echocardiographic	IVC size and collapsibility	Tricuspid regurgitant velocity	Tricuspid regurgitant velocity + RAP, PA acceleration time	E/e′, Strain	E/e′, Strain	
MRI			Phase contrast		Tissue tagging	Phase contrast
Invasive	Direct via RHC	Direct via RHC	Direct via RHC	PCWP, Direct via atrial septum	LHC	Direct

Abbreviations: ANP, atrial natriuretic peptide; BNP, brain natriuretic peptide; IVC, inferior vena cava; RAP, right atrial pressure; RHC, right heart catheterization.

Heart Failure with Reduced Ejection Fraction

The structural characteristics of HFrEF are readily apparent at rest, but EF in particular is not well linked to functional capacity and symptoms. The ability to augment cardiac output in response to exercise challenge can significantly differentiate outcome,[15] particularly when combined with the change in pulmonary pressure. Peak cardiac power, calculated as the product of peak mean arterial blood pressure and cardiac output (divided by a constant), is independently predictive of adverse outcomes.[16]

Heart Failure with Preserved Ejection Fraction

HFpEF is a disease defined by the lack of a single unifying mechanism; the failure of multiple previous drug and device trials has been repeatedly attributed to the marked heterogeneity of the disease. Patients with HFpEF share similar patterns in clinical presentation, including exercise intolerance; however, they display markedly different physiologic phenotypes. Unsupervised machine learning algorithms using cluster analysis have successfully demonstrated the presence of different phenogroups[17]; however, further work is required to expand the factors by which these subgroups are defined (ie, mechanistic pathways vs clinically features[18]).

Exercise testing has been repeatedly demonstrated as the key diagnostic test, because resting measures of diastolic function are often normal.[11] The gold standard for diagnosis is an elevation in pulmonary capillary wedge pressure (PCWP) at a low workload (**Fig. 3**). In a small study of patients

with HFrEF and HFpEF, Obokata and colleagues[19] demonstrated similar changes in afterload, stroke volume, and pulmonary artery systolic pressure (PASP) in both forms of heart failure; there was a markedly abnormal response of ventriculo-arterial coupling in HFpEF, again highlighting the importance of collective relationships rather than isolated variables.

Pulmonary Arterial Hypertension

Both pulmonary pressure and RV function are critical determinants of long-term prognosis in patients with pulmonary arterial (PA) hypertension. At rest, right atrial pressure and cardiac index have been associated with mortality, with inconsistent data around resting mean PA pressure (PAP), particularly because this is dependent on the degree of pulmonary vascular resistance and RV function.[20] Derived parameters capturing the relationship of RV function and pulmonary pressure, therefore, have been proposed to hold greater prognostic value; PA capacitance (measured as the ratio of stroke volume to pulmonary pulse pressure) and pressure-flow (mean PAP to cardiac output) both hold significant predictive value in idiopathic and heritable pulmonary hypertension.[21] The ratio of tricuspid annular plane systolic excursion (TAPSE) to PASP also has been proposed as a measure of RV-PA coupling; in a study of 459 patients with heart failure (either HFrEF or HFpEF), TAPSE/PASP was found a significant predictor of event-free survival.[22]

Clinical measures of exercise capacity, such as the 6-minute walk distance (6MWD), are highly predictive of outcome in PA hypertension. Exercise hemodynamics allow for an earlier evaluation of RV dysfunction and pulmonary vascular remodeling and have been shown to correlate well with improvements in 6MWD, more so than resting parameters.[23] Exercise hemodynamics have also been used to identify patients with exercise-induced pulmonary hypertension, which, although well recognized, remains an area of active research with no guideline-recommended therapy, although several groups have suggested that these patients have an early vasculopathy and may be amenable to treatment.[21]

Valvular Heart Disease

Almost half a century ago, Anderson and colleagues[24] demonstrated that exercise hemodynamics differ in patients with aortic stenosis (AS), particularly in regard to determination of myocardial reserve. AS induces symptoms not only through fixed mechanical obstruction but also through the development of LV hypertrophy, fibrosis, and

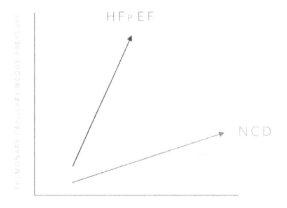

Fig. 3. Hemodynamic response to exercise in patients with HFpEF and controls. NCD, non-cardiac dyspnoea. (*Adapted from* Maeder MT, Thompson BR, Brunner-La Rocca HP, et al. Hemodynamic basis of exercise limitation in patients with heart failure and normal ejection fraction. J Am Coll Cardiol 2010;56(11):855–63; with permission.)

subsequent systolic and diastolic dysfunction. Although treatment guidelines for symptomatic severe AS are clear, recommendations for asymptomatic patients or those who have less than severe stenoses are still evolving, particularly in the era of reduced operative risk for both surgical and transcutaneous aortic valve replacement.

Exercise evaluation allows for quantification of symptoms in seemingly asymptomatic patients and assessment for the development of exercise-induced pulmonary hypertension. In a study of 105 patients with asymptomatic severe AS, Lancellotti and colleagues[25] used stress echocardiography to estimate pulmonary pressure at rest and exercise. Exercise-induced pulmonary hypertension was highly predictive of cardiac event-free survival, independent of changes in the mean aortic pressure gradient.

Exercise-induced pulmonary hypertension in the context of mitral regurgitation may occur due to either a dynamic worsening of mitral regurgitation with increased LV afterload or subclinical pulmonary vascular damage and consequent impaired pulmonary vascular recruitment. Regardless, exercise-induced pulmonary hypertension identifies patients at an increased risk of future major cardiovascular events and death.[25]

Clinical studies assessing the role of exercise hemodynamics in determining intervention are required, particularly for defining appropriate timing of replacement, valvulo-ventricular interactions, and accurately determining functional limitation in the asymptomatic patient.

TECHNIQUES FOR MEASURING HEMODYNAMICS
Cardiac Catheterization

Invasive hemodynamic testing, particularly with exercise, remains the gold standard for the accurate quantification of FP in all forms of heart failure.

Technique
Although exercise methods vary, typically patients are subjected to cycle ergometry in the supine or semisupine position, with right heart catheterization typically performed from the brachial approach to facilitate exercise. The transducer must be zeroed at the midthoracic line, halfway between the anterior sternum and the bed surface, reflecting the level of the left atrium. The balloon catheter is inflated in the right atrium and sequential measurements taken until the wedge position is obtained. Ideally, 3 traces of the wedge pressure should be recorded and the mean value taken; blood sampling from the wedge position can be taken to confirm an arterialized sample. Cardiac output can be measured using either thermodilution or the direct Fick method, although the former is preferred because it is more reliable and more strongly associated with mortality.[26] Simultaneous echocardiography permits the diagnosis of dynamic conditions, such as mitral regurgitation or failure of contractile augmentation. Expired gas analysis also may be performed to quantify exercise capacity and objectify ventilatory dysfunction.

Challenge
Resistance is increased in a stagewise fashion, although the specific protocols vary between centers. Isometric handgrip, leg raising, and arm weights have all also been used. In a study of 26 patients (14 HFpEF and 12 control) undergoing right heart catheterization, HFpEF patients demonstrated a 2-fold greater increase in PCWP with exercise compared with fluid challenge.[10] After resting measures have been taking, graded resistance is applied at prespecified intervals until the patient reaches a symptomatic limit. Peak pressures, including right atrial, PA, PCWP, and cardiac output, are then recorded along with oximetry for the mixed venous oxygen content.

Left heart catheterization using conductance catheterization provides the most accurate measure of LV stiffness. Aside from the LV end-diastolic pressure, tau (the relaxation time constant), LV diastolic elastance, rate of pressure change (LV dP/dt), end-diastolic stiffness, end-systolic elastance, and wall stress can all be directly measured, providing the most accurate load-independent measures of LV function. This is often reserved for the research setting in view of the technical complexity and cost of the procedure as well as additional risk introduced by entering the arterial circulation. Coronary angiography is also recommended if coronary artery disease is suspected as a cause for heart failure.

In the authors' opinion, invasive measurement is the optimal means of identifying both the presence of elevated FP at rest and its increase in response to stress. The problem, however, is the prevalence of the problem of undifferentiated dyspnea and suspected HFpEF in the community. Some form of noninvasive testing is required from the standpoint of feasibility.

Echocardiography

Echocardiography is ubiquitous and often the first imaging test performed to investigate heart failure. The estimation of hemodynamic parameters should be based on the combination of abnormal indices, rather than reliance on an isolated abnormal measurement.[27]

Tricuspid regurgitant velocity

In the presence of an adequate signal of tricuspid regurgitation, continuous-wave Doppler can provide an accurate estimate of both rest and exercise pulmonary pressure. At rest, appropriate gain and contrast adjustment together with the use of contrast or agitated saline can assist with obtaining the modal velocity[28]; however, respiration and swinging on the cardiac axis significantly impede measurement at peak exercise. In a heterogenous cohort of 61 patients, including controls, athletes, and patients with pulmonary hypertension of varying etiology, echocardiographic measures of PASP were possible in 93% of patients at rest, dropping to 69% at peak exercise.[28] The difference in peak exercise invasive and echocardiographically derived PASP was less than 10 mm Hg in 48% of patients; however, there was a significant bias to a higher estimated mean PAP (+5.1 ± 6.9 mm Hg).

Mitral valve Doppler

The E wave and A wave velocities require careful technical attention for resting measures. Positioning of the sample volume, use of the low wall filter setting, and use of low signal gain all improve accuracy. Fusion associated with tachycardia at peak exercise results in the A wave often precluded from measurement.

Tissue Doppler

Tissue Doppler forms the current mainstay in regard to estimating LVFP based on echocardiography. The ratio of peak early diastolic mitral inflow velocity (E) to peak early diastolic mitral annular velocity (e′) strongly suggests elevated FPs but only when treated as a categorical variable at the extremes and not as a continuous estimate. Measuring E/e′ at peak exertion, in particular, has demonstrated reasonable accuracy, although technical challenges, such as cardiac stability within the frame, exaggerated patient respiration, and rapid HR with fusion, can be limiting. Accuracy is limited in patients with mitral valve disease, pericardial disease, and regional wall motion abnormalities.[29]

Although the uptake of diastolic stress echocardiography has been patchy, the test provides 3 pieces of useful information—an objective measure of exercise capacity, a means of identifying silent ischemia (which may be particularly important in diabetes mellitus), and hemodynamic information regarding PAP and LVFP.[30] Despite the imperfections of E/e′ and PCWP,[23] the fact remains that both rest and exercise E/e′ provide prognostic information that is independent of and incremental to standard parameters (**Fig. 4**). Reported accuracies have been in the 70% to 80% range, implying that this screening test is imperfect. Nonetheless, it is not so imperfect as to be

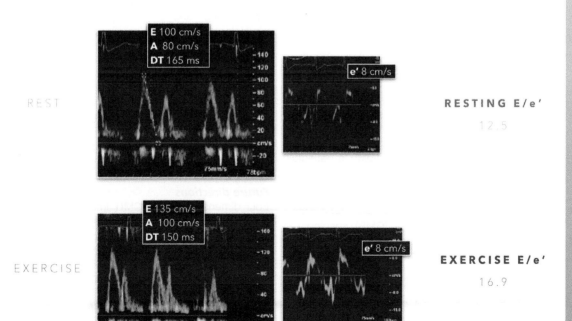

Fig. 4. Mitral inflow Doppler tracings taken from a dyspneic patient at (*A*) rest and (*B*) exercise. Diastolic stress testing can be used to estimate FPs at peak exercise.

useless—patients selected for treatment on the basis of exercise E/e' have shown responses to therapy in a way that has not been shown without this means of selection.[24]

Obokata and colleagues[19] performed deep phenotyping of 74 dyspneic patients using simultaneous echocardiography, cardiac catheterization, and expired gas analysis to determine the role of diastolic stress testing. Exercise was performed using cycle ergometry until subject reported exhaustion. Septal and lateral E/e' ratios modestly correlated with resting PCWP (r = 0.63 and r = 0.58, respectively; P<.001). Peak exercise E/e' underestimated PCWP; although septal E/e' rose in patients who had normal resting pressures, there was no change in E/e' in HFpEF patients who had an elevated resting PCWP.

Speckle tracking

To enhance the ability of resting measures to predict peak exercise FP, various groups have used advanced echocardiographic techniques (such as strain) and biomarkers (atrial natriuretic peptide, brain natriuretic peptide, adrenomedullin, and galectin-3) to improve diagnostic capacity. LV strain, most commonly measured using speckle tracking, reveals subtle systolic dysfunction that can occur in both HFrEF and HFpEF. LV systolic function and diastolic function are tightly coupled. Abnormal strain is associated with worse hemodynamics and holds a modest but significant association with peak exercise wedge pressure. Given the likely relationship between impaired strain and myocardial fibrosis, it follows that patients with more abnormal strain have more significant LV dysfunction and consequently worse hemodynamics. The left atrium faces the brunt of the increased LVFP, and it follows that impairments to left atrial function would correlate. Left atrial strain (**Fig. 5**) has shown promise in both HFrEF and HFpEF[31–33]; however is limited by reproducibility, dependence on adequate image quality, and frame rate and is of limited value in patients with atrial fibrillation.

Magnetic Resonance Imaging

Cardiac magnetic resonance (CMR) imaging is considered the gold standard for anatomic assessment and tissue characterization of the myocardium. In regard to pulmonary hemodynamics, CMR imaging allows for the accurate quantification of LV and RV volumes, mass, EF, and fibrosis.[34]

Phase-contrast techniques

Flow and velocity can also be measured using phase-contrast MRI[35]; in brief, a cross-sectional image of any vessel can be captured and total flow calculated through that vessel lumen. A velocity map is created at a slice and the weighted average obtained. Phase contrast is susceptible to error due to the multitude of variables to be adjusted and due to the time-consuming and inefficient post-processing required.[36] Clinically, such techniques can be applied to valvular heart disease (stenosis or regurgitation), estimation of pulmonary pressure, and quantification of shunts. Nonetheless, although similar measurements can be obtained, the lower temporal resolution of phase-contrast MRI makes it highly likely that peak velocities are underestimated (because sampling may not occur at the exact peak) compared with echocardiography.[37] The provision of measurements analogous to E/e' remains difficult.

Sequential measures along a particular vessel allow for the analysis of a particular pulse wave; consequently, pulse wave velocity and blood vessel compliance can be estimated.[38] Aortic compliance is an important component of ventriculo-arterial coupling. Phase-contrast MRI can similarly provide clinically relevant information regarding pulmonary pressure, compliance, and stiffness, which can be then matched with the RV measures, providing the best noninvasive measure of RV to PA coupling.

Exercise measures

Exercise can be safely performed during CMR imaging with accurate quantification of ventricular volumes[5] and can adequately differentiate physiologic and pathologic remodeling.[39] The ability of CMR imaging to clearly quantify RV volumes and function with exercise highlights a unique role to assess the presystemic circulation, particularly in regard to differentiating impaired RV contractility from increased RV afterload. Further research is required in regard to the feasibility and accuracy compared with invasive hemodynamics in patients with heart failure.

Future directions

Four-dimensional flow CMR imaging uses 3-D spatial encoding and time to visualize the complex flow patterns in a 3-D volume, such as the atria or ventricle, and is not restricted to a certain imaging plane. Such techniques add significant time to the scan, however, and are labor intensive; however, they may be able to identify novel hemodynamic parameters, including wall shear stress and kinetic energy.[40]

As the field rapidly develops, it is clear that CMR imaging offers a promising balance of accurate anatomic evaluation, tissue

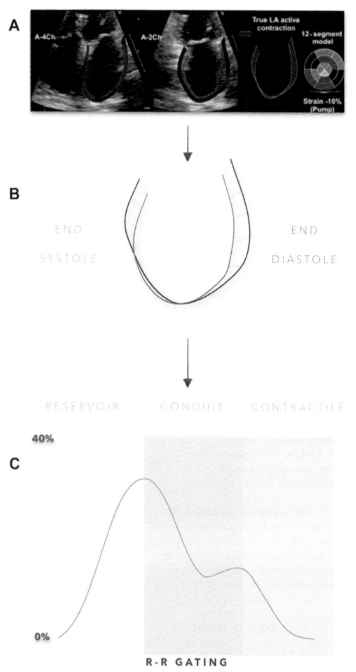

Fig. 5. Typical 4-chamber and 2-chamber left atrial speckle tracking tracings, with derivation to end diastole and end systole. When plotted over the cardiac cycle, the 3 individual components of atrial function can be derived. (A) Measurement of LA strain from original echocardiographic imaging. (B) atrial tracking throughout the cardiac cycle. (c) atrial strain with division of individual components of atrial function, gated to R-R interval. A, atria; CH, chamber; LA, left atrium.

characterization, and hemodynamics. Although favorable, the test is limited by availability and cost, and newer techniques are in need of adequate invasive validation in a diverse range of pathologies.

SUMMARY

Rest and exercise hemodynamics are useful in prognostic and therapeutic decision making across the spectrum of heart failure. Although invasive measurement remains the gold standard, noninvasive parameters are becoming increasingly useful, particularly in regard to quantifying ventriculo-vascular interactions. Currently, significant heterogeneity exists around exercise protocols, and there is a distinct need to develop consensus methodology and to validate these noninvasive measures in all forms of heart failure.

REFERENCES

1. Houstis NE, Lewis GD. Causes of exercise intolerance in heart failure with preserved ejection fraction: searching for consensus. J Card Fail 2014;20(10): 762–78.
2. Guazzi M, Adams V, Conraads V, et al. Clinical recommendations for cardiopulmonary exercise testing data assessment in specific patient populations. Circulation 2016;126(18):2261–74.
3. Cotsamire DL, Sullivan MJ, Bashore TM, et al. Position as a variable for cardiovascular responses during exercise. Clin Cardiol 1987;10(3):137–42.
4. Maeder MT, Thompson BR, Brunner-La Rocca H-P, et al. Hemodynamic basis of exercise limitation in patients with heart failure and normal ejection fraction. J Am Coll Cardiol 2010;56(11):855–63.
5. La Gerche A, Claessen G, Van De Bruaene A, et al. Cardiac MRI: a new gold standard for ventricular volume quantification during high-intensity exercise. Circ Cardiovasc Imaging 2013;6(2):329–38.
6. Kramer B, Massie B, Topic N. Hemodynamic differences between supine and upright exercise in patients with congestive heart failure. Circulation 1982;66(4 I):820–5.
7. Thadani U, Parker JO. Hemodynamics at rest and during supine and sitting bicycle exercise in normal subjects. Am J Cardiol 1978;41(1):52–9.
8. Erdei T, Smiseth OA, Marino P, et al. A systematic review of diastolic stress tests in heart failure with preserved ejection fraction, with proposals from the EU-FP7 MEDIA study group. Eur J Heart Fail 2014; 16(12):1345–61.
9. Fujimoto N, Borlaug BA, Lewis GD, et al. Hemodynamic responses to rapid saline loading: the impact of age, sex, and heart failure. Circulation 2013; 127(1):55–62.
10. Andersen MJ, Olson TP, Melenovsky V, et al. Differential hemodynamic effects of exercise and volume expansion in people with and without heart failure. Circ Heart Fail 2015;8(1):41–8.
11. Borlaug BA, Nishimura RA, Sorajja P, et al. Exercise hemodynamics enhance diagnosis of early heart failure with preserved ejection fraction. Circ Heart Fail 2010;3(5):588–95.
12. Zhou H-L, Ding L, Mi T, et al. Values of hemodynamic variation in response to passive leg raising in predicting exercise capacity of heart failure with preserved ejection fraction. Medicine (Baltimore) 2016;95(44):e5322.
13. Dorfs S, Zeh W, Hochholzer W, et al. Pulmonary capillary wedge pressure during exercise and long-term mortality in patients with suspected heart failure with preserved ejection fraction. Eur Heart J 2014;35(44):3103–12.
14. Chirinos JA. Ventricular–arterial coupling: invasive and non-invasive assessment. Artery Res 2013; 7(1):2–14.
15. Rieth A, Richter MJ, Gall H, et al. Hemodynamic phenotyping based on exercise catheterization predicts outcome in patients with heart failure and reduced ejection fraction. J Heart Lung Transplant 2017;36(8):880–9.
16. Lang CC, Karlin P, Haythe J, et al. Peak cardiac power output, measured noninvasively, is a powerful predictor of outcome in chronic heart failure. Circ Heart Fail 2009;2(1):33–8.
17. Shah SJ, Katz DH, Selvaraj S, et al. Phenomapping for novel classification of heart failure with preserved ejection fraction. Circulation 2014;131(3):269–79.
18. Parikh KS, Sharma K, Fiuzat M, et al. Heart failure with preserved ejection fraction expert panel report. JACC Heart Fail 2018;6(8):619–32.
19. Obokata M, Nagata Y, Kado Y, et al. Ventricular-arterial coupling and exercise-induced pulmonary hypertension during low-level exercise in heart failure with preserved or reduced ejection fraction. J Card Fail 2017;23(3). https://doi.org/10.1016/j.cardfail. 2016.10.001.
20. Galiè N, Humbert M, Vachiery J-L, et al. 2015 ESC/ ERS guidelines for the diagnosis and treatment of pulmonary hypertension. Eur Heart J 2016;37(1): 67–119.
21. Saggar R, Sitbon O. Hemodynamics in pulmonary arterial hypertension: current and future perspectives. Am J Cardiol 2012;110(6 SUPPL):S9–15.
22. Guazzi M, Naeije R, Arena R, et al. Echocardiography of right ventriculoarterial coupling combined with cardiopulmonary exercise testing to predict outcome in heart failure. Chest 2015;148(1): 226–34.
23. Provencher S, Hervé P, Sitbon O, et al. Changes in exercise haemodynamics during treatment in pulmonary arterial hypertension. Eur Respir J 2008; 32(2):393–8.
24. Anderson FL, Tsagaris TJ, Tikoff G, et al. Hemodynamic effects of exercise in patients with aortic stenosis. Am J Med 1969;46(6):872–85.
25. Lancellotti P, Magne J, Dulgheru R, et al. Clinical significance of exercise pulmonary hypertension in secondary mitral regurgitation. Am J Cardiol 2015; 115(10):1454–61.
26. Opotowsky AR, Hess E, Maron BA, et al. Thermodilution vs estimated Fick cardiac output measurement in clinical practice: an analysis of mortality

from the Veterans Affairs Clinical Assessment, Reporting, and Tracking (VA CART) program and Vanderbilt University. JAMA Cardiol 2017;2(10): 1090–9.

27. Nagueh SF, Smiseth O a, Appleton CP, et al. Recommendations for the evaluation of left ventricular diastolic function by echocardiography: an update from the American Society of Echocardiography and the European Association of Cardiovascular Imaging. J Am Soc Echocardiogr 2016;29(4): 277–314.

28. Claessen G, La Gerche A, Voigt JU, et al. Accuracy of echocardiography to evaluate pulmonary vascular and RV function during exercise. JACC Cardiovasc Imaging 2016;9(5):532–43.

29. Park J, Marwick TH. Use and limitations of E/e ' to assess left ventricular filling pressure by echocardiography. J Cardiovasc Ultrasound 2011;19: 169–73.

30. Burgess MI, Jenkins C, Sharman JE, et al. Diastolic stress echocardiography: hemodynamic validation and clinical significance of estimation of ventricular filling pressure with exercise. J Am Coll Cardiol 2006;47(9):1891–900.

31. Santos ABS, Roca GQ, Claggett B, et al. Prognostic relevance of left atrial dysfunction in heart failure with preserved ejection fraction. Circ Heart Fail 2016;9(4):1–12.

32. Sugimoto T, Bandera F, Generati G, et al. Left atrial function dynamics during exercise in heart failure: pathophysiological implications on the right heart and exercise ventilation inefficiency. JACC Cardiovasc Imaging 2017;10(10):1253–64.

33. Hewing B, Theres L, Spethmann S, et al. Left atrial strain predicts hemodynamic parameters in cardiovascular patients. Echocardiography 2017;34(8): 1170–8.

34. Ellims AH, Shaw JA, Stub D, et al. Diffuse myocardial fibrosis evaluated by post-contrast T1 mapping correlates with left ventricular stiffness. J Am Coll Cardiol 2014;63(11):1112–8.

35. Nayak KS, Nielsen J-F, Bernstein MA, et al. Cardiovascular magnetic resonance phase contrast imaging. J Cardiovasc Magn Reson 2015;17(1):71.

36. Oh JK, Chang SA, Choe YH, et al. CMR imaging for diastolic hemodynamic assessment: fantasy or reality? JACC Cardiovasc Imaging 2012;5(1):25–7.

37. Lee VS, Spritzer CE, Carroll BA, et al. Flow quantification using fast cine phase-contrast MR imaging, conventional cine phase-contrast MR imaging, and Doppler sonography: in vitro and in vivo validation. Am J Roentgenol 1997;169(4):1125–31.

38. Srichai MB, Lim RP, Wong S, et al. Cardiovascular applications of phase-contrast MRI. Am J Roentgenol 2009;192(3):662–75.

39. Claessen G, Schnell F, Bogaert J, et al. Exercise cardiac magnetic resonance to differentiate athlete's heart from structural heart disease. Eur Heart J Cardiovasc Imaging 2018;19(9):1062–70.

40. Dyverfeldt P, Bissell M, Barker AJ, et al. 4D flow cardiovascular magnetic resonance consensus statement. J Cardiovasc Magn Reson 2015;17(1):72.

The Role of Echocardiography in Heart Failure with Preserved Ejection Fraction
What Do We Want from Imaging?

Masaru Obokata, MD, PhD, Yogesh N.V. Reddy, MBBS, MSc,
Barry A. Borlaug, MD*

KEYWORDS

• Diagnosis • Diastolic function • Echocardiography • Filling pressure • Heart failure • Phenotyping
• Risk stratification

KEY POINTS

- Echocardiography is essential in the evaluation and management of HFpEF.
- Elevated left heart filling pressure represents the final common effect of diastolic dysfunction and echocardiography can be useful to identify increased filling pressure.
- Diastolic stress echocardiography may improve the diagnosis of HFpEF, but requires additional confirmation.
- Echocardiography also plays a crucial role in categorizing patients with HFpEF based on underlying pathophysiologic phenotypes.
- Echocardiographic parameters provide prognostic information reflecting specific pathophysiologic abnormalities in HFpEF.

INTRODUCTION

Heart failure with preserved ejection fraction (HFpEF) is a common clinical syndrome that is increasing in prevalence coupled with the growing population burden of aging and comorbidities.[1,2] More than half of patients with unexplained exertional dyspnea referred for invasive evaluation are ultimately found to have HFpEF, and more than 70% of patients with prevalent heart failure (HF) more than the age of 65 years have normal ejection fraction (EF).[3,4] Cardiovascular imaging plays a key role in the evaluation and management of HFpEF, particularly echocardiography.[5]

Echocardiography provides essential information on cardiac structure, function, and hemodynamics and is performed in essentially all patients in whom there is clinical suspicion for HFpEF.[6] From a practical standpoint, the most important questions that can be addressed center on (1) diagnosis, determining whether a patient with unexplained dyspnea truly has HFpEF or an alternate cardiac or noncardiac cause of dyspnea; (2) management, in which imaging can be used to evaluate hemodynamic status and determine underlying pathophysiologic phenotypes; and (3) risk stratification for outcomes. This article

Disclosure: The authors have nothing to disclose.
Department of Cardiovascular Medicine, Mayo Clinic and Foundation, 200 First Street Southwest, Rochester, MN 55906, USA
* Corresponding author.
E-mail address: borlaug.barry@mayo.edu

Heart Failure Clin 15 (2019) 241–256
https://doi.org/10.1016/j.hfc.2018.12.004
1551-7136/19/© 2018 Elsevier Inc. All rights reserved.

provides a critical appraisal of the role of echocardiography crossing these 3 categories involved in the care of patients with, or suspected of having, HFpEF.

CASE

A 72-year-old man was referred for evaluation of a 2-year history of progressive exertional dyspnea with fatigue. He was obese (body mass index [BMI], 36.2 kg/m^2) and had chronic systemic hypertension treated with lisinopril and chlorthalidone. Jugular venous pressure was 8 cm H$_2$O, and there was no lower edema. N-terminal pro-B-type natriuretic peptide was 80 pg/mL. Transthoracic echocardiography revealed normal left ventricular (LV) EF (62%), LV size (LV end-diastolic dimension, 51 mm), left atrial (LA) volume (LA volume index [LAVI], 22 mL/m^2), and right ventricular (RV) size, with normal systolic function. Transmitral inflow Doppler showed an E/A ratio of 1.0 with medial E/e' (ratio of early diastolic transmitral inflow velocity to mitral annular tissue velocity) of 12.9 and estimated right ventricular systolic pressure (RVSP) was 36 mm Hg (peak tricuspid regurgitation velocity, 2.8 m/s). LV global longitudinal strain (GLS) was mildly reduced at −16.8%. A prominent epicardial fat pad was seen on echocardiography.

This common clinical presentation should raise clinical suspicion for HFpEF, and, if present, it raises the question of what the underlying drivers of this patient's HFpEF syndrome are. This question is used here to frame what is sought from echocardiography in the evaluation of suspected HFpEF.

Diastolic Dysfunction and Heart Failure with Preserved Ejection Fraction

Although the two terms are often used interchangeably, it is important to remember that diastolic dysfunction is not equivalent to HFpEF. HFpEF by definition requires the presence of increased filling pressures either at rest or with exertion, without which systemic perfusion cannot be maintained.[7] Although diastolic dysfunction is a central feature in HFpEF, the pathophysiology is complex, with variable contributions from diastolic dysfunction, impaired contractile reserve, impaired atrial function, relative pericardial restraint, and abnormal ventricular vascular coupling, which all contribute to the increase in pulmonary venous and left-sided filling pressures.[8–10] Increases in LV filling pressures promote symptoms of dyspnea,[11] impair exercise capacity,[11,12] and increase risk for HF hospitalization and mortality in HFpEF.[13,14] Thus diastolic

dysfunction is considered to be the cornerstone of HFpEF pathophysiology.[8]

Diastolic dysfunction is defined by prolongation of relaxation in early diastole, an increase in viscoelastic LV diastolic chamber stiffness, or some combination of the two.[15] Declines in LV relaxation and compliance are part of normal aging, and accordingly not all patients with diastolic dysfunction have or will go on to develop clinical HFpEF.[16–18] In one prospective cohort study, only 12% of subjects with severe diastolic dysfunction at initial evaluation developed clinical HFpEF over 6 years of follow-up.[19] Approximately one-third of patients with HFpEF enrolled in clinical trials lack echocardiographic evidence of diastolic dysfunction.[20–22] Thus, although echocardiographic categorization of diastolic dysfunction is prognostic[23] and useful to predict incident HFpEF,[19] recent studies have suggested that they should not be used in isolation for diagnostic purposes.[3,24]

Echocardiography to Identify Increased Filling Pressure

The ultimate expression of abnormalities in diastolic function is an increase in LV filling pressures. There are several echocardiographic indices that have been applied for the estimation of filling pressures, but the most studied (by far) is the E/e'.[24–28] The diagnostic accuracy of the E/e' ratio in HFpEF has recently been questioned, because a recent meta-analysis reported only a modest correlation between E/e' and invasively obtained resting filling pressures across studies (pooled $r = 0.56$).[5] Correlations between E/e' and invasive filling pressure in patients with preserved EF have been reported in 30 studies and vary widely in the strength of correlation ($r = 0.02–0.87$) (**Table 1**). Despite its variable and often modest correlation with filling pressure, E/e' has been reported to have prognostic value in patients with HFpEF.[5,21,29]

Transmitral flow (TMF) is driven by the LA-LV pressure gradient during diastole and can be used for identification of increased filling pressure in patients with normal sinus rhythm. TMF is often graded as normal, impaired relaxation, pseudonormal, and restrictive filling patterns. Because TMF is influenced by LA pressure, E/A ratio shows a U-shaped relationship with LV filling pressure. The biphasic relationship of E/A ratio makes it difficult to differentiate normal and pseudonormal patterns, and clinicians must rely on other echocardiographic indices, such as E/e' ratio.[6]

Other indices have also been related to LV filling pressures.[6] Pulmonary vein (PV) Doppler flow

Table 1
Correlations between E/e' and invasive filling pressure in patients with preserved ejection fraction

Study	n	Patients' Characteristics	Time Frame	Echo	Invasive	r	P	Cutoff Cath (mm Hg)	Cutoff Echo	Sens (%)	Spec (%)	Feasibility (%)	Reproducibility Intra/inter (%)[a]
Nagueh 1997[25]	60	45 ICU, 15 Cath laboratory	Simultaneous	E/e' (sep)	PCWP	0.87	<.001	>15	>10	97	78	—	5 ± 4/6 ± 5
Ommen 2000[27]	64	73% suspicious CAD	Simultaneous	E/e' (avg)	MDP	0.45	—	—	—	—	—	100	—
				E/e' (sep)	MDP	0.47	—	>12	>15	22	100	100	—
Poerner 2003[36]	85	Patients referred to CAG and E/A>0.9	Mean 3 h	E/e' (sep)	LVEDP	0.40	<.01	—	—	—	—	—	—
				E/e' (lat)	LVEDP	0.49	<.01	—	—	—	—	—	—
				E/e' (avg)	LVEDP	0.57	<.01	—	—	—	—	—	—
Mansencal 2004[65]	20	CAD	<1 h	E/e' (lat)	Pre-A	0.18	—	>15	>12	0	100	100	—
Hadano 2005[37]	65	UA 6%, AS 5%	<3 h	E/e' (lat)	PCWP	0.54	<.001	>15	>12	42	92	—	—
Kidawa 2005[38]	50	Patients referred to CAG	Simultaneous	E/e' (lat)	LVEDP	0.58	<.01	>15	>11	28	92	—	—
				E/e' (sep)	LVEDP	0.29	NS	—	—	—	—	—	—
Kasner 2007[43]	55	43 HFpEF and 12 controls	3–5 h	E/e' (lat)	LVEDP	0.71	.001	—	—	—	—	—	—
Min 2007[103]	55	Patients referred to cath and E/e' 8–15	Simultaneous	E/e' (sep)	LVEDP	0.03	.8	—	—	—	—	—	—
Dokanish 2008[58]	32	Patients with dyspnea	Immediately after cath	E/e' (avg)	Pre-A	0.39	<.001	>15	>15	73	77	—	—
Rudko 2008[104]	39	Increased filling pressure or DD (77% CAD)	Simultaneous	E/e' (sep)	LVEDP	0.47	<.001	—	—	—	—	—	—
Dokanish 2010[44]	122	Patients referred to CAG	<20 min	E/e' (avg)	Pre-A	0.63	<.001	>15	>13	70	93	—	—

(continued on next page)

Table 1
(continued)

Study	n	Patients' Characteristics	Time Frame	Echo	Invasive	r	P	Cutoff Cath (mm Hg)	Cutoff Echo	Sens (%)	Spec (%)	Feasibility (%)	Reproducibility (%)[a]
Kasner 2010[57]	33	21 HFpEF and 11 controls	Simultaneous	E/e' (avg)	LVEDP	0.57	<.001	—	—	—	—	—	—
Maeder 2010[79]	22	14 HFpEF and 8 controls	Simultaneous	E/e' (sep) E/e' (lat) E/e' (avg)	PCWP PCWP PCWP	0.19 0.04 0.12	.39 .87 .59	—	—	—	—	—	—
Hsiao 2011[105]	100	Stable CAD	Immediately after cath	E/e' (sep) E/e' (lat)	Pre-A Pre-A	0.31 0.23	.002 .02	—	—	—	—	—	—
Maeder 2011[106]	36	15 HFpEF, 11 PAH, 10 healthy controls	Immediately after cath	E/e' (sep) E/e' (lat) E/e' (avg)	PCWP PCWP PCWP	0.23 −0.04 0.13	.2 .8 .5	—	—	—	—	—	—
Bhella 2011[67]	11	11 HFpEF	Simultaneous	E/e' (avg)	PCWP	0.64	.04	—	—	59	92	—	—
Previtali 2012[107]	57	Patients referred to CAG	<1 h	E/e' (lat) E/e' (avg)	LVEDP LVEDP	0.1 —	.4 NS	— >15	— >12.1 (optimal)	— 44	— 71	—	Intra/inter <10/20 Intra/inter <10/20
Manouras 2013[68]	38	Patients with angina/ dyspnea	Simultaneous	E/e' (sep) E/e' (lat) E/e' (avg)	Pre-A Pre-A Pre-A	0.02 0.40 0.21	NS <.05 <.05	—	—	—	—	—	—
Tatsumi 2014[108]	22	Patients underwent 3D echo and cath	0.1 ± 5.8 d	E/e' (sep)	PCWP	0.64	.001	>12	>13	8	91	—	—
Kasner 2015[109]	23	HFpEF	Simultaneous	E/e' (avg)	LVEDP	0.84	<.001	—	—	—	—	—	—
Matsushita 2015[110]	16	Inpatient HFpEF	Same hospitalization	E/e' (avg)	PCWP	0.56	.01	>15	>10	71	56	—	—

Study	n	Population	Timing	E/e'	Reference	r	P						
Ma 2015[111]	114	84 CAD and 30 controls	< 24 h	E/e' (sep)	LVEDP	0.60	<.01	—	—	—	—	—	—
Santos 2015[78]	118	Patients with dyspnea	Immediately after cath	E/e' (sep)	PCWP	0.41	<.001	>15	≥15	6	92	79	—
				E/e' (lat)	PCWP	0.30	<.001	>15	≥12	13	92	75	—
				E/e' (avg)	PCWP	0.36	<.001	>15	≥13	6	90	75	—
Cameli 2016[45]	20	39% UA, 25% angina with positive stress test	1 h	E/e' (avg)	LVEDP	0.72	<.001	—	—	—	—	100	—
Rommel 2016[112]	36	24 HFpEF and 12 controls	N/R	E/e' (N/R)	LVEDP	0.63	<.001	—	—	—	—	—	—
Ma 2016[62]	114	84 CAD and 30 controls	—	E/e' (sep)	LVEDP	0.60	<.01	>15	>10.9	91	68	—	—
				E/e' (lat)	LVEDP	0.29	<.01	—	—	—	—	—	—
				E/e' (avg)	LVEDP	0.41	<.01	—	—	—	—	—	—
Hayashi 2016[61]	47	Cardiac diseases (eg, CAD, OMI, HCM, HFpEF)	<3 h	E/e' (avg)	MDP	0.56	<.001	—	—	—	—	—	—
Obokata 2016[24]	74	50 HFpEF and 24 controls	Simultaneous	E/e' (sep)	PCWP	0.63	<.001	—	—	—	—	99	—
				E/e' (lat)	PCWP	0.58	<.001	—	—	—	—	95	—
Lancellotti 2017[46]	120	Suspicious CAD	Simultaneous	E/e' (avg)	LVEDP	0.17	.07	≥15	≥14	2.4	96	—	—
				E/e' (sep)	LVEDP	0.08	.36	≥15	≥15	4.8	96	—	—
Andersen 2017[28,b]	450	Patients referred to right or left cath (EF<50% n = 209)	Simultaneous or immediately after cath	E/e' (avg)	PCWP	0.65	<.001	—	—	—	—	—	—

Abbreviations: 3D, three-dimensional; A, late diastolic mitral inflow velocity; AS, aortic stenosis; Avg, average; CAD, coronary artery disease; CAG, coronary angiography; Cath, catheterization; DD, diastolic dysfunction; E, early diastolic mitral inflow velocity; e', early diastolic mitral annular tissue velocity; Echo, echocardiography; EF, ejection fraction; HCM, hypertrophic cardiomyopathy; ICU, intensive care unit; lat, lateral; LVEDP, LV end-diastolic pressure; MDP, left ventricular mean diastolic pressure; N/R, not reported; NS, not significant; OMI, old myocardial infarction; PAH, pulmonary arterial hypertension; PCWP, pulmonary capillary wedge pressure; Pre-A, LV pressure during preatrial contraction; Sens, sensitivity; sep, septal; Spec, specificity; UA, unstable angina.

a Reproducibility represents percentage variability, intraclass correlation coefficient, or mean difference.

b This study pooled together both patients with HFpEF and HF with reduced EF.

reversals during atrial contraction provide a measure of end-diastolic LV operative compliance and LV end-diastolic pressure (LVEDP). With increased impedance to end-diastolic atrial contraction, there is a prolongation of flow reversal into the PV relative to the duration of forward flow. Differences in these durations exceeding 20 to 30 milliseconds have been correlated with increased LVEDP,[30–33] with a diagnostic sensitivity of 87% and specificity of 85%.[34] Six studies have reported reasonable correlations between backward and forward PV flow duration and invasively measured LV filling pressure in patients with preserved EF ($r = 0.39–0.70$).[27,34–38] Although these data seem favorable, diagnostic-quality recordings of the PV Doppler flow are often not technically feasible, and other PV parameters, such as systolic and diastolic flow velocities, are less robust.[25,27,35] As such, PV Doppler indices have not gained substantial traction as indicators of filling pressure.

An alternative method of assessing the impact of increased left-sided filling pressures chronically is to determine their downstream effects on the LA. Atrial operating compliance and atrial volume are linked to LV diastolic function through atrioventricular coupling, whereby chronic impedance to LA emptying secondary to LV diastolic dysfunction causes LA remodeling and dysfunction.[39–42] LA volume is thought to reflect the chronic effects of LV filling pressure increase over time, rather than instantaneous pressures.

Because this is a chronic marker, correlations between LA volume index and ambient LV filling pressures are lower than what has been reported for other indices, such as E/e' and PV Doppler ($r = 0.10–0.49$).[28,43–46] In contrast with E/e', LA volume index is not strongly associated with outcome in HFpEF,[21,47–49] which does not mean that cumulative effects of filling pressure does not contribute to outcome in HFpEF but emphasizes the need for an alternative parameter to evaluate LA burden, such as LA reservoir strain, which is discussed later.

Earlier studies suggested that patients with HFpEF show concentric hypertrophy, which leads to increased passive chamber stiffness and thus increased filling pressure.[50] LV mass index has been reported to be modestly correlated with invasively measured LV filling pressure ($r = 0.41–0.48$; $P<.001$).[43,44] Current European Society of Cardiology (ESC) guidelines include increased LV mass index as one of the criteria for the diagnosis of HFpEF.[51] However, community-based studies, as well as trial ancillary studies, have shown that many patients with HFpEF have concentric remodeling in the absence of hypertrophy, or even normal LV geometry.[22,52,53]

Consistent with this observation, it was recently shown that LV hypertrophy was highly specific (88%) but poorly sensitive (26%) for the diagnosis of HFpEF and therefore its absence cannot be used to rule out the diagnosis.[3] When evaluating LV morphology, care should be taken to exclude other differential diagnoses that mimic HFpEF (Table 2). Whenever significant LV hypertrophy is identified, the diagnosis of amyloidosis must be considered, particularly in the presence of a pericardial effusion or apical sparing pattern of LV strain.[54] In a series of consecutive patients with LV hypertrophy greater than or equal to 12 mm, amyloidosis represented 13% of hospitalized "HFpEF."[55] This distinction from HFpEF is particularly important now that new treatments are becoming available for cardiac amyloid.[56]

Strain and strain rate imaging have also been evaluated to estimate LV filling pressure. The ratio of mitral E velocity to longitudinal diastolic strain rate during early diastole (E/SR$_E$) correlated moderately with invasively obtained filling pressure, with high sensitivity and specificity (E/SR$_E$ >11.5, 91%, and 78%, respectively).[57–59] One study reported that E/SR$_E$ predicted cardiovascular outcomes better than E/e'.[60] Smaller studies have shown correlations between LV GLS and filling pressures.[57,61,62] Left atrial longitudinal strain during ventricular systole represents atrial reservoir function and is reduced in HFpEF.[63] One study has shown a high correlation between LA reservoir strain and invasive filling pressure ($r = -0.79$) in patients with preserved EF,[45] but its discriminatory ability to diagnose HFpEF from noncardiac dyspnea remains unexplored. In contrast, decreased GLS (>−16%) has been reported to be associated with adverse outcomes in HFpEF.[29]

Optimal Use of Echocardiography in Diagnosis of Heart Failure with Preserved Ejection Fraction

The diagnosis of HFpEF is obvious in patients with overt congestion at rest, in whom jugular vein distention, peripheral edema and pulmonary congestion are present, and echocardiography is not necessary to establish the clinical diagnosis. In contrast, evaluation of euvolemic patients with exertional dyspnea presents a greater diagnostic challenge.[3,24,64] Correlative analyses are important to show strength of association between 2 variables, and as described earlier, numerous echocardiographic indices are correlated with filling pressures. However, from a diagnostic perspective, it is more important to consider the

Table 2
Differential diagnoses of heart failure with preserved ejection fraction and their echocardiographic clues

Differential Diagnosis	Echocardiographic Clues
Hypertrophic cardiomyopathy	Asymmetric hypertrophy, ↑↑LV wall thickness, LVOT obstruction, SAM
Restrictive cardiomyopathy	Small LV cavity, ↑LV wall thickness, sparkling myocardium, apical sparing, severely reduced tissue Doppler, PE
Pulmonary arterial hypertension	↑RVSP with no sign of increased LV filling pressure, isolated right heart dilatation, PA dilatation, RVOT Doppler midsystolic notch
Constrictive pericarditis	Pericardial thickening, septal bounce, annulus paradoxus and annulus reversus, ↑respiratory variation in mitral/tricuspid flow, absence of IVC collapse
Valvular heart disease	Morphologic valvular abnormalities, color Doppler
Coronary artery disease	Regional wall motion abnormality and thinning
Chronic thromboembolic pulmonary hypertension	↑RVSP with no sign of increased LV filling pressure, isolated right heart dilatation, PA dilatation, RVOT Doppler midsystolic notch
High-output HF	↑Doppler-derived cardiac output

Abbreviations: IVC, inferior vena cava; LVOT, left ventricular outflow obstruction; PA, pulmonary artery; PE, pericardial effusion; RVOT, right ventricular outflow; SAM, systolic anterior motion of the mitral valve.

ability of a test to discriminate cases from controls rather than simple correlative analyses.

In this regard, an increased E/e' ratio has been reported to have excellent specificity for identifying high LV filling pressure (77%–100%), suggesting that it may be useful to rule in the diagnosis of HFpEF when increased.[3,24,37,38,44,46,58,65–68] However, the E/e' ratio shows poor sensitivity (range

0%–73%), meaning it is not an effective test to exclude HFpEF.[24,37,38,44,46,65–68] Because impaired relaxation is expected to accompany high filling pressures, it has been proposed that increase in E/e' be coupled with an impairment in the e' velocity.[51] This more stringent requirement may improve specificity, but will only further compromise sensitivity.[24]

Expert consensus guidelines have recommended use of an increased LA volume index at a cut point of greater than 34 mL/m^2 as another indicator of diastolic dysfunction.[69–71] When prospectively evaluated, an enlarged LA volume index (>34 mL/m^2) is specific (83%) for HFpEF but, like E/e', it is poorly sensitive (49%).[3,46] One potential concern is the appropriate method of allometrically scaling LA volume to body size in obese patients, who represent most of the HFpEF population.[72] With obesity, a linear adjustment of LA volume index to body surface area may result in underestimation of LA remodeling, because the quotient becomes lower as body mass increases. Another complicating issue in the evaluation of LA volume is the presence of atrial fibrillation.[73] Despite this, recent data have shown that the presence of atrial fibrillation in patients with dyspnea is highly predictive of the presence of underlying HFpEF, making this less of an issue, at least as it pertains to diagnosis.[3,74]

The current guidelines have recommended a combination of different indices of diastolic function to diagnose HFpEF. Although these approaches have been found to show high specificity, sensitivity is poor.[3,24] The authors recently developed a simple score to predict the presence of HFpEF among more than 500 patients with unexplained dyspnea.[3] Although many echocardiographic variables were predictive of HFpEF diagnosis in isolation (**Table 3**), the combination of increased E/e' (>9) and RVSP (>35 mm Hg) were additive to clinical characteristics, including older age, larger BMI, number of antihypertensive drugs, and history of atrial fibrillation in multivariable analyses (H$_2$FPEF score; **Fig. 1**).[3] This scheme was then validated in an independent test cohort in which it retained excellent discriminatory capacity (area under the curve, 0.886; P<.0001). Thus, although numerous echocardiographic indicators are related to the presence or absence of HFpEF (see **Table 3**), it seems that the combination of E/e' and RVSP is optimal to inform the noninvasive diagnosis.

According to the approach,[3] the findings in this case on echocardiography (increased E/e' and RVSP) along with older age, obesity, and use of 2 antihypertensive drugs indicate HFpEF is the

Table 3
Operating characteristics of echocardiographic parameters for the diagnosis of heart failure with preserved ejection fraction

	AUC	P	Sensitivity (%)	Specificity (%)
Ejection Fraction <55%	0.52	.09	8	96
LV Hypertrophy	0.57	.0006	26	88
LA Volume Index >34 mL/m^2	0.66	<.0001	49	83
E/e' Ratio (septal) >9	0.69	<.0001	78	59
E/e' Ratio (septal) >13	0.66	<.0001	46	86
Septal e' Velocity <7 cm/s	0.62	<.0001	48	76
Right atrial pressure >10 mm Hg	0.56	<.0001	16	97
RV Systolic Pressure >35mm Hg	0.66	<.0001	46	86
RV Fractional Area Change <48%	0.64	<.0001	39	88
Tricuspid Annular Plane Systolic Excursion <16 mm	0.54	.0008	9	99
Visual RV Dysfunction	0.58	<.0001	22	94
Visual RV Dilatation	0.60	<.0001	32	88

Abbreviation: AUC, area under the curve.

Data from Reddy YNV, Carter RE, Obokata M, et al. A simple, evidence-based approach to help guide diagnosis of heart failure with preserved ejection fraction. Circulation 2018;138(9):861–70.

likely cause of exertional dyspnea with 92% probability.

In contrast, patients with very low probability can be excluded and work-up for other causes is required. Dynamic stress testing to evaluate abnormal increase in filling pressure is required to establish the cause of exertional dyspnea, as discussed later (**Fig. 2**).[24] In this case, an exercise

	Clinical Variable	Values	Points
H$_2$	**H**eavy	Body mass index >30 kg/m^2	2
	Hypertensive	2 or more antihypertensive medicines	1
F	Atrial **F**ibrillation	Paroxysmal or persistent	3
P	**P**ulmonary Hypertension	Doppler echocardiographic estimated right ventricular systolic pressure >35 mm Hg	1
E	**E**lder	Age >60 y	1
F	**F**illing Pressure	Doppler echocardiographic E/e' >9	1
	H$_2$FPEF score		Sum (0–9)

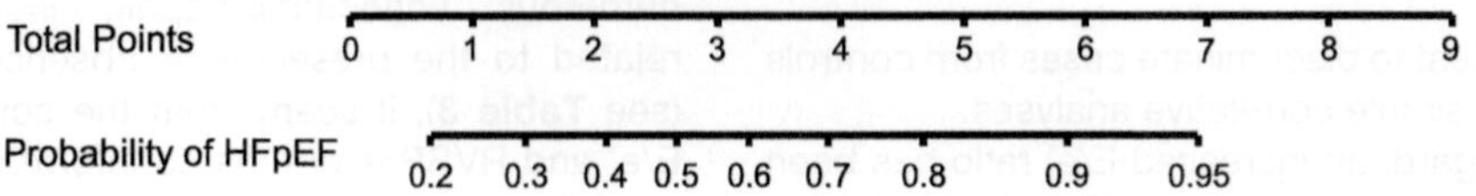

Total Points: 0 1 2 3 4 5 6 7 8 9

Probability of HFpEF: 0.2 0.3 0.4 0.5 0.6 0.7 0.8 0.9 0.95

Fig. 1. The H$_2$FPEF score to aid in diagnosis HFpEF. In this score, the echocardiographic parameters that were independently predictive for HFpEF (E/e' >9 and RVSP >35 mm Hg) are incorporated in tandem with clinical characteristics to determine the probability that HFpEF is present in patients presenting with unexplained dyspnea. (*Adapted from* Reddy YNV, Carter RE, Obokata M, et al. A simple, evidence-based approach to help guide diagnosis of heart failure with preserved ejection fraction. Circulation. 2018;138(9):861–70; with permission.)

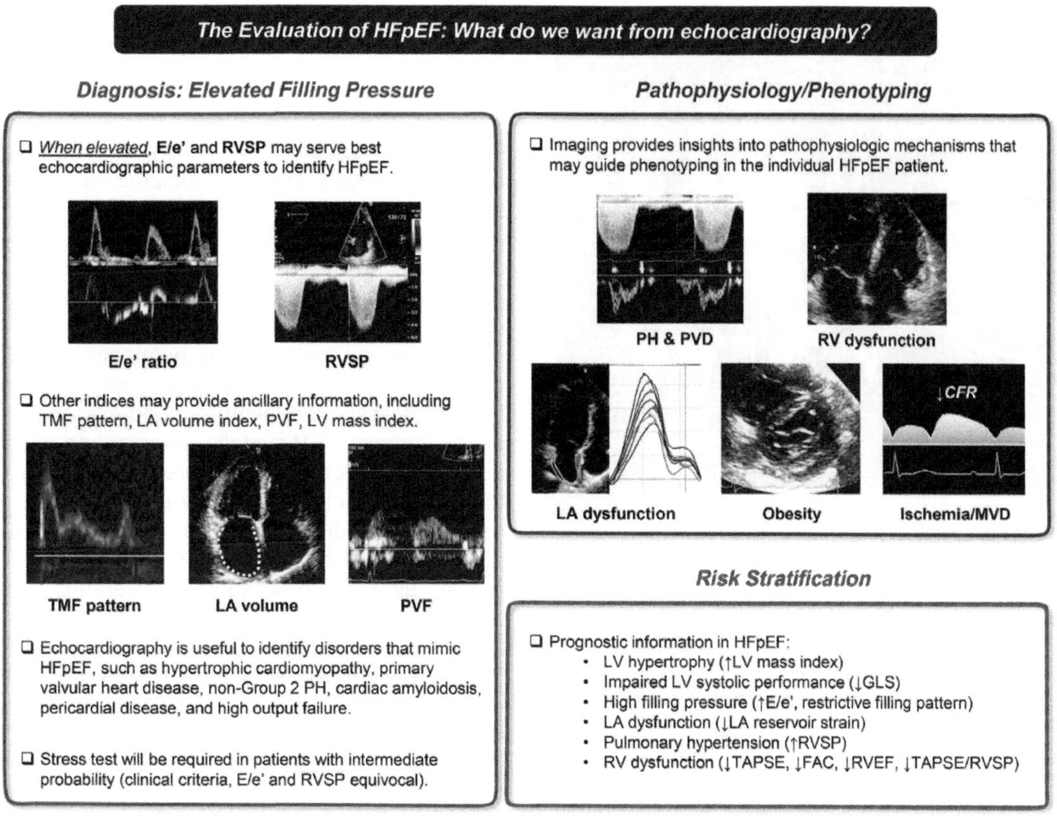

The Evaluation of HFpEF: What do we want from echocardiography?

Diagnosis: Elevated Filling Pressure

☐ *When elevated*, **E/e'** and **RVSP** may serve best echocardiographic parameters to identify HFpEF.

E/e' ratio   RVSP

☐ Other indices may provide ancillary information, including TMF pattern, LA volume index, PVF, LV mass index.

TMF pattern   LA volume   PVF

☐ Echocardiography is useful to identify disorders that mimic HFpEF, such as hypertrophic cardiomyopathy, primary valvular heart disease, non-Group 2 PH, cardiac amyloidosis, pericardial disease, and high output failure.

☐ Stress test will be required in patients with intermediate probability (clinical criteria, E/e' and RVSP equivocal).

Pathophysiology/Phenotyping

☐ Imaging provides insights into pathophysiologic mechanisms that may guide phenotyping in the individual HFpEF patient.

PH & PVD   RV dysfunction

LA dysfunction   Obesity   Ischemia/MVD

Risk Stratification

☐ Prognostic information in HFpEF:
  • LV hypertrophy (↑LV mass index)
  • Impaired LV systolic performance (↓GLS)
  • High filling pressure (↑E/e', restrictive filling pattern)
  • LA dysfunction (↓LA reservoir strain)
  • Pulmonary hypertension (↑RVSP)
  • RV dysfunction (↓TAPSE, ↓FAC, ↓RVEF, ↓TAPSE/RVSP)

Fig. 2. Summary of the role of noninvasive imaging in the evaluation of HFpEF. FAC, RV fractional area change; MVD, microvascular dysfunction; PH, pulmonary hypertension; PVD, pulmonary vascular disease; PVF, pulmonary venous flow; TAPSE, tricuspid annular plane systolic excursion.

catheterization study showed a normal pulmonary capillary wedge pressure (PCWP) at rest (11 mm Hg) but markedly increased filling pressures during exertion (30 mm Hg), which confirmed the diagnosis of HFpEF.

Diastolic stress echocardiography for the diagnosis of heart failure with preserved ejection fraction

Part of the difficulty in diagnosing HFpEF is related to the fact that filling pressures are often normal at rest, but become increased only during the stress of exercise.[3,24,64] Because of this, invasive cardiopulmonary exercise testing has emerged as the gold standard to definitively identify or exclude HFpEF as the cause of dyspnea.[3,24,64,75,76] Recent studies have evaluated whether similar data can be obtained noninvasively using diastolic stress echocardiography (**Fig. 3**).[24]

A recent study using simultaneous catheterization-echocardiographic evaluation at rest and during exercise in patients being evaluated for exertional dyspnea (EF ≥50%) showed that addition of E/e' during exercise improved

sensitivity for diagnosis of HFpEF compared with resting assessment alone, but at the cost of a decreased specificity.[24] However, only 74 patients were enrolled in this single-center study, and other groups have not observed such favorable results in HFpEF with exercise echocardiography.[67,77–79] Some studies have raised questions with the ability of E/e' to track changes in filling pressure during exercise, particularly because E/e' increases far less than directly measured filling pressures.[24,67,79] Given the discrepant results in the totality of studies published to date and the lack of reproducibility, additional validation, preferably using multicenter designs, is required to clarify the role for noninvasive diastolic stress echocardiography in the evaluation of HFpEF.[80]

Abnormal LV systolic and diastolic responses to exercise assessed by LV longitudinal strain or strain rate and E/e' have been reported to improve risk prediction compared with clinical and resting measurements in HFpEF, although this usage also requires additional confirmation in larger, multicenter studies.[81,82]

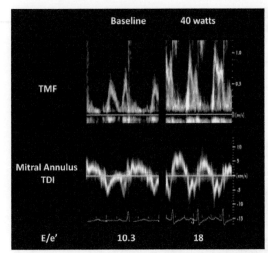

Fig. 3. Typical case of diastolic stress echocardiography. TMF and mitral annular tissue Doppler velocities at rest and during 40 W supine ergometer exercise in a patient with invasively proven HFpEF (PCWP during exercise, 27 mm Hg). At baseline, transthoracic echocardiography shows normal EF (70%), LA volume index (30 mL/m^2), normal E/e' (average 10.3), and an estimated RVSP of 28 mm Hg. With exercise up to 40 W, mitral E increases dramatically without significant change in e', resulting in an increased E/e' ratio. Tricuspid regurgitant velocity increases from 2.5 to 3.5 m/s during exercise. TDI, tissue Doppler imaging.

Echocardiography to Identify Heart Failure with Preserved Ejection Fraction Phenotypes

It has recently been recognized that HFpEF is a heterogeneous syndrome, and treatments applying the one-size-fits-all approach have uniformly failed to date when tested in clinical trials.[83] Accordingly, there is an unmet need to categorize different phenotypes within the broader spectrum of HFpEF into pathophysiologically homogenous groups, and cardiac imaging may be a very useful tool to enable this characterization. Candidate phenotypes that might be used for deeper characterization by echocardiography in HFpEF are described later.

Left Atrial Dysfunction Phenotype

LA remodeling and dysfunction secondary to increased LV filling pressure are associated with worse symptoms of dyspnea, more pulmonary vascular disease, greater RV dysfunction, depressed exercise capacity, and adverse outcomes in HFpEF.[39,42,84,85] Thus, LA hypertension/dysfunction can be a potential subphenotype of HFpEF. Multiple recent studies have shown the utility of LA reservoir strain assessed by speckle-tracking echocardiography to identify LA

dysfunction, help diagnosis, and predict outcomes in HFpEF.[42,63,85,86]

Pulmonary Hypertension and Pulmonary Vascular Disease Phenotype

Pulmonary hypertension (PH) is common in patients with HFpEF and is associated with worse exercise capacity and clinical outcomes.[48,87,88] Although PH is predominantly related to LA hypertension in most patients with HFpEF, some patients develop pulmonary vascular disease, manifest by increase in pulmonary vascular resistance and reduction in pulmonary arterial compliance.[89] HFpEF with pulmonary vascular disease is associated with reduced exercise capacity, impaired RV systolic reserve, and worse outcomes, suggesting a different phenotype in the HFpEF spectrum.[90] The presence of pulmonary vascular disease can be suspected from midsystolic notching in the RV outflow Doppler profile, along with a short acceleration time caused by increased pulmonary arterial impedance with enhanced early wave reflection.[91,92] There is increasing recognition of the importance of RV and pulmonary vascular (RV-PA) coupling and a recent study reported that RV-PA coupling assessed by tricuspid annular plane systolic excursion (TAPSE) to RVSP (<0.36 mm/mm Hg) predicts pulmonary vascular disease in HFpEF.[93]

Right Ventricular Dysfunction Phenotype

The presence of PH causes RV systolic dysfunction in HFpEF, but recent data have shown that RV-PA coupling is even more important.[87,88] TAPSE, RV fractional area change, free wall strain, tricuspid annular s' velocity, and RV index of myocardial performance can be measured as indices of RV systolic function.[94,95] RV-PA coupling can then be assessed by the ratio of RV function to RVSP,[94,95] and lower TAPSE/RVSP ratio (<0.36 mm/mm Hg) is associated with adverse outcomes in HFpEF.[93,94,96]

RV dysfunction is associated with RV remodeling. Echocardiography allows for assessments of RV dilatation (RV basal, mid, and longitudinal dimensions and areas), RV hypertrophy, as well as right atrial (RA) dilatation. Increased RV diameter, area, and wall thickness have been shown to predict adverse outcome in HFpEF.[47,87] RV and RA dilatation leads to tricuspid annular dilatation and resultant tricuspid insufficiency, which may further promote systemic venous congestion and impair left heart filling, particularly during exercise.[97] Thus, the severity of tricuspid insufficiency should be assessed in all patients with HFpEF.

Obesity Phenotype

Obesity is now recognized as an important phenotype of HFpEF.[72] Compared with patients with nonobese HFpEF, patients with the obese phenotype show several key differences, including greater relationships between body weight and cardiac filling pressures, greater plasma volume expansion, more ventricular remodeling, more adverse hemodynamics, altered RV-pulmonary artery coupling, worse exercise capacity, and enhanced pericardial restraint.[72] Assessments of septal configuration in the short axis can provide noninvasive estimates of the degree of relative pericardial restraint, which contributes to the PCWP increase in the HFpEF obese phenotype as well as patients with pulmonary vascular phenotype and those with severe tricuspid insufficiency (**Fig. 4**).[72,89,97]

Visceral adiposity and ectopic fat deposits can contribute to the obesity phenotype by altering hemodynamics, inducing systemic and local inflammation, and causing mechanistic compression exaggerating pericardial restraint. Abdominal obesity is associated with epicardial fat and has recently been found to be associated with increased mortality in HFpEF.[98] Measurements of epicardial thickness are feasible by echocardiography (**Fig. 5**) but are more accurately performed using other modalities, such as computed tomography and MRI.

Ischemia/microvascular dysfunction phenotype

The presence of epicardial coronary artery disease identifies a distinct HFpEF phenotype in view of its high prevalence; worse prognosis; and, importantly, a possibility of improving outcomes through

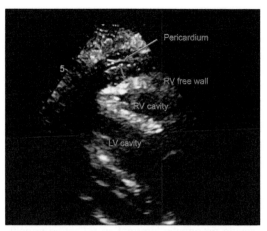

Fig. 5. Prominent epicardial fat in obese HFpEF. Parasternal long-axis view at end-systole in an obese patient with HFpEF (BMI, 38 kg/m²). Note the increased epicardial fat thickness (14 mm) identified between the RV free wall and the pericardium.

revascularization.[99] Stress imaging, including echocardiography, has been shown to be less accurate in patients with HFpEF, with high rates of false-positive and false-negative tests.[99] This finding may reflect that subendocardial ischemia may also develop in the absence of epicardial coronary stenosis in HFpEF, caused by the combination of coronary microvascular dysfunction and hemodynamic derangements that compromise subendocardial perfusion.[100]

Patients with HFpEF developing greater myocardial injury during exercise in tandem with myocardial supply-demand mismatch, and those with greater burden of ischemia and injury show the most profound limitations in LV systolic and diastolic reserve, higher filling pressures during exercise, and more impaired exercise capacity.[100] A recent study has shown that adenosine stress echocardiography can be used to assess coronary flow reserve in these patients, and this may be an important noninvasive phenotyping tool, particularly if new treatments are developed targeting microvascular function.[101] Other groups have used nuclear and MRI-based imaging to evaluate for coronary microvascular dysfunction in HFpEF,[102] and there is hope that novel therapies targeted to microvascular dysfunction may be properly targeted to the right patients using the different imaging modalities.

SUMMARY AND FUTURE DIRECTIONS

Echocardiography is clearly essential in the evaluation for HFpEF and provides valuable information to estimate LV filling pressure and understand pathophysiology and improve both evaluation for

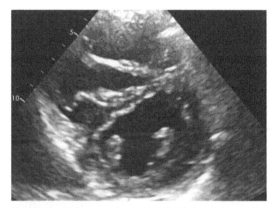

Fig. 4. Typical case of obese HFpEF. An echocardiographic parasternal short-axis view at end-diastole shows the D-shaped septum in a patient with obese HFpEF (BMI, 44 kg/m²). Cardiac catheterization reveals severely increased RA pressure (17 mm Hg) relative to PCWP (21 mm Hg).

both diagnosis and prognosis. Together with clinical characteristics, echocardiography can help determine the likelihood that HFpEF is present and allow more informed decision making regarding the need for more advanced testing. However, echocardiography alone is often insufficient to make or refute the diagnosis of HFpEF, and, in many cases, invasive hemodynamic exercise testing is required. Categorizing patients with HFpEF based on underlying pathophysiologic phenotypes represents a key next step in providing individualized medicine, and echocardiography plays a crucial role in this regard, although the optimal ways to categorize patients remain unknown. In addition, echocardiographic parameters provide prognostic information reflecting specific pathophysiologic abnormalities in HFpEF. Further study is required to standardize diagnostic criteria for HFpEF, determine roles for different modalities in its evaluation, establish the potential value for diastolic stress echocardiography, and identify the optimal roles of noninvasive imaging along with other clinical markers for HFpEF phenotyping.

ACKNOWLEDGMENTS

Dr. Borlaug is supported by the National Institutes of Health (R01 HL128526, R01 HL 126638, U01 HL125205, and U10 HL110262). Dr. Obokata is supported by a research fellowship from the Uehara Memorial Foundation, Japan.

REFERENCES

1. Owan TE, Hodge DO, Herges RM, et al. Trends in prevalence and outcome of heart failure with preserved ejection fraction. N Engl J Med 2006;355:251–9.
2. Chang PP, Wruck LM, Shahar E, et al. Trends in hospitalizations and survival of acute decompensated heart failure in four US communities (2005-2014): ARIC study community surveillance. Circulation 2018;138:12–24.
3. Reddy YNV, Carter RE, Obokata M, et al. A simple, evidence-based approach to help guide diagnosis of heart failure with preserved ejection fraction. Circulation 2018;138(9):861–70.
4. Shah AM, Claggett B, Loehr LR, et al. Heart failure stages among older adults in the community: The Atherosclerosis Risk in Communities study. Circulation 2017;135:224–40.
5. Nauta JF, Hummel YM, van der Meer P, et al. Correlation with invasive left ventricular filling pressures and prognostic relevance of the echocardiographic diastolic parameters used in the 2016 ESC heart failure guidelines and in the 2016 ASE/EACVI recommendations: a systematic review in patients with heart failure with preserved ejection fraction. Eur J Heart Fail 2018; 20(9):1303–11.
6. Nagueh SF, Smiseth OA, Appleton CP, et al. Recommendations for the evaluation of left ventricular diastolic function by echocardiography: an update from the American Society of Echocardiography and the European Association of Cardiovascular Imaging. J Am Soc Echocardiogr 2016;29:277–314.
7. Abudiab MM, Redfield MM, Melenovsky V, et al. Cardiac output response to exercise in relation to metabolic demand in heart failure with preserved ejection fraction. Eur J Heart Fail 2013;15:776–85.
8. Borlaug BA. The pathophysiology of heart failure with preserved ejection fraction. Nat Rev Cardiol 2014;11:507–15.
9. Borlaug BA, Kane GC, Melenovsky V, et al. Abnormal right ventricular-pulmonary artery coupling with exercise in heart failure with preserved ejection fraction. Eur Heart J 2016;37:3293–302.
10. Borlaug BA, Olson TP, Lam CS, et al. Global cardiovascular reserve dysfunction in heart failure with preserved ejection fraction. J Am Coll Cardiol 2010;56:845–54.
11. Obokata M, Olson TP, Reddy YN, et al. Hemodynamics, dyspnea, and pulmonary reserve in heart failure with preserved ejection fraction. Eur Heart J 2018;39:2810–21.
12. Reddy YNV, Olson TP, Obokata M, et al. Hemodynamic correlates and diagnostic role of cardiopulmonary exercise testing in heart failure with preserved ejection fraction. JACC Heart Fail 2018;6:665–75.
13. Adamson PB, Abraham WT, Bourge RC, et al. Wireless pulmonary artery pressure monitoring guides management to reduce decompensation in heart failure with preserved ejection fraction. Circ Heart Fail 2014;7:935–44.
14. Dorfs S, Zeh W, Hochholzer W, et al. Pulmonary capillary wedge pressure during exercise and long-term mortality in patients with suspected heart failure with preserved ejection fraction. Eur Heart J 2014;35:3103–12.
15. Borlaug BA, Kass DA. Invasive hemodynamic assessment in heart failure. Cardiol Clin 2011;29:269–80.
16. Nayor M, Cooper LL, Enserro DM, et al. Left ventricular diastolic dysfunction in the community: impact of diagnostic criteria on the burden, correlates, and prognosis. J Am Heart Assoc 2018;7 [pii: e008291].
17. Shah AM, Claggett B, Kitzman D, et al. Contemporary assessment of left ventricular diastolic function in older adults: the Atherosclerosis Risk in Communities study. Circulation 2017;135:426–39.

18. Reddy YNV, Borlaug BA. What do you want from your echocardiogram? J Am Heart Assoc 2018;7 [pii: e009462].

19. Kane GC, Karon BL, Mahoney DW, et al. Progression of left ventricular diastolic dysfunction and risk of heart failure. JAMA 2011;306:856–63.

20. Persson H, Lonn E, Edner M, et al. Diastolic dysfunction in heart failure with preserved systolic function: need for objective evidence: results from the CHARM echocardiographic substudy–CHARMES. J Am Coll Cardiol 2007;49:687–94.

21. Shah AM, Claggett B, Sweitzer NK, et al. Cardiac structure and function and prognosis in heart failure with preserved ejection fraction: findings from the echocardiographic study of the Treatment of Preserved Cardiac Function Heart Failure with an Aldosterone Antagonist (TOPCAT) Trial. Circ Heart Fail 2014;7:740–51.

22. Zile MR, Gottdiener JS, Hetzel SJ, et al. Prevalence and significance of alterations in cardiac structure and function in patients with heart failure and a preserved ejection fraction. Circulation 2011;124:2491–501.

23. Aljaroudi W, Alraies MC, Halley C, et al. Impact of progression of diastolic dysfunction on mortality in patients with normal ejection fraction. Circulation 2012;125:782–8.

24. Obokata M, Kane GC, Reddy YN, et al. Role of diastolic stress testing in the evaluation for heart failure with preserved ejection fraction: a simultaneous invasive-echocardiographic study. Circulation 2017;135:825–38.

25. Nagueh SF, Middleton KJ, Kopelen HA, et al. Doppler tissue imaging: a noninvasive technique for evaluation of left ventricular relaxation and estimation of filling pressures. J Am Coll Cardiol 1997;30:1527–33.

26. Nagueh SF, Mikati I, Kopelen HA, et al. Doppler estimation of left ventricular filling pressure in sinus tachycardia. A new application of tissue Doppler imaging. Circulation 1998;98:1644–50.

27. Ommen SR, Nishimura RA, Appleton CP, et al. Clinical utility of Doppler echocardiography and tissue Doppler imaging in the estimation of left ventricular filling pressures: a comparative simultaneous Doppler-catheterization study. Circulation 2000;102:1788–94.

28. Andersen OS, Smiseth OA, Dokainish H, et al. Estimating left ventricular filling pressure by echocardiography. J Am Coll Cardiol 2017;69:1937–48.

29. Shah AM, Claggett B, Sweitzer NK, et al. Prognostic importance of impaired systolic function in heart failure with preserved ejection fraction and the impact of spironolactone. Circulation 2015;132:402–14.

30. Yamamoto K, Nishimura RA, Burnett JC Jr, et al. Assessment of left ventricular end-diastolic pressure by Doppler echocardiography: contribution of duration of pulmonary venous versus mitral flow velocity curves at atrial contraction. J Am Soc Echocardiogr 1997;10:52–9.

31. Buffle E, Kramarz J, Elazar E, et al. Added value of pulmonary venous flow Doppler assessment in patients with preserved ejection fraction and its contribution to the diastolic grading paradigm. Eur Heart J Cardiovasc Imaging 2015;16:1191–7.

32. Appleton CP, Galloway JM, Gonzalez MS, et al. Estimation of left ventricular filling pressures using two-dimensional and Doppler echocardiography in adult patients with cardiac disease. Additional value of analyzing left atrial size, left atrial ejection fraction and the difference in duration of pulmonary venous and mitral flow velocity at atrial contraction. J Am Coll Cardiol 1993;22:1972–82.

33. Kuecherer HF, Muhiudeen IA, Kusumoto FM, et al. Estimation of mean left atrial pressure from transesophageal pulsed Doppler echocardiography of pulmonary venous flow. Circulation 1990;82:1127–39.

34. Poerner TC, Goebel B, Unglaub P, et al. Non-invasive evaluation of left ventricular filling pressures in patients with abnormal relaxation. Clin Sci 2004;106:485–94.

35. Yamamoto K, Nishimura RA, Chaliki HP, et al. Determination of left ventricular filling pressure by Doppler echocardiography in patients with coronary artery disease: critical role of left ventricular systolic function. J Am Coll Cardiol 1997;30:1819–26.

36. Poerner TC, Goebel B, Unglaub P, et al. Detection of a pseudonormal mitral inflow pattern: an echocardiographic and tissue Doppler study. Echocardiography 2003;20:345–56.

37. Hadano Y, Murata K, Liu J, et al. Can transthoracic Doppler echocardiography predict the discrepancy between left ventricular end-diastolic pressure and mean pulmonary capillary wedge pressure in patients with heart failure? Circ J 2005;69:432–8.

38. Kidawa M, Coignard L, Drobinski G, et al. Comparative value of tissue Doppler imaging and m-mode color Doppler mitral flow propagation velocity for the evaluation of left ventricular filling pressure. Chest 2005;128:2544–50.

39. Melenovsky V, Hwang SJ, Redfield MM, et al. Left atrial remodeling and function in advanced heart failure with preserved or reduced ejection fraction. Circ Heart Fail 2015;8:295–303.

40. Zakeri R, Moulay G, Chai Q, et al. Left atrial remodeling and atrioventricular coupling in a canine model of early heart failure with preserved ejection fraction. Circ Heart Fail 2016;9 [pii: e003238].

41. von Roeder M, Rommel KP, Kowallick JT, et al. Influence of left atrial function on exercise capacity

and left ventricular function in patients with heart failure and preserved ejection fraction. Circ Cardiovasc Imaging 2017;10 [pii: e005467].

42. Freed BH, Daruwalla V, Cheng JY, et al. Prognostic utility and clinical significance of cardiac mechanics in heart failure with preserved ejection fraction: importance of left atrial strain. Circ Cardiovasc Imaging 2016;9 [pii: e003754].

43. Kasner M, Westermann D, Steendijk P, et al. Utility of Doppler echocardiography and tissue Doppler imaging in the estimation of diastolic function in heart failure with normal ejection fraction: a comparative Doppler-conductance catheterization study. Circulation 2007;116:637–47.

44. Dokainish H, Nguyen JS, Sengupta R, et al. Do additional echocardiographic variables increase the accuracy of e/e' for predicting left ventricular filling pressure in normal ejection fraction? An echocardiographic and invasive hemodynamic study. J Am Soc Echocardiogr 2010;23:156–61.

45. Cameli M, Sparla S, Losito M, et al. Correlation of left atrial strain and Doppler measurements with invasive measurement of left ventricular end-diastolic pressure in patients stratified for different values of ejection fraction. Echocardiography 2016;33:398–405.

46. Lancellotti P, Galderisi M, Edvardsen T, et al. Echo-Doppler estimation of left ventricular filling pressure: results of the multicentre EACVI Euro-Filling study. Eur Heart J Cardiovasc Imaging 2017;18: 961–8.

47. Burke MA, Katz DH, Beussink L, et al. Prognostic importance of pathophysiologic markers in patients with heart failure and preserved ejection fraction. Circ Heart Fail 2014;7:288–99.

48. Lam CS, Roger VL, Rodeheffer RJ, et al. Pulmonary hypertension in heart failure with preserved ejection fraction: a community-based study. J Am Coll Cardiol 2009;53:1119–26.

49. Donal E, Lund LH, Oger E, et al. Importance of combined left atrial size and estimated pulmonary pressure for clinical outcome in patients presenting with heart failure with preserved ejection fraction. Eur Heart J Cardiovasc Imaging 2017; 18:629–35.

50. Zile MR, Baicu CF, Gaasch WH. Diastolic heart failure–abnormalities in active relaxation and passive stiffness of the left ventricle. N Engl J Med 2004;350:1953–9.

51. Ponikowski P, Voors AA, Anker SD, et al. 2016 ESC guidelines for the diagnosis and treatment of acute and chronic heart failure: The Task Force for the Diagnosis and Treatment of Acute and Chronic Heart Failure of the European Society of Cardiology (ESC) developed with the special contribution of the Heart Failure Association (HFA) of the ESC. Eur Heart J 2016;37:2129–200.

52. Borlaug BA, Lam CS, Roger VL, et al. Contractility and ventricular systolic stiffening in hypertensive heart disease insights into the pathogenesis of heart failure with preserved ejection fraction. J Am Coll Cardiol 2009;54:410–8.

53. Lam CS, Roger VL, Rodeheffer RJ, et al. Cardiac structure and ventricular-vascular function in persons with heart failure and preserved ejection fraction from Olmsted County, Minnesota. Circulation 2007;115:1982–90.

54. Phelan D, Collier P, Thavendiranathan P, et al. Relative apical sparing of longitudinal strain using two-dimensional speckle-tracking echocardiography is both sensitive and specific for the diagnosis of cardiac amyloidosis. Heart 2012;98: 1442–8.

55. Gonzalez-Lopez E, Gallego-Delgado M, Guzzo-Merello G, et al. Wild-type transthyretin amyloidosis as a cause of heart failure with preserved ejection fraction. Eur Heart J 2015;36:2585–94.

56. Maurer MS, Schwartz JH, Gundapaneni B, et al. Tafamidis treatment for patients with transthyretin amyloid cardiomyopathy. N Engl J Med 2018;379: 1007–16.

57. Kasner M, Gaub R, Sinning D, et al. Global strain rate imaging for the estimation of diastolic function in HFNEF compared with pressure-volume loop analysis. Eur J Echocardiogr 2010;11:743–51.

58. Dokainish H, Sengupta R, Pillai M, et al. Usefulness of new diastolic strain and strain rate indexes for the estimation of left ventricular filling pressure. Am J Cardiol 2008;101:1504–9.

59. Wang J, Khoury DS, Thohan V, et al. Global diastolic strain rate for the assessment of left ventricular relaxation and filling pressures. Circulation 2007;115:1376–83.

60. Lassen MCH, Biering-Sorensen SR, Olsen FJ, et al. Ratio of transmitral early filling velocity to early diastolic strain rate predicts long-term risk of cardiovascular morbidity and mortality in the general population. Eur Heart J 2018. https://doi.org/10.1093/eurheartj/ehy164.

61. Hayashi T, Yamada S, Iwano H, et al. Left ventricular global strain for estimating relaxation and filling pressure –a multicenter study. Circ J 2016;80: 1163–70.

62. Ma H, Wu WC, Xie RA, et al. Correlation of global strain rate and left ventricular filling pressure in patients with coronary artery disease: a 2-D speckle-tracking study. Ultrasound Med Biol 2016;42: 413–20.

63. Obokata M, Negishi K, Kurosawa K, et al. Incremental diagnostic value of LA strain with leg lifts in heart failure with preserved ejection fraction. JACC Cardiovasc Imaging 2013;6:749–58.

64. Borlaug BA, Nishimura RA, Sorajja P, et al. Exercise hemodynamics enhance diagnosis of early heart

failure with preserved ejection fraction. Circ Heart Fail 2010;3:588–95.

65. Mansencal N, Bouvier E, Joseph T, et al. Value of tissue Doppler imaging to predict left ventricular filling pressure in patients with coronary artery disease. Echocardiography 2004;21:133–8.

66. Penicka M, Bartunek J, Trakalova H, et al. Heart failure with preserved ejection fraction in outpatients with unexplained dyspnea: a pressure-volume loop analysis. J Am Coll Cardiol 2010;55:1701–10.

67. Bhella PS, Pacini EL, Prasad A, et al. Echocardiographic indices do not reliably track changes in left-sided filling pressure in healthy subjects or patients with heart failure with preserved ejection fraction. Circ Cardiovasc Imaging 2011;4:482–9.

68. Manouras A, Nyktari E, Sahlen A, et al. The value of e/em ratio in the estimation of left ventricular filling pressures: impact of acute load reduction: a comparative simultaneous echocardiographic and catheterization study. Int J Cardiol 2013;166:589–95.

69. Lang RM, Badano LP, Mor-Avi V, et al. Recommendations for cardiac chamber quantification by echocardiography in adults: an update from the American Society of Echocardiography and the European Association of Cardiovascular Imaging. Eur Heart J Cardiovasc Imaging 2015;16:233–70.

70. Kou S, Caballero L, Dulgheru R, et al. Echocardiographic reference ranges for normal cardiac chamber size: results from the NORRE study. Eur Heart J Cardiovasc Imaging 2014;15:680–90.

71. Nistri S, Galderisi M, Ballo P, et al. Determinants of echocardiographic left atrial volume: implications for normalcy. Eur J Echocardiogr 2011;12:826–33.

72. Obokata M, Reddy YN, Pislaru SV, et al. Evidence supporting the existence of a distinct obese phenotype of heart failure with preserved ejection fraction. Circulation 2017;136:6–19.

73. Lam CS, Rienstra M, Tay WT, et al. Atrial fibrillation in heart failure with preserved ejection fraction: association with exercise capacity, left ventricular filling pressures, natriuretic peptides, and left atrial volume. JACC Heart Fail 2017;5:92–8.

74. Reddy YNV, Obokata M, Gersh BJ, et al. High prevalence of occult heart failure with preserved ejection fraction among patients with atrial fibrillation and dyspnea. Circulation 2018;137:534–5.

75. Maron BA, Cockrill BA, Waxman AB, et al. The invasive cardiopulmonary exercise test. Circulation 2013;127:1157–64.

76. Givertz MM, Fang JC, Sorajja P, et al. Executive summary of the SCAI/HFSA clinical expert consensus document on the use of invasive hemodynamics for the diagnosis and management of cardiovascular disease. J Card Fail 2017;23:487–91.

77. Sharifov OF, Gupta H. What is the evidence that the tissue Doppler index e/e' reflects left ventricular filling pressure changes after exercise or pharmacological intervention for evaluating diastolic function? A systematic review. J Am Heart Assoc 2017;6 [pii: e004766].

78. Santos M, Rivero J, McCullough SD, et al. E/e' ratio in patients with unexplained dyspnea: lack of accuracy in estimating left ventricular filling pressure. Circ Heart Fail 2015;8:749–56.

79. Maeder MT, Thompson BR, Brunner-La Rocca HP, et al. Hemodynamic basis of exercise limitation in patients with heart failure and normal ejection fraction. J Am Coll Cardiol 2010;56:855–63.

80. Obokata M, Borlaug BA. The strengths and limitations of e/e' in heart failure with preserved ejection fraction. Eur J Heart Fail 2018;20(9):1312–4.

81. Wang J, Fang F, Wai-Kwok Yip G, et al. Left ventricular long-axis performance during exercise is an important prognosticator in patients with heart failure and preserved ejection fraction. Int J Cardiol 2015;178:131–5.

82. Kosmala W, Przewlocka-Kosmala M, Rojek A, et al. Association of abnormal left ventricular functional reserve with outcome in heart failure with preserved ejection fraction. JACC Cardiovasc Imaging 2017;11(12):1737–46.

83. Shah SJ, Kitzman DW, Borlaug BA, et al. Phenotype-specific treatment of heart failure with preserved ejection fraction: a multiorgan roadmap. Circulation 2016;134:73–90.

84. Melenovsky V, Borlaug BA, Rosen B, et al. Cardiovascular features of heart failure with preserved ejection fraction versus nonfailing hypertensive left ventricular hypertrophy in the urban Baltimore community: the role of atrial remodeling/dysfunction. J Am Coll Cardiol 2007;49:198–207.

85. Santos AB, Kraigher-Krainer E, Gupta DK, et al. Impaired left atrial function in heart failure with preserved ejection fraction. Eur J Heart Fail 2014;16:1096–103.

86. Santos AB, Roca GQ, Claggett B, et al. Prognostic relevance of left atrial dysfunction in heart failure with preserved ejection fraction. Circ Heart Fail 2016;9:e002763.

87. Melenovsky V, Hwang SJ, Lin G, et al. Right heart dysfunction in heart failure with preserved ejection fraction. Eur Heart J 2014;35:3452–62.

88. Mohammed SF, Hussain I, Abou Ezzeddine OF, et al. Right ventricular function in heart failure with preserved ejection fraction: a community-based study. Circulation 2014;130:2310–20.

89. Gorter TM, Obokata M, Reddy YN, et al. Exercise unmasks distinct pathophysiologic features in heart failure with preserved ejection fraction and pulmonary vascular disease. Eur Heart J 2018;39(30):2825–35.

90. Borlaug BA, Obokata M. Is it time to recognize a new phenotype? Heart failure with preserved ejection fraction with pulmonary vascular disease. Eur Heart J 2017;38:2874–8.

91. Arkles JS, Opotowsky AR, Ojeda J, et al. Shape of the right ventricular Doppler envelope predicts hemodynamics and right heart function in pulmonary hypertension. Am J Respir Crit Care Med 2011; 183:268–76.

92. Takahama H, McCully RB, Frantz RP, et al. Unraveling the RV ejection Doppler envelope: insight into pulmonary artery hemodynamics and disease severity. JACC Cardiovasc Imaging 2017;10: 1268–77.

93. Gorter TM, van Veldhuisen DJ, Voors AA, et al. Right ventricular-vascular coupling in heart failure with preserved ejection fraction and pre- vs. post-capillary pulmonary hypertension. Eur Heart J Cardiovasc Imaging 2018;19:425–32.

94. Guazzi M, Bandera F, Pelissero G, et al. Tricuspid annular plane systolic excursion and pulmonary arterial systolic pressure relationship in heart failure: an index of right ventricular contractile function and prognosis. Am J Physiol Heart Circ Physiol 2013;305:H1373–81.

95. Rudski LG, Lai WW, Afilalo J, et al. Guidelines for the echocardiographic assessment of the right heart in adults: a report from the American Society of Echocardiography endorsed by the European Association of Echocardiography, a registered branch of the European Society of Cardiology, and the Canadian Society of Echocardiography. J Am Soc Echocardiogr 2010;23:685–713 [quiz: 786-8].

96. Guazzi M, Dixon D, Labate V, et al. RV contractile function and its coupling to pulmonary circulation in heart failure with preserved ejection fraction: stratification of clinical phenotypes and outcomes. JACC Cardiovasc Imaging 2017;10:1211–21.

97. Andersen MJ, Nishimura RA, Borlaug BA. The hemodynamic basis of exercise intolerance in tricuspid regurgitation. Circ Heart Fail 2014;7: 911–7.

98. Tsujimoto T, Kajio H. Abdominal obesity is associated with an increased risk of all-cause mortality in patients with HFpEF. J Am Coll Cardiol 2017; 70:2739–49.

99. Hwang SJ, Melenovsky V, Borlaug BA. Implications of coronary artery disease in heart failure with preserved ejection fraction. J Am Coll Cardiol 2014;63: 2817–27.

100. Obokata M, Reddy YNV, Melenovsky V, et al. Myocardial injury and cardiac reserve in patients with heart failure and preserved ejection fraction. J Am Coll Cardiol 2018;72:29–40.

101. Shah SJ, Lam CSP, Svedlund S, et al. Prevalence and correlates of coronary microvascular dysfunction in heart failure with preserved ejection fraction: PROMIS-HFpEF. Eur Heart J 2018; 39(37):3439–50.

102. Mohammed SF, Majure DT, Redfield MM. Zooming in on the microvasculature in heart failure with preserved ejection fraction. Circ Heart Fail 2016;9 [pii: e003272].

103. Min PK, Ha JW, Jung JH, et al. Incremental value of measuring the time difference between onset of mitral inflow and onset of early diastolic mitral annulus velocity for the evaluation of left ventricular diastolic pressures in patients with normal systolic function and an indeterminate E/E'. Am J Cardiol 2007;100:326–30.

104. Rudko R, Przewlocki T, Pasowicz M, et al. IVRT'/IVRT index is a useful tool for detection of elevated left ventricular filling pressure in patients with preserved ejection fraction. Echocardiography 2008; 25:473–81.

105. Hsiao SH, Chiou KR, Lin KL, et al. Left atrial distensibility and E/e' for estimating left ventricular filling pressure in patients with stable angina. -A comparative echocardiography and catheterization study-. Circ J 2011;75:1942–50.

106. Maeder MT, Karapanagiotidis S, Dewar EM, et al. Accuracy of Doppler echocardiography to estimate key hemodynamic variables in subjects with normal left ventricular ejection fraction. J Card Fail 2011;17:405–12.

107. Previtali M, Chieffo E, Ferrario M, et al. Is mitral E/E' ratio a reliable predictor of left ventricular diastolic pressures in patients without heart failure? Eur Heart J Cardiovasc Imaging 2012;13:588–95.

108. Tatsumi K, Tanaka H, Matsumoto K, et al. Global endocardial area change rate for the assessment of left ventricular relaxation and filling pressure: using 3-dimensional speckle-tracking study. Int J Cardiovasc Imaging 2014;30:1473–81.

109. Kasner M, Sinning D, Burkhoff D, et al. Diastolic pressure-volume quotient (DPVQ) as a novel echocardiographic index for estimation of LV stiffness in HFpEF. Clin Res Cardiol 2015;104:955–63.

110. Matsushita K, Minamishima T, Goda A, et al. Comparison of the reliability of E/E' to estimate pulmonary capillary wedge pressure in heart failure patients with preserved ejection fraction versus those with reduced ejection fraction. Int J Cardiovasc Imaging 2015;31:1497–502.

111. Ma H, Xie RA, Gao LJ, et al. Prediction of left ventricular filling pressure by 3-dimensional speckle-tracking echocardiography in patients with coronary artery disease. J Ultrasound Med 2015;34: 1809–18.

112. Rommel KP, von Roeder M, Latuscynski K, et al. Extracellular volume fraction for characterization of patients with heart failure and preserved ejection fraction. J Am Coll Cardiol 2016;67:1815–25.

Intraventricular Flow
More than Pretty Pictures

In-Cheol Kim, MD, PhD[a], Geu-Ru Hong, MD, PhD[b],*

KEYWORDS

- Heart failure • Intraventricular flow • Vortex

KEY POINTS

- Intraventricular flow pattern forms vortices allowing movement of blood from the mitral inlet to the aortic outlet for efficient energy preservation.
- Myocardial, valvular, electrical dysfunction in heart failure causes chamber enlargement, volume/pressure overload in conjunction with flow dynamic distortion.
- Currently, vorticial flow analysis is available with echo particle image velocimetry, echo vector flow mapping, and velocity-encoded phase contrast cardiac magnetic resonance.
- Flow dynamics in diverse disease conditions, which can manifest as heart failure, are well validated and continuously on the way of development.
- With conventional structural and functional parameters, vortex flow analysis–guided treatment in HF might be a novel option.

INTRAVENTRICULAR FLOW ANALYSIS OF NORMAL HEART

Intraventricular flow pattern is characterized by the formation of vortices allowing movement of blood from the mitral inlet to the aortic outlet, which efficiently preserves energy during the cardiac cycle. Diastolic filling accompanies an initial rapid flowing transmitral jet, which decelerates and is subsequently redirected toward the left ventricular (LV) outflow tract. The formation of vortices can store a part of the kinetic energy of the incoming flow in a rotary motion.[1–4] Vortices have different formation time, size, shape, strength, depth, and direction depending on the cardiac structure and function. Thus, vorticial characteristics are considered a signature of myocardial health and disease.[3–7]

FLOW ANALYSIS IN FAILING HEART

Heart failure (HF) is a clinical syndrome characterized by typical symptoms and accompanying signs and is caused by structural and/or functional cardiac abnormality that results in a reduced cardiac output and/or elevated intracardiac pressures at rest or during stress.[8,9]

Patients with HF typically show myocardial, valvular, and electrical dysfunction, which result in enlarged cardiac chambers and increased intracardiac volume and pressure. Traditional cardiac function evaluation focuses on these familiar parameters. However, we often encounter patients with different degrees of compensation despite similar echocardiographic parameters of cardiac dysfunction. Despite the development of new cardiovascular imaging technology that reconstructs anatomic information precisely, there are still discrepancies between patient's symptoms and imaging parameters. Good structural parameters do not always indicate better patient performance and vice versa. Intracardiac flow analysis can provide explanation of such discrepancies.[7,10] New technologies that aid in visualizing and quantifying flow dynamic information during the cardiac cycle

Disclosure: The authors have nothing to disclose.
[a] Division of Cardiology, Keimyung University Dongsan Medical Center, 56 Dalsung-ro Jung-gu, Daegu 41931, Republic of Korea; [b] Division of Cardiology, Severance Cardiovascular Hospital, Yonsei University College of Medicine, 50 Yonsei-ro, Seodae mun-gu, Seoul 03722, Republic of Korea
* Corresponding author.
E-mail address: GRHONG@yuhs.ac

Heart Failure Clin 15 (2019) 257–265
https://doi.org/10.1016/j.hfc.2018.12.005
1551-7136/19/© 2018 Elsevier Inc. All rights reserved.

help expand the options to understand complex cardiac diseases in conjunction with patients' symptoms and to predict cardiovascular outcomes.[6,11] In this review, we describe the details of the current method for analyzing ventricular intracardiac flow in HF and its clinical applications.

INTRACARDIAC FLOW VISUALIZATION METHODS IN HEART FAILURE

Vorticial flow analysis is available in several means: echo particle image velocimetry (PIV) using contrast agent, echo vector flow mapping (VFM) using Doppler, and velocity-encoded phase contrast (PC) cardiac magnetic resonance (CMR) (**Table 1**).[3,7,12] Recently, new tools that can measure three-dimensional (3D) flow throughout the cardiac cycle noninvasively are becoming available, and reconstruction of more detailed intracardiac blood flow can enhance understanding of cardiac diseases. It is possible to investigate the routes, behaviors, and interactions of the blood transiting the ventricles in normal and failing hearts

and to consider the possible impact of flow characteristics on the efficiency of ventricular function.[13–18]

Cardiac Magnetic Resonance

Velocity-encoded PC-CMR is the most frequently used CMR technique for acquiring blood flow in the cardiac chambers and major vessels.[19–21] Although real-time PC-CMR is possible for two-dimensional (2D) measurements, better quality data are obtained by combining the information from several heartbeats using electrocardiogram gating.[3,7,12] The acquired 2D PC-CMR data are used for flow quantification, which enables the calculations of flowtime curves, net flow, mean velocities, peak velocities, and retrograde fraction.[22] Currently, via electrocardiogram and respiratory gating, the complete time-resolved, 3D, and 3D velocity field are measured over a volume that covers the complete heart or large vessels.[16,23] This 3D cine PC-CMR technique enables the measurement of the intracardiac blood flow with a

Table 1
Comparison of intracardiac flow visualization methods

	CE-PIV	Color Doppler VFM	Phase Contrast CMR
Signal source	Tracking of contrast microbubbles	Color Doppler-based flow mapping	Velocity-encoded phase contrast MRI
Resolution	Good spatial resolution in 2D, limited 3D	Good spatial resolution in 2D and 3D	Good spatial resolution in 2D and 3D
Advantages	1. Bedside, lower cost, short process time 2. Accurate visualized vortex 3. Validated quantitative parameters	1. Bedside, lower cost, short process time 2. Does not require contrast microbubbles	1. Unrestricted access 2. Full 3D capability 3. Higher spatial resolution
Limitations	1. Need contrast agent 2. Need higher frame rate 3. Acoustic shadowing	1. Lacking validated parameters 2. Need manual dealiasing 3. Lower temporal resolution 4. Acoustic shadowing	1. Need several cardiac cycles 2. Longer examination time 3. Limitation in intracardiac devices
Accuracy	1. Limited in high-velocity flow 2. Accurate in low-velocity flow	1. Accurate in high velocity 2. Underestimation in low velocity	1. Accurate in high and low velocity
Applications	1. Measure for LV, RV function 2. LA, aorta flow	1. LV function analysis 2. Valve function analysis	1. Measurement of flow in cardiac chambers and aorta

Abbreviations: 2D, two-dimensional; 3D, three-dimensional; CE, contrast echocardiography; CMR, cardiac magnetic resonance; LA, left atrium; PIV, particle image velocimetry; RV, right ventricular; VFM, vector flow mapping.
Data from Refs.[3,7,22]

higher resolution and a shorter acquisition time (**Fig. 1**). To visualize complex, three-directional blood flow within a 3D volume, various visualization tools, including 2D vector-fields, 3D streamlines, and time resolved 3D particle traces, have been proposed.[24,25] Limitations associated with CMR flow visualization are longer test duration, high cost, lower temporal resolution, and unavailable bedside examination.[26,27]

Echocardiography

Intracardiac flow visualization using ultrasound technique has definite advantages with a lower cost, shorter post-processing time, higher temporal resolution, and availability in real-time clinical setting. VFM based on color-Doppler and contrast echocardiography (CE) using PIV is currently being used for visualizing the intracardiac flow using ultrasound.[3,7,12]

Color Doppler–based flow analysis
Color-Doppler technique is a simple and reliable method to visualize intracardiac unidirectional flow along the line of each ultrasound beam.[6] VFM technique based on color Doppler data has recently been developed and has shown reasonable accuracy in in vitro and in vivo settings.[28,29] VFM solves angle-dependency problem through mathematical calculations based on echodynamography. This consists of a series of equations aimed at converting a 2D distribution of measured axial velocities (parallel to the ultrasound beam) and estimated radial velocities (perpendicular to the former ones) into a plane of vortical and nonvortical flow vectors. However, color Doppler derived flow method has several limitations to note: (1) lower temporal and spatial resolution, (2) underestimation of low velocity flow, and (3) the need for dealiasing process.[7]

Contrast echocardiography particle image velocimetry technique
Vorticity imaging by CE using PIV (CE-PIV) is a novel approach to visualize the intracardiac flow. Recent advances in contrast media and ultrasound tissue harmonic imaging techniques have made it possible to visualize and record the movements of single microbubbles in the cardiac chambers (**Fig. 2**).[6] To this extent, CE may be a better and more convenient modality to investigate the complex flow field in the heart.[30,31] PIV is an optical method used to measure velocities and related properties in fluids. The fluid is seeded with particles, which, for the purposes of PIV, are generally assumed to faithfully follow the flow dynamics. It is the motion of these seeding particles that is used to calculate information on velocity.[32] Using PIV, velocity is estimated based on displacement of contrast bubbles. From the whole velocity vector, the vorticity (the curl of velocity) is computed. Vortex depth is defined as the vertical position of the center of the vortex relative to the LV long axis. Vortex transverse position refers to the transverse position relative to the posteroseptal axis. Vortex length is measured by the longitudinal length of the vortex relative to the LV length. Vortex width is calculated by the horizontal length of the vortex relative to the LV length. Vortex sphericity index is defined as a ratio of length to width of the vortex. Relative strength represents the strength of the pulsatile component of vorticity with respect to the average vorticity in the whole LV. The vortex

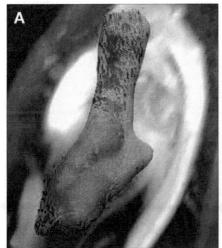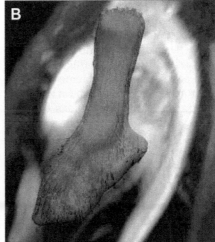

Fig. 1. Four-dimensional flow MRI and visualization of three-dimensional flow. Four-dimensional cine MRI views of left ventricle and ascending aorta in normal subject in diastole (*A*) and systole (*B*).

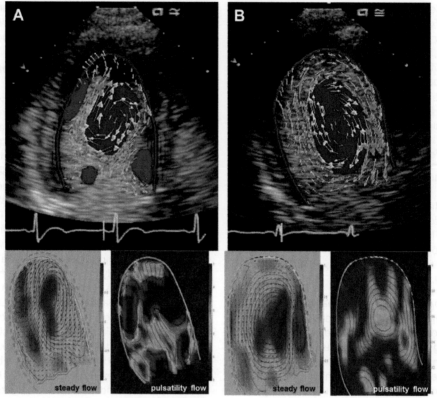

Fig. 2. Difference in vortex flow pattern in normal subject (*A*) and heart failure (*B*) in CE-PIV. The echo freeze frames (*top*), and parametric representation of steady streaming field and the pulsatile strength field (*bottom*) in normal (*A*) and LV systolic dysfunction groups (*B*). The vortex in normal subjects showed an elliptical and strong pulsatility, whereas spherical and weak pulsatility vortex was observed in patients with systolic heart failure.

relative strength represents the same ratio accounting for the pulsatile vorticity of the vortex only, instead of the entire LV. Kinetic energy fluctuation is defined as the standard deviation of kinetic energy normalized with corresponding mean values, and it represents the degree of regularity in flow or turbulence. Energy dissipation is the amount of kinetic energy dissipated as friction during the entire heartbeat and was normalized by using the mean kinetic energy to provide a dimensionless index.[10,33] The CE-PIV technique is noninvasive, and its latest developments allow a high degree of accuracy in in vitro and in vivo settings.[32,34,35] However, several limitations exist in the detection of high velocities because of the need for very high frame rates and microbubbles.[7]

APPLICATION OF FLOW DYNAMICS IN SPECIAL CONDITIONS RELATED WITH HEART FAILURE

HF is a consequence of various cardiac diseases. Thus, it is important to evaluate flow dynamics in diverse disease conditions that can manifest as HF.

Dilated Cardiomyopathy

Dilated cardiomyopathy is characterized by chamber enlargement and systolic dysfunction.[36] Dilated cardiomyopathy is often considered as a clinical interest for intracardiac flow analysis because low systolic function defined as conventional ejection fraction is often not directly correlated with patients' symptoms and functional status. Vortex flow analysis may show different patterns even when the conventional echocardiographic parameters are similar. A recent study showed that a decreased echo-PIV energy parameter is related with poor exercise capacity in patients with severe LV systolic dysfunction.[10] Figs. 3 and 4 are examples of HF patients with severe LV dysfunction with different symptoms. Even though they have similar ejection fraction (ejection fraction 21% and 19%, respectively), the symptoms of each patient were markedly different.

Ischemic Heart Disease

Intraventricular blood flow dynamic is related with different stages of LV dysfunction in acute

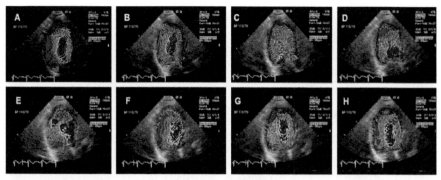

Fig. 3. Ejection fraction 21%, New York Heart Association functional class I patient with kinetic energy fluctuation 0.80. (*A–H*) Sequential echo-PIV mapping images show consistently preserved major (*blue*) and minor vortex (*red*) flow in left ventricle throughout the cardiac cycle.

ST-segment elevation myocardial infarction and is useful in evaluating the future risk of thrombus formation in acute anterior myocardial infarction.[33,37] In acute ST-segment elevation myocardial infarction, the highest energy dissipation was observed in patients with preserved global LV systolic function. Increased energy dissipation indicates that extra effort is required to maintain adequate pump efficiency.[33] Patients with decreased value of vortex depth and pulsatility power had strong association with LV apical thrombus (**Fig. 5**) and prospective investigation also proved higher incidence of LV thrombus among patients who showed poor vorticial flow pattern at the diagnosis of anterior myocardial infarction, which reflects possibility of vortex-guided anticoagulation therapy in this field.

Hypertrophic Cardiomyopathy

Hypertrophic cardiomyopathy is another interesting subject to apply flow dynamics because complex structures in a narrow cardiac chamber result in flow disturbance and are related to pathophysiologic mechanisms in LV remodeling. In the normal left ventricle, the formation of a transmitral vortex helps to maintain the position of the mitral leaflets close to the posterior wall and assists in directing the upcoming systolic stream toward the outflow tract. However, in hypertrophic cardiomyopathy, the anterior displacement of the papillary muscles moves the entire mitral apparatus adjacent to the outflow tract, which reverses the direction of the transmitral vortex and promotes the anterior motion of the mitral leaflets during systole because of the creation of drag forces.[3,38]

Valvular Heart Disease and Cardiac Surgery

Surgical treatment in mitral and aortic valve disease for the correction of hemodynamic cardiac overload can improve symptoms and survival rates. Moreover, applying appropriate surgical strategies at optimal timing is important for better clinical outcome.[39,40] Surgical procedures should be focused on preventing or reversing LV remodeling. Thus, perioperative assessment of the impaired blood flow might have an important role in the LV remodeling process and long-term

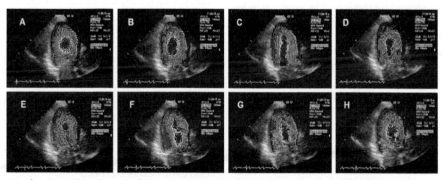

Fig. 4. Ejection fraction 19%, New York Heart Association functional class III patient with kinetic energy fluctuation 0.57. Sequential echo-PIV mapping images during cardiac cycle (*A–H*) show collided and weakened major (*blue*) and minor (*red*) vortex flow in left ventricle.

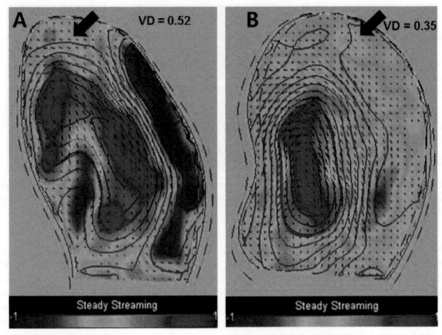

Fig. 5. Comparison of the location and morphology of the average LV vortex flow pattern between patient without thrombus (*A*) and with thrombus (*B*). The center of the average vortex flow was located near the apex in a patient without thrombus (*A*). However, in a patient with thrombus, the vortex was located in the center of the LV, much farther from the apex and did not reach to the LV apex (*B*). An *arrow* indicates different vortex flow pattern in the apex between the two patients. VD, Vortex depth.

outcomes.[11] Impaired fluid dynamics has been documented in patients after successful prosthetic valve replacement, with varying flow patterns depending on the type, orientation, and position of the valve prosthesis.[41,42] The reversed vorticial motion pattern is associated with a significant increase in energy dissipation and a modification of pressure distribution on the LV wall that deviates from the longitudinal orientation.[41,42] By contrast, preserving the native valve apparatus with mitral repair maintains normal flow rotation, thus avoiding the development of turbulence. Therefore, mitral valve repair should be designed to treat valve lesions, achieving a physiologic flow pattern to attempt the ultimate curative effect. Although it is not widely performed, surgical ventricular reconstruction may be performed in selected patients by vortex flow analysis who might benefit after the procedure.[43–45] Intraventricular flow analysis is used to assess the quality of blood flow immediately after surgery, when maladaptive fluid dynamics are the preliminary indicator of suboptimal cardiac function and a high risk of adverse outcome. A natural flow with a regular, stable vortex and aligned intraventricular pressure gradient might lead to favorable outcome.[11]

Cardiac Resynchronization Therapy and Left Ventricular Assist Device

One can also investigate the effect of cardiac device therapies, such as cardiac resynchronization therapy or LV assist device (LVAD), by flow analysis.[46–48] Cardiac resynchronization therapy has been used extensively to reverse the progression of advanced HF and to reverse cardiac remodeling.[49] Vortex flow analysis also gives an insight into the role of optimization.[47] Flow analysis can also be used to prove improved response of specific pacing method.[50] LVADs are mechanical pumps surgically connected to the LV and aorta to increase aortic flow and end-organ perfusion, which can improve patient health and quality of life, and to significantly reduce the mortality of cardiac failure.[51–55] However, there are concerns that LVAD may disrupt the natural blood flow path through the heart introducing flow patterns associated with thrombosis. A previous study revealed that vortex formation was unchanged, although vortex circulation and kinetic energy increased with LVAD speed, particularly in systole.[48]

FUTURE PERSPECTIVES

There are growing interests in the clinical applications of intracardiac flow analysis in HF with various causes. Representative methods for flow analysis were useful for the evaluation of current disease status, selection of therapeutic strategy, assessment of response after treatment, and prediction of future clinical outcomes. Several therapeutic strategies for HF could be expected to have implications with respect to flow; thus, flow parameters could potentially be used to select best therapies, pacing modes, and surgical interventions for patients with HF. It is expected to elucidate cardiologic unmet area by flow analysis with the assist of technical improvement in diagnostic methodologies.

SUMMARY

Intracardiac flow analysis can provide information regarding the shape and wall properties, chamber dimensions, and flow efficiency throughout the cardiac cycle. CMR and echocardiography are main modalities to acquire intraventricular flow data. HF can develop from multiple disease etiologies and thus, various therapeutic options are needed. In conjunction with the conventional structural and functional parameters, vortex flow analysis–guided treatment in HF might be a novel option for cardiac physicians.

REFERENCES

1. Pedrizzetti G, Sengupta PP. Vortex imaging: new information gain from tracking cardiac energy loss. Eur Heart J Cardiovasc Imaging 2015;16(7): 719–20.
2. Pedrizzetti G, Domenichini F. Nature optimizes the swirling flow in the human left ventricle. Phys Rev Lett 2005;95(10):108101.
3. Sengupta PP, Pedrizzetti G, Kilner PJ, et al. Emerging trends in CV flow visualization. JACC Cardiovasc Imaging 2012;5(3):305–16.
4. Sengupta PP, Narula J, Chandrashekhar Y. The dynamic vortex of a beating heart: wring out the old and ring in the new! J Am Coll Cardiol 2014; 64(16):1722–4.
5. Kheradvar A, Milano M, Gharib M. Correlation between vortex ring formation and mitral annulus dynamics during ventricular rapid filling. ASAIO J 2007;53(1):8–16.
6. Hong GR, Pedrizzetti G, Tonti G, et al. Characterization and quantification of vortex flow in the human left ventricle by contrast echocardiography using vector particle image velocimetry. JACC Cardiovasc Imaging 2008;1(6):705–17.
7. Hong GR, Kim M, Pedrizzetti G, et al. Current clinical application of intracardiac flow analysis using echocardiography. J Cardiovasc Ultrasound 2013;21(4): 155–62.
8. Yancy CW, Jessup M, Bozkurt B, et al. 2013 ACCF/AHA guideline for the management of heart failure: executive summary: a report of the American College of Cardiology Foundation/American Heart Association Task Force on practice guidelines. Circulation 2013;128(16):1810–52.
9. Ponikowski P, Voors AA, Anker SD, et al. 2016 ESC guidelines for the diagnosis and treatment of acute and chronic heart failure: the Task Force for the diagnosis and treatment of acute and chronic heart failure of the European Society of Cardiology (ESC) Developed with the special contribution of the Heart Failure Association (HFA) of the ESC. Eur Heart J 2016;37(27):2129–200.
10. Kim IC, Hong GR, Pedrizzetti G, et al. Usefulness of left ventricular vortex flow analysis for predicting clinical outcomes in patients with chronic heart failure: a quantitative vorticity imaging study using contrast echocardiography. Ultrasound Med Biol 2018;44(9):1951–9.
11. Pedrizzetti G, La Canna G, Alfieri O, et al. The vortex: an early predictor of cardiovascular outcome? Nat Rev Cardiol 2014;11(9):545–53.
12. Abe H, Caracciolo G, Kheradvar A, et al. Contrast echocardiography for assessing left ventricular vortex strength in heart failure: a prospective cohort study. Eur Heart J Cardiovasc Imaging 2013;14(11):1049–60.
13. Kilner PJ, Yang GZ, Wilkes AJ, et al. Asymmetric redirection of flow through the heart. Nature 2000; 404(6779):759–61.
14. Richter Y, Edelman ER. Cardiology is flow. Circulation 2006;113(23):2679–82.
15. Yang GZ, Merrifield R, Masood S, et al. Flow and myocardial interaction: an imaging perspective. Philos Trans R Soc Lond B Biol Sci 2007; 362(1484):1329–41.
16. Toger J, Arvidsson PM, Bock J, et al. Hemodynamic forces in the left and right ventricles of the human heart using 4D flow magnetic resonance imaging: phantom validation, reproducibility, sensitivity to respiratory gating and free analysis software. PLoS One 2018;13(4):e0195597.
17. Pedrizzetti G, Domenichini F. Left ventricular fluid mechanics: the long way from theoretical models to clinical applications. Ann Biomed Eng 2015;43(1):26–40.
18. Carlhall CJ, Bolger A. Passing strange: flow in the failing ventricle. Circ Heart Fail 2010;3(2):326–31.
19. Pelc NJ, Herfkens RJ, Shimakawa A, et al. Phase contrast cine magnetic resonance imaging. Magn Reson Q 1991;7(4):229–54.
20. Bryant DJ, Payne JA, Firmin DN, et al. Measurement of flow with NMR imaging using a gradient pulse and phase difference technique. J Comput Assist Tomogr 1984;8(4):588–93.
21. Moran PR. A flow velocity zeugmatographic interlace for NMR imaging in humans. Magn Reson Imaging 1982;1(4):197–203.

22. Rodriguez Munoz D, Markl M, Moya Mur JL, et al. Intracardiac flow visualization: current status and future directions. Eur Heart J Cardiovasc Imaging 2013;14(11):1029–38.

23. Wigstrom L, Sjoqvist L, Wranne B. Temporally resolved 3D phase-contrast imaging. Magn Reson Med 1996;36(5):800–3.

24. Buonocore MH. Visualizing blood flow patterns using streamlines, arrows, and particle paths. Magn Reson Med 1998;40(2):210–26.

25. Napel S, Lee DH, Frayne R, et al. Visualizing three-dimensional flow with simulated streamlines and three-dimensional phase-contrast MR imaging. J Magn Reson Imaging 1992;2(2):143–53.

26. Shandas R, Gharib M, Sahn DJ. Nature of flow acceleration into a finite-sized orifice: steady and pulsatile flow studies on the flow convergence region using simultaneous ultrasound Doppler flow mapping and laser Doppler velocimetry. J Am Coll Cardiol 1995;25(5):1199–212.

27. Ishizu T, Seo Y, Ishimitsu T, et al. The wake of a large vortex is associated with intraventricular filling delay in impaired left ventricles with a pseudonormalized transmitral flow pattern. Echocardiography 2006; 23(5):369–75.

28. Uejima T, Koike A, Sawada H, et al. A new echocardiographic method for identifying vortex flow in the left ventricle: numerical validation. Ultrasound Med Biol 2010;36(5):772–88.

29. Garcia D, Del Alamo JC, Tanne D, et al. Two-dimensional intraventricular flow mapping by digital processing conventional color-Doppler echocardiography images. IEEE Trans Med Imaging 2010;29(10):1701–13.

30. Thanigaraj S, Chugh R, Schechtman KB, et al. Defining left ventricular segmental and global function by echocardiographic intraventricular contrast flow patterns. Am J Cardiol 2000;85(1):65–8.

31. Mulvagh SL, DeMaria AN, Feinstein SB, et al. Contrast echocardiography: current and future applications. J Am Soc Echocardiogr 2000;13(4): 331–42.

32. Mukdadi OM, Kim HB, Hertzberg J, et al. Numerical modeling of microbubble backscatter to optimize ultrasound particle image velocimetry imaging: initial studies. Ultrasonics 2004;42(10):1111–21.

33. Agati L, Cimino S, Tonti G, et al. Quantitative analysis of intraventricular blood flow dynamics by echocardiographic particle image velocimetry in patients with acute myocardial infarction at different stages of left ventricular dysfunction. Eur Heart J Cardiovasc Imaging 2014;15(11):1203–12.

34. Sengupta PP, Pedrizzetti G, Narula J. Multiplanar visualization of blood flow using echocardiographic particle imaging velocimetry. JACC Cardiovasc Imaging 2012;5(5):566–9.

35. Domenichini F, Querzoli G, Cenedese A, et al. Combined experimental and numerical analysis of the flow structure into the left ventricle. J Biomech 2007;40(9):1988–94.

36. Pinto YM, Elliott PM, Arbustini E, et al. Proposal for a revised definition of dilated cardiomyopathy, hypokinetic non-dilated cardiomyopathy, and its implications for clinical practice: a position statement of the ESC working group on myocardial and pericardial diseases. Eur Heart J 2016;37(23):1850–8.

37. Son JW, Park WJ, Choi JH, et al. Abnormal left ventricular vortex flow patterns in association with left ventricular apical thrombus formation in patients with anterior myocardial infarction: a quantitative analysis by contrast echocardiography. Circ J 2012;76(11):2640–6.

38. Ro R, Halpern D, Sahn DJ, et al. Vector flow mapping in obstructive hypertrophic cardiomyopathy to assess the relationship of early systolic left ventricular flow and the mitral valve. J Am Coll Cardiol 2014; 64(19):1984–95.

39. Ross J Jr. Afterload mismatch in aortic and mitral valve disease: implications for surgical therapy. J Am Coll Cardiol 1985;5(4):811–26.

40. Nishimura RA, Otto CM, Bonow RO, et al. 2014 AHA/ACC guideline for the management of patients with valvular heart disease: a report of the American College of Cardiology/American Heart Association Task Force on practice guidelines. Circulation 2014; 129(23):e521–643.

41. Faludi R, Szulik M, D'Hooge J, et al. Left ventricular flow patterns in healthy subjects and patients with prosthetic mitral valves: an in vivo study using echocardiographic particle image velocimetry. J Thorac Cardiovasc Surg 2010;139(6):1501–10.

42. Pedrizzetti G, Domenichini F, Tonti G. On the left ventricular vortex reversal after mitral valve replacement. Ann Biomed Eng 2010;38(3):769–73.

43. Adhyapak SM, Parachuri VR. Architecture of the left ventricle: insights for optimal surgical ventricular restoration. Heart Fail Rev 2010;15(1):73–83.

44. George TJ, Arnaoutakis GJ, Shah AS. Surgical treatment of advanced heart failure: alternatives to heart transplantation and mechanical circulatory assist devices. Prog Cardiovasc Dis 2011;54(2):115–31.

45. Doenst T, Spiegel K, Reik M, et al. Fluid-dynamic modeling of the human left ventricle: methodology and application to surgical ventricular reconstruction. Ann Thorac Surg 2009;87(4):1187–95.

46. Siciliano M, Migliore F, Badano L, et al. Cardiac resynchronization therapy by multipoint pacing improves response of left ventricular mechanics and fluid dynamics: a three-dimensional and particle image velocimetry echo study. Europace 2017;19(11): 1833–40.

47. Goliasch G, Goscinska-Bis K, Caracciolo G, et al. CRT improves LV filling dynamics: insights from echocardiographic particle imaging velocimetry. JACC Cardiovasc Imaging 2013;6(6):704–13.

48. Wong K, Samaroo G, Ling I, et al. Intraventricular flow patterns and stasis in the LVAD-assisted heart. J Biomech 2014;47(6):1485–94.

49. Mullens W, Verga T, Grimm RA, et al. Persistent hemodynamic benefits of cardiac resynchronization therapy with disease progression in advanced heart failure. J Am Coll Cardiol 2009; 53(7):600–7.

50. Wildemann TM, Siciliano SD, Weber LP. The mechanisms associated with the development of hypertension after exposure to lead, mercury species or their mixtures differs with the metal and the mixture ratio. Toxicology 2016;339:1–8.

51. Slaughter MS, Pagani FD, Rogers JG, et al. Clinical management of continuous-flow left ventricular assist devices in advanced heart failure. J Heart Lung Transplant 2010;29(4 Suppl):S1–39.

52. Raju S, MacIver J, Foroutan F, et al. Long-term use of left ventricular assist devices: a report on clinical outcomes. Can J Surg 2017;60(4):236–46.

53. Lietz K, Long JW, Kfoury AG, et al. Outcomes of left ventricular assist device implantation as destination therapy in the post-REMATCH era: implications for patient selection. Circulation 2007;116(5):497–505.

54. Rose EA, Gelijns AC, Moskowitz AJ, et al. Long-term use of a left ventricular assist device for end-stage heart failure. N Engl J Med 2001;345(20):1435–43.

55. Rogers JG, Pagani FD, Tatooles AJ, et al. Intrapericardial left ventricular assist device for advanced heart failure. N Engl J Med 2017;376(5):451–60.

Ventricular Stiffness and Ventricular-Arterial Coupling in Heart Failure
What Is It, How to Assess, and Why?

Chi Young Shim, MD, PhD*, Geu-Ru Hong, MD, PhD, Jong-Won Ha, MD, PhD

KEYWORDS

- Heart failure • Ventricular stiffness • Arterial stiffness • Ventricular-arterial coupling • Uncoupling

KEY POINTS

- Ventricular-arterial coupling is a central determinant of net cardiovascular performance.
- Ventricular-arterial coupling and uncoupling are key concepts for understanding the pathogenesis of heart failure.
- Both ventricular stiffness and arterial stiffness are common features of aging and are exacerbated by cardiovascular risk factors such as hypertension, diabetes mellitus, obesity, and renal failure.
- Diverse noninvasive imaging methods have been proposed for assessing ventricular stiffness, arterial stiffness, and ventricular-arterial coupling.
- Assessment of ventricular-arterial coupling provides important information on the development and prognosis of heart failure in addition to established risk factors for heart failure.

INTRODUCTION

The heart and blood vessels are constantly interfering with each other in a closed system. However, the concept of ventricular-arterial coupling (VAC) is often overlooked in understanding the pathophysiology of heart failure (HF). The first reason for this is a poor understanding of ventricular stiffness, arterial stiffness, and their coupling and uncoupling. Second, this is probably due to the lack of simple noninvasive measures such as left ventricular (LV) ejection fraction that can be intuitively used in clinical practice. For a few decades, the concept of VAC based on the stiffness has been considered as a key pathogenesis of HF with preserved ejection fraction. Moreover, there is a growing interest in the aging society and the development of various therapies as it can preserve LV ejection fraction.

Recently, various methods of evaluating VAC and its components have been suggested by several investigators, and it has been found that a few indicators can predict the progression from subclinical status to HF syndrome. This article reviews the concept, interpretation of various indices obtained using noninvasive methods of VAC, and clinical relevance among patients at risk for HF and for patients with established HF.

Basic Understanding of Ventricular-Arterial Coupling and Its Components

VAC is a physiologic interaction between the heart and the systemic vasculature and is considered as

Disclosure: The authors have nothing to disclose.
Division of Cardiology, Severance Cardiovascular Hospital, Yonsei University College of Medicine, Seoul, Republic of Korea
* Corresponding author. 50-1 Yonsei-ro, Seodaemun-gu, Seoul 03722, Republic of Korea.
E-mail address: cysprs@yuhs.ac

Heart Failure Clin 15 (2019) 267–274
https://doi.org/10.1016/j.hfc.2018.12.006
1551-7136/19/© 2018 Elsevier Inc. All rights reserved.

a key determinant of net cardiovascular performance.[1–5] To understand the components of VAC, it is necessary to start with an understanding of the pressure-volume loop generated through the cardiac cycle. **Fig. 1**A schematically displays a pressure-volume loop according to the opening and closure of aortic and mitral valves. Within one cardiac cycle, the LV undergoes changes in pressure and volume through the 4 phases of isovolumic relaxation, diastole, isovolumic contraction, and ventricular systole.

In a pressure-volume relationship, elastance generally represents a change in pressure over a volume change. Thus, as shown in **Fig. 1**B, ventricular systolic elastance (Ees) can be derived from the ratio of end-systolic pressure (ESP) to end-systolic volume.[5,6] In addition, effective arterial elastance (Ea) is defined as the ratio of ESP to stroke volume (SV).[5,7] Finally, the VAC index is defined as the ratio of Ea to Ees, which correlates well with the operating mechanical efficacy of a given heart operating at a given heart rate and contractile state.[3–5,8] The value of this coupling index is usually in the range of 0.3 to 1.3.[3] Importantly, the VAC index is closely related to ejection fraction (ejection fraction = 1/[1 + VAC index]).[1,9] Therefore, markedly inefficient ratios are closely associated with the reduced ejection fraction and poor mechanical efficiency.[1–3]

It is well known that there is an adaptation process in which the ventricular stiffness and arterial stiffness increases proportionally to maintain maximal cardiac work, before the ventricular arterial coupling is broken. This is a phenomenon that occurs even in the normal aging process as shown in **Fig. 1**B. In young subjects, both ventricle and arterial systems are compliant. In the elderly, however, arterial stiffness according to vascular aging induces ventricular adaptation such as ventricular hypertrophy, systolic, and diastolic stiffness. As a result, both Ea and Ees change steeply, but VAC

is maintained. However, combined ventricular and vascular stiffness can influence cardiovascular performance in several ways as shown in **Fig. 2**A.[10] First, a high ventricular stiffness at rest cannot increase further during exercise or stressful condition, so this limits a proper ventricular arterial coupling. Second, enhanced sensitivity of blood pressure to circulating volume and diuretics is common and may trigger rapid onset pulmonary edema. As a consequence, cardiac energy expenditure will increase. Therefore, it is prone to develop overt HF accompanied by ventricular-arterial uncoupling in any direction as shown in **Fig. 2**B.

The VAC index with exercise shows diverse changes in each individual. The index at rest is not different according to age and gender. A noticeable decrease in the VAC index during exercise is a normal response because the ventricular-arterial system should do its work more efficiently. However, age-associated differences in VAC indices occur in both genders during exercise in healthy adults although resting VAC index was not age related.[11] Thus, old subjects demonstrated a blunted response in decreasing VAC during exercise compared with young subjects, accompanied by a less increase in Ees in older subjects. Therefore, assessment of VAC and its components during exercise can give us additional information regarding cardiac reserve and capacity.

Arterial Stiffening and Its Dynamic Changes

Arterial stiffness is not only a cardinal feature in normal aging but also exacerbated by cardiovascular risk factors or disease.[12–16] Normally, the aorta supplies blood from the heart to the capillaries, acting as a highly efficient conduit and a highly efficient cushion. Because young subjects have good pressure amplification from the central to the peripheral, and old subjects do not, their

A　　　　　　　　**B**

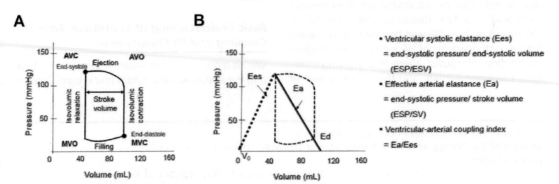

Fig. 1. (A) A pressure-volume loop. AVC, aortic valve closure; AVO, aortic valve opening; MVC, mitral valve closure; MVO, mitral valve opening. (B) Ventricular-arterial coupling index and its key components.

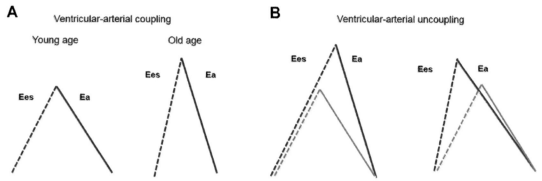

Fig. 2. (*A*) Ventricular-arterial coupling. (*B*) Ventricular-arterial uncoupling. Ees, ventricular systolic elastance; Ea, effective arterial elastance.

central blood pressures differ even when they have the same brachial pressures. As the aorta ages and stiffens, however, blood travels faster, returns earlier, and boosts pressure in late systole. Thus, in old adults, wave reflections travel quickly, arriving back in the proximal aorta while the LV is still ejecting blood in systolic phase. Therefore, vascular stiffening results in elevation of augmentation pressure and augmentation index (AIx), widening of the arterial pulse pressure (PP), and increase in pulse wave velocities (PWV).[5] Recent studies have demonstrated that noninvasively assessed PP amplification from central to peripheral arteries might be a mechanical biomarker of cardiovascular risk.[17,18]

Furthermore, dynamic changes in arterial stiffness during exercise might be diverse according to the individual characteristics. With increasing age, exercise PP amplification is significantly attenuated because of increased wave reflection.[19] These effects are exacerbated by hypercholesterolemia and may contribute to cardiovascular risk by mechanisms associated with central hypertension.[19] In a previous study, the authors investigated a gender-related difference in Ea during exercise in patients with hypertension.[20] It was demonstrated that a steeper increase in Ea during exercise was significant in hypertensive women compared with age-matched hypertensive men.[20] Moreover, exercise arterial stiffening was an independent determinant of exercise intolerance even after controlling the confounding factors.[20] This finding suggested that dynamic increases in Ea, reflecting increased dynamic pulsatile load during exercise, may be one of the mechanisms of the gender difference in diastolic dysfunction and HF incidence in hypertensive subjects. In another study, the authors also suggested that being overweight is related to impaired dynamic arterial compliance by presenting the differences in wave reflection after exercise in overweight women compared with lean women.[21] Body mass index was an independent determinant of dynamic arterial stiffening in women, suggesting being overweight is related to dynamic changes in arterial compliance with exercise in women.[21] In conclusion, arterial compliance is not static but dynamic in its nature. Therefore, dynamic arterial stiffness might act as LV afterloads and contribute to HF in relation to well-known risk factors of HF with preserved ejection fraction, such as age, women, and obesity.

Assessment of Arterial Stiffness

Fig. 3 shows relatively easy and practical methods to evaluate arterial stiffness or central hemodynamic variables that reflect it.[5] Diverse methods for assessing arterial stiffness have their own advantages and pitfalls. Therefore, it is necessary to understand the technical assumptions and formulas of noninvasive measurement tools of arterial stiffness. PWV is the speed at which the forward pressure wave is transmitted in the aorta and arteries.[14] Therefore, it is calculated by measuring the time taken for the arterial waveform to pass between 2 points a measured distance apart. PWV has been validated and is reproducible and has been widely applied as the gold standard of assessing arterial stiffness.[22,23] Pulse waveform analysis permits measurement of central systolic blood pressure, central PP, and AIx. AIx is calculated as the ratio between augmentation pressure and central PP expressed as a percentage.[15,23] The age-related changes in central AIx and aortic PWV follow different patterns.[14] AIx might provide a more sensitive marker of arterial aging in younger individuals, whereas aortic PWV might be a more sensitive marker in older individuals.[15] PP amplification has been suggested as a mechanical biomarker of cardiovascular risk by accumulating

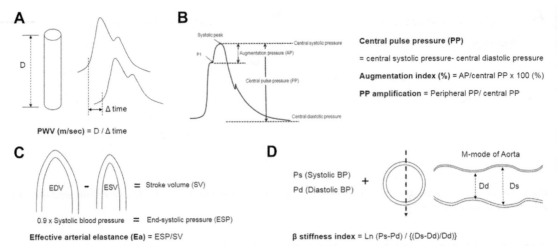

Fig. 3. Indices representing arterial stiffness. (*A*) Pulse wave velocity. (*B*) Variables derived from pulse wave analysis. (*C*) Effective arterial elastance. (*D*) β stiffness index.

a lot of clinical evidences regarding the association with LV function and occurrence of HF.[17,18] In terms of echocardiographic assessments of arterial stiffness, Ea can be calculated by evaluating ESP and SV by applying a simple formula.[5] It is necessary to simultaneously measure blood pressure. Carotid stiffness index β, recently carotid artery strain, has been used to assess arterial stiffness in various cardiovascular diseases.[24–28]

Assessment of Ventricular Stiffness

To assess ventricular stiffness and VAC, invasive hemodynamic assessment with pressure-volume loop analysis obtained by cardiac catheterization may be most accurate. However, the invasive method has many limitations to be repeatedly used for the diagnosis and monitoring of HF. Therefore, various noninvasive imaging techniques have been developed to meet both feasibility and accuracy to evaluate ventricular stiffness. **Fig. 4** displays representative methods for evaluating ventricular stiffness using 2-dimensional, Doppler echocardiography, exercise stress echocardiography, or speckle tracking echocardiography.

As an index to evaluate the relaxation of the LV, e 'velocity, which is early diastolic annular velocity in tissue Doppler imaging of the mitral annulus, is validated as a value showing a linear correlation with tau measured by invasive methods.[29] Similarly, S' velocity in tissue Doppler imaging reflects the speed of ventricular contraction, so that it reflects ventricular systolic stiffness as shown in **Fig. 4**A. E/e' is a well-known and widely used variable for estimating LV filling pressure.[30] Supine exercise stress echocardiography can detect early

or subclinical changes in ventricular stiffness using diastolic reserve indices.[31,32] A few previous studies have demonstrated different diastolic functional reserve according to the baseline characteristics and proposed prognostic implications in a few specific group.[33,34] In addition, Ees can be estimated by volumetric assessment and hemodynamic evaluation.[5,6] Nowadays, global longitudinal strain can be obtained from the segmental longitudinal strains and has been used for evaluation of LV mechanical function and ventricular stiffness.[35,36] Moreover, some investigators also attempted three-dimensional volumetric assessment for calculating Ees.[37]

Pathophysiologic Mechanisms of Ventricular Stiffness Related with Arterial Stiffness

For more than a decade, the relationship between arterial stiffness and ventricular stiffness has been studied in various populations.[38–45] In hypertensive subjects with dyspnea on exertion, e' velocity on mitral annulus tissue Doppler imaging showed a significant correlation with arterial compliance.[38] A similar correlation study demonstrated that AIx gradually increased according to the severity of LV diastolic dysfunction.[42] **Fig. 5**A shows the possible relationship between arterial stiffness and ventricular stiffness.[38] Increased central systolic blood pressure results in increasing LV afterload and makes myocyte hypertrophy and impaired relaxation. Simultaneously, central aortic diastolic blood pressure decreases. It reduces coronary perfusion and induces subendocardial ischemia and fibrosis. These adverse effects finally lead to LV stiffness and diastolic dysfunction. Nowadays, increased arterial stiffness has been

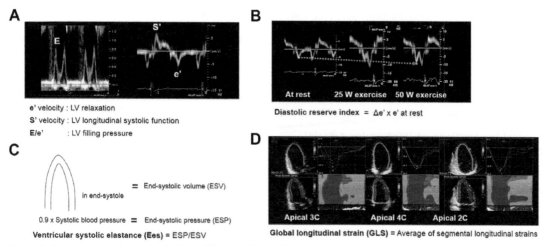

e' velocity : LV relaxation
S' velocity : LV longitudinal systolic function
E/e' : LV filling pressure

Diastolic reserve index = Δe' x e' at rest

= End-systolic volume (ESV)
in end-systole

0.9 x Systolic blood pressure = End-systolic pressure (ESP)

Ventricular systolic elastance (Ees) = ESP/ESV

Global longitudinal strain (GLS) = Average of segmental longitudinal strains

Fig. 4. Indices representing ventricular stiffness. (*A*) Variables derived from tissue Doppler imaging. (*B*) Diastolic reserve index. (*C*) Ventricular systolic elastance. (*D*) Global longitudinal strain.

considered a principal contributor to the pathophysiology of HF with normal ejection fraction as shown in **Fig. 5**B. Moreover, these pathophysiologic findings become more apparent during exercise than at rest.[35] Based on this mechanical linkage between arterial stiffness and HF with preserved ejection fraction, future risks for HF can be predicted.

The relationship between arterial stiffness and LV mechanical function has been verified for risk factors of HF with preserved ejection fraction. It is well known that women are more likely to develop HF with preserved ejection fraction than men. In a previous study, the authors assessed central hemodynamics simultaneously with echocardiogram in age-matched men and women without apparent cardiovascular disease.[43] They demonstrated gender differences in central hemodynamics and their relationship to LV diastolic function.[43] Because central hemodynamics reflecting arterial stiffness are different between men and women despite similar peripheral pressures, the effects of earlier wave reflection on central pressure may contribute to greater susceptibility to HF with preserved ejection fraction in women. Thus, it was suggested that women may display greater load-related diastolic dysfunction. Gender differences in arterial stiffness and influence on LV function have been reaffirmed through subsequent studies by other investigators.[44,45] The mechanical link between aortic mechanical function and LV function has

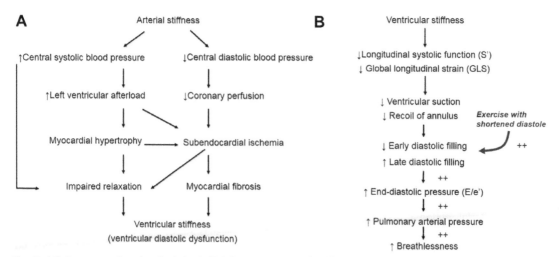

Fig. 5. (*A*) A proposed pathophysiologic link between arterial stiffness and ventricular stiffness. (*B*) Association between ventricular stiffness and occurrence of heart failure.

been suggested not only at rest but also with exercise. In a previous study, exercise PP amplification, as a marker of dynamic arterial compliance, was significantly correlated with variables for ventricular stiffness in subjects who showed exaggerated blood pressure response to exercise.[46]

Clinical Implications of Ventricular-Arterial Coupling

There have been several studies to evaluate clinical implications of VAC in HF.[47–49] VAC at rest and during exercise has been associated with increased risk for HF hospitalization in various populations. Previous investigators demonstrated the association of VAC parameters with a few surrogate markers of ventricular function and/or cardiovascular outcomes. Because hypertension is one of the most important risk factors for HF, the authors investigated the VAC response with exercise in 216 hypertensive patients by using supine bicycle exercise echocardiography.[41] It was found that considerable numbers of hypertensive patients showed a paradoxic increase in VAC index during exercise.[41] This phenomenon was significantly associated with decreased LV diastolic and systolic functional reserve assessed by tissue Doppler imaging.[41]

Several studies have shown that VAC was associated with cardiovascular outcomes in various populations such as diabetes mellitus, HF, end-stage renal disease on hemodialysis, and documented coronary artery disease.[47–49] Particularly, recent data from a prospective cohort study of 815 patients with stable coronary artery disease demonstrated that Ees and the Ea/Ees ratio as measured by echocardiography are strongly associated with future HF hospitalization in patients with coronary artery disease who are largely free of HF at baseline.[50]

In addition, VAC index and its components have been used for monitoring of therapeutic response after modulation of HF risk factors. In a recent randomized, sham-controlled study to investigate the effects of continuous positive airway pressure on LV diastolic function in patients with severe obstructive sleep apnea, treatment with continuous positive airway pressure for 3 months improved LV diastolic function more than sham treatment and was accompanied by improvements in arterial stiffness assessed by pulse wave velocity, Ea, and the VAC index.[51] Thus, pulsatile arterial load represents a promising therapeutic target for risk modification and preventing HF.

SUMMARY

Noninvasive assessment and monitoring of arterial stiffness, ventricular stiffness, and their interactions are useful for understanding the pathophysiologic mechanism of HF and detecting vulnerable subjects for future HF. In the future, a simple and intuitive marker representing VAC is warranted to be widely applied in clinical practice.

REFERENCES

1. Sunagawa K, Maughan WL, Burkhoff D, et al. Left ventricular interaction with arterial load studied in isolated canine ventricle. Am J Physiol 1983;245: H773–80.
2. Starling MR. Left ventricular-arterial coupling relations in the normal human heart. Am Heart J 1993; 125:1659–66.
3. Kass DA. Age-related changes in ventricular-arterial coupling: pathophysiologic implications. Heart Fail Rev 2002;7:51–62.
4. Borlaug BA, Kass DA. Ventricular-vascular interaction in heart failure. Heart Fail Clin 2008;4:23–36.
5. Shim CY. Arterial-cardiac interaction: the concept and implications. J Cardiovasc Ultrasound 2011; 19:62–6.
6. Chen CH, Fetics D, Nevo E, et al. Noninvasive single-beat determination of left ventricular ene-systolic elastance in human. J Am Coll Cardiol 2001;38:2028–34.
7. Kelly RP, Ting CT, Yang TM, et al. Effective arterial elastance as index of arterial vascular load in humans. Circulation 1992;86:513–21.
8. Senzaki H, Chen CH, Kass DA. Single-beat estimation of end-systolic pressure-volume relation in humans. A new method with the potential for noninvasive application. Circulation 1996;94: 2497–506.
9. Kass DA. Ventricular arterial stiffening: integrating the pathophysiology. Hypertension 2005;46:85–93.
10. Kawaguchi M, Hay I, Fetics B, et al. Combined ventricular systolic and arterial stiffening in patients with heart failure and preserved ejection fraction: implications for systolic and diastolic reserve limitations. Circulation 2003;107:714–20.
11. Najjar SS, Schulman SP, Gerstenblith G, et al. Age and gender affect ventricular-vascular coupling during aerobic exercise. J Am Coll Cardiol 2004;44: 611–7.
12. O'Rourke MF, Hashimoto J. Mechanical factors in arterial aging: a clinical perspective. J Am Coll Cardiol 2007;50:1–13.
13. Smulyan H, Asmar RG, Rudnicki A, et al. Comparative effects of aging in men and women on the properties of the arterial tree. J Am Coll Cardiol 2001;37: 1374–80.

14. Choi CU, Kim EJ, Kim SH, et al. Differing effects of aging on central and peripheral blood pressures and pulse wave velocity: a direct intraarterial study. J Hypertens 2010;28:1252–60.

15. McEniery CM, Yasmin, Hall IR, et al. Normal vascular aging: differential effects on wave reflection and aortic pulse wave velocity: the Anglo-Cardiff Collaborative Trial (ACCT). J Am Coll Cardiol 2005;46:1753–60.

16. Kelly R, Hayward C, Avolio A, et al. Noninvasive determination of age-related changes in the human arterial pulse. Circulation 1989;80:1652–9.

17. Benetos A, Thomas F, Joly L, et al. Pulse pressure amplification a mechanical biomarker of cardiovascular risk. J Am Coll Cardiol 2010;55:1032–7.

18. Nijdam ME, Plantinga Y, Hulsen HT, et al. Pulse pressure amplification and risk of cardiovascular disease. Am J Hypertens 2008;21:388–92.

19. Sharman JE, McEniery CM, Dhakam ZR, et al. Pulse pressure amplification during exercise is significantly reduced with age and hypercholesterolemia. J Hypertens 2007;25:1249–54.

20. Park S, Ha JW, Shim CY, et al. Gender-related difference in arterial elastance during exercise in patients with hypertension. Hypertension 2008;51:1163–9.

21. Shim CY, Yang WI, Park S, et al. Overweight and its association with aortic pressure wave reflection after exercise. Am J Hypertens 2011;24:1136–42.

22. Sutton-Tyrrell K, Najjar SS, Boudreau RM, et al. Elevated aortic pulse wave velocity, a marker of arterial stiffness, predicts cardiovascular events in well-functioning older adults. Circulation 2005;111:3384–90.

23. Lauremt S, Cpclcrpft K, Vam Bprtel L, et al. Expert consensus document on arterial stiffness: methodological issues and clinical applications. Eur Heart J 2006;27:2588–605.

24. Hirai T, Sasayama S, Kawasaki T, et al. Stiffness of systemic arteries in patients with myocardial infarction. A noninvasive method to predict severity of coronary atherosclerosis. Circulation 1989;80:78–86.

25. Yang WI, Shim CY, Bang WD, et al. Asynchronous arterial systolic expansion as a marker of vascular aging: assessment of the carotid artery with velocity vector imaging. J Hypertens 2011;29:2404–12.

26. Kim M, Shim CY, You SC, et al. Characteristics of carotid artery structure and mechanical function and their relationships with aortopathy in patients with bicuspid aortic valves. Front Physiol 2017;8:622.

27. Kim SA, Park SH, Jo SH, et al. Alterations of carotid arterial mechanics preceding the wall thickening in patients with hypertension. Atherosclerosis 2016;248:84–90.

28. Yang WI, Kang KW, Lee HY, et al. Incremental predictive value of carotid arterial strain in patients with stroke. Int J Cardiovasc Imaging 2018;34:893–902.

29. Sohn DW, Chai IH, Lee DJ, et al. Assessment of mitral annulus velocity by Doppler tissue imaging in the evaluation of left ventricular diastolic function. J Am Coll Cardiol 1997;30:474–80.

30. Nagueh SF, Middleton KJ, Kopelen HA, et al. Doppler tissue imaging: a noninvasive technique for evaluation of left ventricular relaxation and estimation of filling pressures. J Am Coll Cardiol 1997;30:1524–33.

31. Ha JW, Oh JK, Pellikka P, et al. Diastolic stress echocardiography: a novel noninvasive diagnostic test for diastolic dysfunction using supine bicycle exercise Doppler echocardiography. J Am Soc Echocardiogr 2005;18:63–8.

32. Ha JW, Choi D, Park S, et al. Left ventricular diastolic functional reserve during exercise in patients with impaired myocardial relaxation at rest. Heart 2009;95:399–404.

33. Shim CY, Kim SA, Choi D, et al. Clinical outcomes of exercise-induced pulmonary hypertension in subjects with preserved left ventricular ejection fraction: implication of an increase in left ventricular filling pressure during exercise. Heart 2011;97:1417–24.

34. Kim SA, Shim CY, Kim JM, et al. Impact of left ventricular longitudinal diastolic functional reserve on clinical outcome in patients with type 2 diabetes mellitus. Heart 2011;97(15):1233–8.

35. Tan YT, Wenzelburger F, Lee E, et al. The pathophysiology of heart failure with normal ejection fraction: exercise echocardiography reveals complex abnormalities of both systolic and diastolic ventricular function involving torsion, untwist, and longitudinal motion. J Am Coll Cardiol 2009;54:36–46.

36. Reisner SA, Lysyansky P, Agmon Y, et al. Global longitudinal strain: a novel index of left ventricular systolic function. J Am Soc Echocardiogr 2004;17:630–3.

37. Aubert R, Venner C, Huttin O, et al. Three-dimensional echocardiography for the assessment of right ventriculo-arterial coupling. J Am Soc Echocardiogr 2018;31:905–15.

38. Mottram PM, Haluska BA, Leano R, et al. Relation of arterial stiffness to diastolic dysfunction in hypertensive heart disease. Heart 2005;91:1551–6.

39. Kim D, Shim CY, Hong GR, et al. Differences in left ventricular functional adaptation to arterial stiffness and neurohormonal activation in patients with hypertension: a study with two-dimensional layer-specific speckle tracking echocardiography. Clin Hypertens 2017;23:21.

40. Lee SY, Shim CY, Hong GR, et al. Association of aortic phenotypes and mechanical function with left ventricular diastolic function in subjects with normally functioning bicuspid aortic valves and comparison to subjects with tricuspid aortic valves. Am J Cardiol 2015;116:1547–54.

41. Shim CY, Park S, Choi EY, et al. The relationship between ventricular-vascular coupling during exercise and impaired left ventricular longitudinal functional reserve in hypertensive patients. J Am Soc Hypertens 2013;7:198–205.

42. Weber T, Auer J, O'Rourke MF, et al. Prolonged mechanical systole and increased arterial wave reflections in diastolic dysfunction. Heart 2006;92:1616–22.

43. Shim CY, Park S, Choi D, et al. Sex differences in central hemodynamics and their relationship to left ventricular diastolic function. J Am Coll Cardiol 2011;57:1226–33.

44. Gori M, Lam CS, Gupta DK, et al. Sex-specific cardiovascular structure and function in heart failure with preserved ejection fraction. Eur J Heart Fail 2014;16:535–42.

45. Coutinho T, Borlaug BA, Pellikka PA, et al. Sex differences in arterial stiffness and ventricular-arterial interactions. J Am Coll Cardiol 2013;61:96–103.

46. Shim CY, Hong GR, Park S, et al. Impact of central haemodynamics on left ventricular function in individuals with an exaggerated blood pressure response to exercise. J Hypertens 2015;33:612–20.

47. Cortigiani L, Bombardini T, Corbisiero A, et al. The additive prognostic value of end-systolic pressure-volume relation in patients with diabetes mellitus having negative dobutamine stress echocardiography by wall motion criteria. Heart 2009;95:1429–35.

48. Ky B, French B, May Khan A, et al. Ventricular-arterial coupling, remodeling, and prognosis in chronic heart failure. J Am Coll Cardiol 2013;62:1165–72.

49. Obokata M, Kurosawa K, Ishida H, et al. Incremantal prognostic value of ventricular-arterial coupling over ejection fraction in patients with maintenance hemodialysis. J Am Soc Echocardiogr 2014;30:444–53.

50. Fitzpatrick JK, Meyer CS, Schiller NB, et al. Ventricular-vascular coupling at rest and after exercise is associated with heart failure hospitalizations in patients with coronary artery disease. J Am Soc Echocardiogr 2018;31:1212–20.

51. Shim CY, Kim D, Park S, et al. Effects of continuous positive airway pressure therapy on left ventricular diastolic function: a randomized, sham-controlled clinical trial. Eur Respir J 2018;51 [pii:1701774].

Imaging-Specific Cardiomyopathies
A Practical Guide

Kate Rankin, FRACP, Babitha Thampinathan, BSc, RDCS,
Paaladinesh Thavendiranathan, MD, SM, FRCPC*

KEYWORDS

- Ischemic cardiomyopathy • Nonischemic cardiomyopathy • Multimodality imaging
- Echocardiography • Cardiovascular magnetic resonance • Computed tomography
- Nuclear imaging

KEY POINTS

- Cardiovascular imaging techniques such as echocardiography, cardiovascular magnetic resonance (CMR), computed tomography (CT), and nuclear imaging play a crucial role in diagnosis and management of cardiomyopathies and also provide important prognostic information.
- Echocardiography remains the primary modality for initial assessment with strengths in determining wall motion abnormalities, valvular disease, subclinical myocardial dysfunction, and diastolic function. Its major limitation is in the interobserver and intraobserver variability of the measurements.
- CMR has excellent reproducibility in the measurement of myocardial function; however, its major strength is in tissue characterization, with specific strength in the assessment of infiltrative cardiomyopathies, myocarditis, iron overload, and hypertrophic cardiomyopathy.
- The primary role of cardiac CT in cardiomyopathies is to rule out coronary artery disease as the potential cause.
- Nuclear/positron emission tomography imaging is particularly useful in the assessment of myocardial perfusion and metabolism. Its primary clinical application today is in the assessment of sarcoidosis and myocarditis.

INTRODUCTION - APPROACH TO THE FAILING HEART

Heart failure is a clinical syndrome with a broad spectrum of presentations. In addition to clinical history and physical examination, cardiovascular imaging techniques such as echocardiography, cardiovascular magnetic resonance (CMR), computed tomography (CT), and nuclear imaging play a crucial role in diagnosis, guiding management, and providing prognostic information. An important goal of imaging with techniques such as CMR and nuclear imaging is to identify potentially reversible causes of cardiomyopathy that may not have otherwise been recognized.

This article aims to discuss each of the imaging modalities currently available for clinical use in the assessment of cardiomyopathies and their respective strengths and weaknesses (**Table 1**). The focus will be on nonischemic cardiomyopathies. An approach will be discussed for specific cardiomyopathies, with a focus on the role of integrated imaging in their diagnosis, prognosis, and management.

Disclosure: The authors have nothing to disclose.
Division of Cardiology, Peter Munk Cardiac Center, Ted Rogers Program in Cardiotoxicity Prevention, Toronto General Hospital, University Health Network, University of Toronto, 4N-490, 585 University Avenue, Toronto, Ontario M5G 2N2, Canada
* Corresponding author.
E-mail address: dinesh.thavendiranathan@utoronto.ca

Heart Failure Clin 15 (2019) 275–295
https://doi.org/10.1016/j.hfc.2018.12.007

Table 1
Most commonly used cardiac imaging techniques

Imaging Modality	Strength	Weakness
Two-dimensional echocardiography	• Bedside access • Low cost • Rapid and noninvasive assessment of regional wall motion • Detailed assessment of diastolic function/LV filling pressures • Identification of concomitant valvular disease • Echo enhancing agent can be used to optimize LV function/wall motion assessment and identify complications including LV thrombus	• Operator-dependent • Inter- and intra- observer variability • Accuracy heavily reliant on image quality and reader experience • Relies on geometric assumptions
Three-dimensional echocardiography	• Improved accuracy and reproducibility in the assessment of LV and RV ejection fraction and volumes • Superior ability to identify spatio-temporal relationships between structures • True real time 3-dimensional data	• Operator-dependent • Reliant on image quality • Work flow challenges
Speckle-tracking strain	• Angle-independent • Ability to detect subtle wall motion abnormalities leading to earlier diagnosis • Incremental prognostic value in cardiomyopathies	• Vendor variability • Reliance on excellent image quality for adequate tracking
MRI	• Excellent reproducibility • High resolution/spatial definition • Reference method for LV and RV volume and function assessment, LV mass • Tissue characterization – evaluation of myocardial inflammation, edema and fibrosis • Accurate ischemia assessment • No radiation exposure	• Increased cost • Less readily available • Multiple contraindications including certain implanted cardiac devices
Cardiac CT	• Noninvasive assessment of CAD with high sensitivity • Workup of chest pain in low-intermediate risk population	• Radiation exposure, although levels with contemporary scanners well below invasive coronary angiography
PET	• Myocardial metabolic and perfusion evaluation	• Limited availability • Radiation exposure

ISCHEMIC CARDIOMYOPATHY

Cardiomyopathies can be practically divided into ischemic and nonischemic categories based on presence or absence of coronary artery disease (CAD). Cardiac imaging can help differentiate between these cardiomyopathies. Echocardiography and strain imaging can identify the presence of regional wall motion abnormalities in coronary territories. The presence of subendocardial late gadolinium enhancement (LGE) by CMR demonstrates prior myocardial infarction. Furthermore, CMR and

Table 2
Distinguishing features of ischemic and nonischemic cardiomyopathy on multimodality imaging

	Ischemic CM	Non-ischemic CM
Echocardiography	• Regional LV dysfunction in infarcted myocardial territory • Myocardial perfusion defect on echo-enhancement agent imaging • WMA with stress testing • Biphasic response on DSE indicative of hibernating myocardium	• Global LV dysfunction • RV dysfunction/enlargement more common
Cardiac CT	• Coronary artery calcification • Coronary artery stenosis on gated CT	• Absence of coronary calcification does not rule out CAD • Absence of atherosclerosis on coronary CTA significantly reduces the chance of CAD as the cause of cardiomyopathy
Nuclear	• Perfusion defects in coronary artery distribution	• Homogeneous tracer uptake • Perfusion defects in non-coronary distribution
CMR	• Subendocardial LGE	• Varied distribution patterns of LGE without primary subendocardial involvement

nuclear imaging including positron emission tomography (PET) can help identify ischemia and the extent of myocardial infarction. Finally, cardiac CT provides a comprehensive, noninvasive assessment of coronary anatomy and the presence of epicardial coronary artery stenosis. In addition, imaging techniques play an important role in guiding management decisions and prognostication in ischemic cardiomyopathy. In particular, echocardiography and CMR-based assessment of left ventricular ejection fraction (LVEF) is used to determine candidacy for certain medical therapies and device therapies (eg, implantable cardioverter-defibrillator [ICD]).[1] The degree of LGE by CMR can help determine viability and the chances of myocardial recovery after revascularization.[2] PET myocardial perfusion imaging (MPI) demonstrates high diagnostic accuracy for detection of CAD.[3] Additionally, perfusion abnormalities demonstrated on PET MPI are associated with adverse cardiovascular outcomes. A 10% increase in ischemic and scarred myocardium on PET MPI is associated with a significantly increased risk of cardiac death.[4] Findings that can differentiate ischemic from nonischemic cardiomyopathy using different imaging modalities are summarized in **Table 2**.

NONISCHEMIC CARDIOMYOPATHIES
Hypertrophic Cardiomyopathy

Hypertrophic cardiomyopathy (HCM) is an inherited cardiac condition with a variable clinical course, ranging from asymptomatic individuals to patients with limiting symptoms. HCM is characterized by left ventricular (LV) hypertrophy, usually involving the interventricular septum, although various patterns have been described.[5] Two-thirds of patients with HCM have dynamic LV outflow tract obstruction, secondary to a combination of septal hypertrophy, a narrow LV outflow tract, and systolic anterior motion of the mitral valve (SAM).[5] Such features are readily diagnosed on transthoracic echocardiography, the mainstay of HCM diagnosis (**Fig. 1**). Alternative imaging modalities such as CMR play a role in providing vital additional information to inform clinical decision making and aid in risk stratification.

Echocardiography

The echocardiographic evaluation of patients with HCM includes: determination of the presence of hypertrophy, its severity, and its distribution; LVEF; degree of dynamic left ventricular

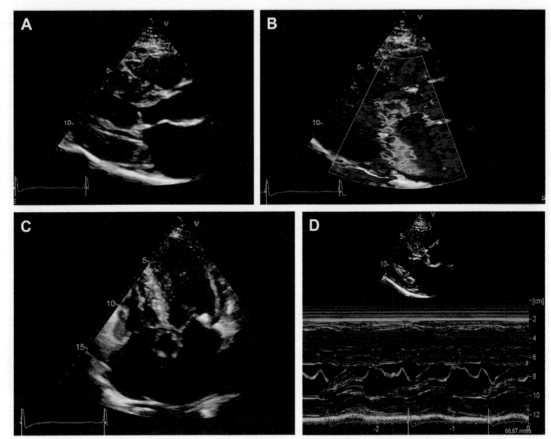

Fig. 1. Hypertrophic cardiomyopathy and the mitral valve. (*A, C*) Systolic anterior motion of the anterior mitral valve leaflet seen in parasternal long axis and apical 5-chamber view and (*B*) associated posteriorly directed mitral regurgitation. (*D*) M-mode echocardiography demonstrating systolic anterior motion of the anterior mitral valve leaflet.

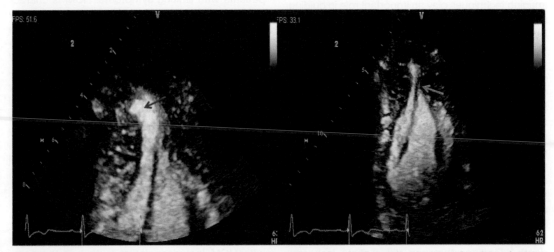

Fig. 2. Hypertrophic cardiomyopathy (apical variant). Two-dimensional echocardiography with echo enhancing agent demonstrates typical findings in apical HCM including marked hypertrophy of apical LV wall segments, presence of apical pouch (*red arrow*), and apically displaced papillary muscle (*yellow arrow*).

outflow tract (LVOT) obstruction at rest and with Valsalva maneuver; evaluation of the mitral valve and papillary muscles including papillary muscle displacement; degree and direction of MR and severity of SAM; presence of right ventricular (RV) hypertrophy/RVOT obstruction and apical aneurysm; LV diastolic function; and estimation of pulmonary artery systolic pressure (see **Fig. 1; Fig. 2**).[5]

Two-dimensional echocardiography is currently the recommended screening test for HCM in patients with a family history. It is recommended that adolescents are screened on a yearly basis and adults screened every 5 years.[6] Doppler methods can be used to assess for presence of subclinical LV dysfunction. Reduced s' and e' velocities can occur before hypertrophy is evident.[5] Abnormalities in LV strain have been demonstrated in patients with HCM compared with controls.[7] This includes reduction in average global longitudinal strain, markedly reduced strain in hypertrophied regions,[8] and reduction in LV untwisting. Additionally, strain imaging can be used to identify subclinical LV dysfunction in individuals being screened for HCM, with a finding of reduced global longitudinal strain (GLS) suggesting early disease[9]

With respect to prognosis, LV wall thickness of at least 30 mm, resting LVOT gradient greater than 30 mm Hg, and LA enlargement are all associated with increased risk of HCM-related death.[10] Specifically, maximal wall thickness of at least 30 mm constitutes one of the high-risk criteria for consideration of primary prevention ICD implantation.[11] Exercise stress echocardiography is also of clinical importance in risk stratification and guiding management of HCM patients, assessing exercise-induced LVOT gradient (particularly in symptomatic HCM patients to assess for provocable gradient), hemodynamic response to exercise, and for presence of exercise-induced arrhythmia.[10]

Echocardiography also plays a role in septal reduction techniques. Transesophageal echocardiography (TEE) is utilized to guide the approach for surgical myectomy. The maximal septal thickness and distance of maximal thickness from the aortic annulus guide decisions regarding myectomy, while the presence of mitral valve abnormalities guides the need for concomitant replacement or repair.[12,13] Septal ethanol ablation procedures are performed with transthoracic echocardiography (TTE) guidance. Echo contrast is administered to the septal perforator branch intended for ethanol injection to assess territories it perfuses to ensure the infarct created does not result in other cardiovascular complications.[5]

Cardiovascular magnetic resonance

CMR provides accurate evaluation of LV/RV morphology and function, extent, location, and degree of LV hypertrophy; papillary muscle abnormalities; mitral valve apparatus and regurgitation; the presence of SAM; crypts and apico-basal muscle bundle; and the presence of apical aneurysm. Most importantly, contrast-enhanced CMR with LGE sequences helps establish the presence, location, and degree of focal fibrosis/scar, which has prognostic implications (**Fig. 3**).[5] Although there is no specific distribution pattern of LGE typical for HCM, LGE is more common in hypertrophied segments and also often located at the insertion points of the RV free wall and ventricular septum.[14] The presence of LGE can also be used to differentiate HCM from other causes of myocardial hypertrophy. More contemporary tissue characterization techniques such as myocardial T1 mapping or extracellular volume fraction (ECV) may be more sensitive in identifying myocardial fibrosis (see **Fig. 3**); however, their impact on altering management or determining prognosis remains to be determined.[15]

Cardiac computed tomography

Cardiac CT is an alternate option in patients for whom MRI is contraindicated because of the presence of ICD, or when echocardiography is limited because of suboptimal images. Cardiac CT provides accurate measurements of LV wall thickness, volume, and mass; however, CMR has superior tissue characterization capabilities. Cardiac CT also provides a noninvasive assessment to rule out the presence of CAD in the context of chest pain, a common symptom in these patients.[5]

Restrictive Cardiomyopathies

Restrictive cardiomyopathies constitute a heterogeneous group of heart muscle diseases. Classical features include a small nondilated left ventricle with severe atrial dilatation and normal systolic function with restrictive pattern of LV diastolic filling.[16]

Amyloidosis

The most common cause of restrictive cardiomyopathy, systemic amyloidosis, is a disorder of protein metabolism involving the deposition of abnormal extracellular proteins in different organs. AL amyloidosis affects the heart in 90% of cases, whereas AA amyloid only rarely affects the heart. Amyloid deposition occurs initially in the subendocardium and subsequently extends to the myocardium with interdeposition of amyloid proteins between myocardial fibers. These deposits

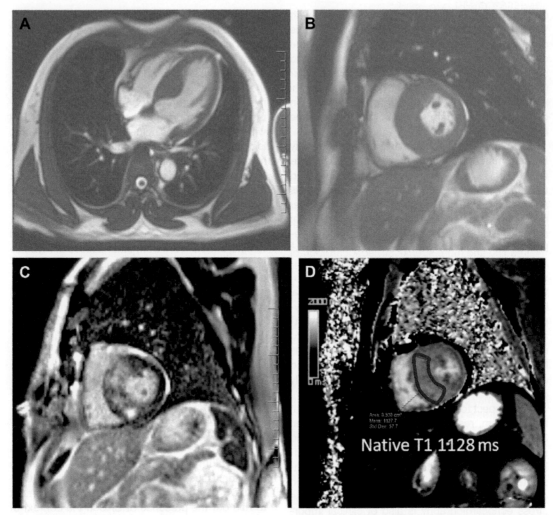

Fig. 3. Hypertrophic cardiomyopathy. (*A*, *B*) Asymmetric hypertrophy of the IVS, shown both in 4-chamber and short-axis view. (*C*) LGE short-axis images showing significant LGE in the interventricular septum in the area of hypertrophy. (*D*) Native T1 mapping on a 1.5 T S magnet demonstrating significantly increased T1 values (1128 ms).

account for the morphologic and functional abnormalities seen in cardiac amyloidosis.[16]

Echocardiography

A primary 2-dimensional feature of cardiac amyloidosis is increased LV wall thickness with a granular/speckle appearance of the LV myocardium. However, with the use of harmonic imaging, the speckle appearance is not specific.[17] There is also a decrease in LV cavity size causing reduction in end-diastolic volumes, although the EF typically remains normal until the late stages of disease progression. Other potential nonspecific 2-dimensional echo findings include; RV wall and valvular thickening, increased left and right atrial volumes, and pericardial effusion (**Fig. 4**).[18] Interatrial septal thickening is a characteristic

feature of cardiac amyloidosis.[19] Tissue Doppler imaging (TDI) demonstrates reduced e' and a' velocities (<5 cm/s) consistent with myocardial dysfunction (see **Fig. 4**). Transmitral Doppler inflow shows restrictive filling pattern (E/A ratio >2, shortened mitral deceleration time) with an increased E/e' ratio suggestive of increased left atrial pressures.[20]

LV GLS is reduced in amyloidosis. A base-to-apex LV peak systolic longitudinal strain gradient has been shown to help differentiate cardiac amyloidosis from other conditions associated with LV hypertrophy (see **Fig. 4**).[21] This relative apical sparing pattern also provides prognostic information and improves concordance among readers in echocardiography laboratories for the diagnosis of cardiac amyloidosis.[22,23]

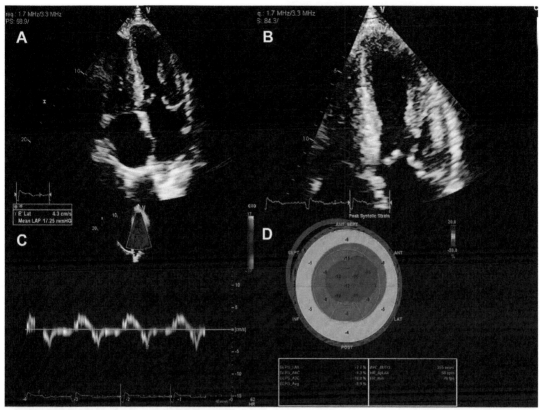

Fig. 4. Cardiac amyloidosis. (*A, B*) Two-dimensional echocardiography apical 4-chamber image demonstrating increased LV wall thickness with granular/speckle appearance, thickening of AV valves, and thickening of interatrial septum. (*C*) Markedly reduced lateral mitral annular tissue Doppler velocity, e′. (*D*) Bull's eye strain map demonstrating relative apical sparing pattern, typical of cardiac amyloidosis.

Cardiovascular magnetic resonance

Typical morphologic features of amyloidosis identified on echocardiography are also appreciated on CMR. LV LGE is a specific finding and tends to occur in multiple potential patterns including global transmural, global/heterogeneous, global subendocardial, focal patchy, and suboptimal nulling.[24] Myocardial LGE can be an early feature of cardiac involvement in patients with normal wall thickness on an echocardiogram (**Fig. 5**).[24] Presence of LGE in the atrial wall is another characteristic feature of cardiac amyloidosis.[19] Other CMR findings specific to amyloidosis include shortened subendocardial T1 relaxation time and expansion of extracellular volume fraction.[19,25,26] Native T1 mapping demonstrating elevated values (see **Fig. 5**) is potentially a useful technique for the diagnosis of cardiac amyloidosis, especially in patients with renal failure in whom administration of gadolinium-based contrast agents is contraindicated.

Nuclear imaging

Bone imaging agents such as Tc-99m pyrophosphate (PYP) appear to be useful in the diagnosis of ATTR amyloidosis.[27] Tc-99 m is taken up by the heart in ATTR amyloid cardiomyopathy.[19] A Tc-99m PYP heart to contralateral lung ratio of greater than 1.5 distinguishes ATTR from AL amyloidosis.[28] A strongly positive Tc-99m PYP suggests ATTR cardiac amyloidosis; however, a negative Tc-99m PYP scan does not rule out AL cardiac amyloid.[19]

Sarcoidosis

Sarcoidosis is a disease of unknown etiology that is characterized by the formation of noncaseating granuloma in various organs.[29] Cardiac granulomas are found in approximately 25% of patients at autopsy. However, cardiac sarcoidosis is clinically apparent in only approximately 5% of patients with common manifestations including cardiomyopathy, tachyarrhythmias, heart block, and sudden cardiac death.[16]

Echocardiography

Echocardiographic findings are nonspecific and can include regional LV systolic dysfunction and impaired diastolic function (ranging from impaired

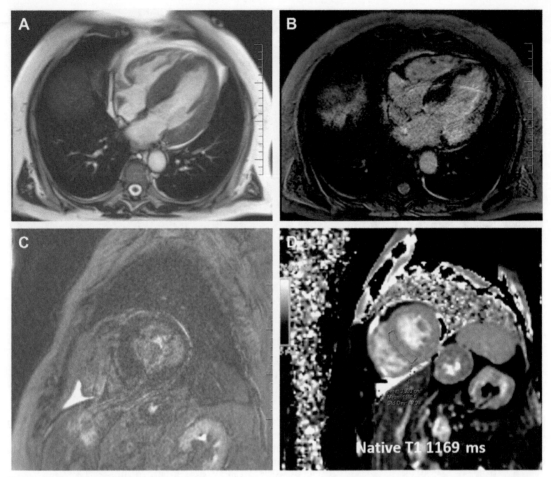

Fig. 5. Cardiac amyloidosis. (*A*) Apical 4-chamber view demonstrating significant global hypertrophy with some asymmetry involving the septum. (*B*) Apical 4-chamber and (*C*) short-axis LGE images in the same patient with significant subendocardial and midmyocardial LGE that is diffuse and low signal from the blood pool. (*D*) Native precontrast T1 mapping short axis view demonstrating high T1 values (1169 ms, 1.5 T S magnet).

relaxation to restrictive filling).[16] Two-dimensional echocardiography can be used for initial screening and assessment of cardiac sarcoid, but it has low sensitivity. Common findings include basal thinning of interventricular septum (thinning, akinetic/dyskinetic) leading to aneurysm formation, other focal areas of wall thinning in a noncoronary distribution, diastolic dysfunction, ventricular dilatation, reduced EF/global hypokinesis, pericardial effusion, and valvular disease. Strain imaging may be helpful in detecting subtle LV changes leading to dysfunction.[30] Reduced GLS with preserved circumferential LV strain has been described in patients with sarcoidosis and preserved LVEF.[31] Additionally, GLS greater than −17% in patients with sarcoidosis has been associated with an increased risk of death and ventricular arrhythmia in a recent cohort study.[32]

Cardiovascular magnetic resonance

The diagnosis of sarcoidosis by CMR is based on the identification of typical patterns of myocardial LGE.[33] Although various patterns of LGE can be seen, the most typical are subepicardial and mid-wall LGE along the basal septum and/or inferolateral wall (**Fig. 6**).[29] The location of scar has been used as a guide for endomyocardial biopsy to maximize diagnostic yield.[34] Because marked edema in the setting of inflammation can increase interstitial space and result in LGE, the size of LGE can decrease following immunosuppressive therapy, potentially providing a method to assess for response to therapy over serial examinations.[35,36] Patients with cardiac sarcoidosis with LGE extent at least 20% of LV mass are at an increased risk of cardiac death, hospitalization for heart failure, and life-threatening arrhythmias.[37] These patients are also less likely to recover myocardial function

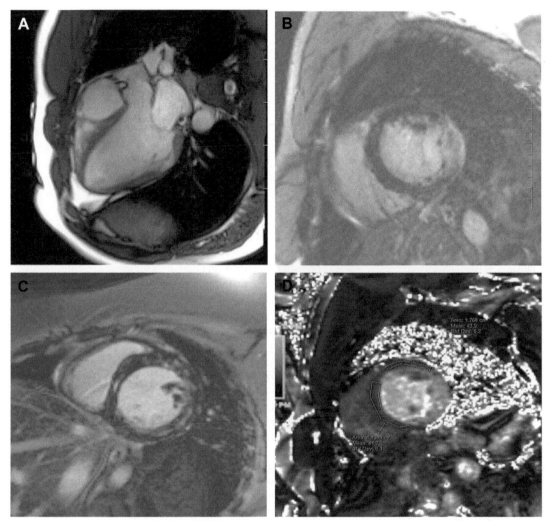

Fig. 6. Cardiac sarcoidosis. (*A*) Apical 3-chamber view cine image with a focal area of thinning involving the basal inferior lateral wall (this wall was akinetic on cine images). (*B, C*) LGE images in the short-axis view with transmural and patchy midmyocardial LGE. (*D*) Myocardial T2 mapping on 3.0 T S magnet with T2 values of 44 ms.

following steroid therapy.[37] In addition to LGE, patchy myocardial edema can also be identified using T2 weighted imaging and tends to localize to the subepicardial regions.[38] The detection of edema may help guide immunosuppressive therapy.[38]

Nuclear/positron emission tomography

18F-fluorodeoxyglucose (^{18}F-FDG) PET is an accurate and effective imaging technique to assess for myocardial inflammation in cardiac sarcoidosis and provides complementary information to CMR (**Fig. 7**).[29] It may also help assess response to and guide immunosuppressive therapy.[29,39] ^{18}F-FDG, a glucose analog, is retained within cells with high metabolic activity, such as granuloma. Several patterns of ^{18}F-FDG uptake have been reported in sarcoidosis: no uptake, diffuse uptake,

focal uptake, and focal on diffuse uptake.[40] These findings, along with resting perfusion data, can be used to categorize disease status, with increasing size of perfusion defect and increased uptake of ^{18}F-FDG associated with advancing disease stage. Fibrous disease is demonstrated by severe perfusion defect with minimal or no ^{18}F-FDG uptake.[41] ^{18}F-FDG PET may have a value in the early diagnosis of cardiac sarcoid; however, limited data exist comparing its accuracy with CMR.[29] Overall, CMR may be more sensitive for initial diagnosis, while ^{18}F-FDG PET more effective for monitoring inflammation and response to anti-inflammatory therapy.[29,39,42] An important limitation of FDG-PET imaging is the difficulty in appropriate suppression of physiologic glucose utilization due to challenges with patient compliance with high-fat and low-

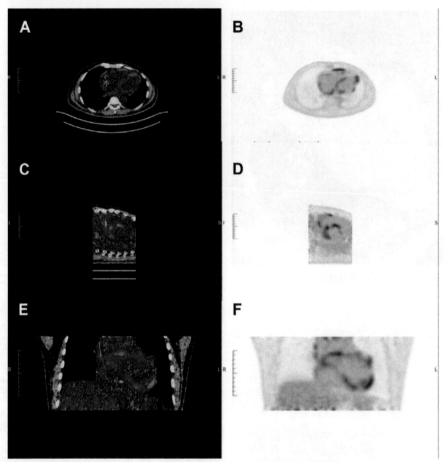

Fig. 7. CT-FDG PET fusion and FDG-PET in cardiac sarcoidosis. (*A*) Axial CT-FDG PET fusion image and (*B*) axial FDG-PET image demonstrate FDG uptake in the interventricular septum and apex. There is also FDG uptake in the right ventricle. (*C*, *D*) Sagittal images demonstrate FDG uptake in the right ventricle and in the LV apex. (*E*, *F*) Coronal views show FDG uptake in the inferior wall, apex, and basal interventricular septum. (*Courtesy of* Dr. R.M Iwanochko, Ontario, Canada).

carbohydrate diet prior to the test. This can result in a high proportion of nondiagnostic studies[43] emphasizing the importance of careful preparation.

Anderson-Fabry disease

Anderson-Fabry disease (AFD) is an X-linked, lysosomal storage disorder caused by mutations in the alpha-galactosidase gene. The diagnosis is confirmed with genetic testing, although cardiac imaging also plays a role in the assessment. AFD is a common mimic of hypertrophic cardiomyopathy with similar morphologic features on echocardiography.[44]

Two-dimensional echocardiography

The most common feature seen on 2-dimensional echocardiography is increased LV wall thickness, specifically concentric LV hypertrophy (LVH). It is considered the hallmark feature of the glycolipid deposits found in the ventricular muscle fibers.[45]

Although not a specific finding in patients with AFD, the LV endocardial borders can have hyperechogenic (thickened endocardium) and hypoechogenic components (middle and outer layers of myocardium) (**Fig. 8**).[45,46] Other morphologic characteristics include atrial enlargement, aortic dilatation, valvular heart disease (mitral and aortic regurgitation), and regional wall motion/ventricular function impairment. TDI may identify early stages of AFD (with or without overt LVH), demonstrating reduced mitral annular velocities and increased E/e' ratio.[45]

In patients with AFD, regional myocardial dysfunction may be better assessed by strain imaging.[47] Global longitudinal strain is typically reduced even in the presence of a normal EF.[48] Interestingly, in the context of papillary muscle involvement with glycolipid deposits, two studies have demonstrated reduced longitudinal strain in the mid lateral and posterior walls.[46,47] Later

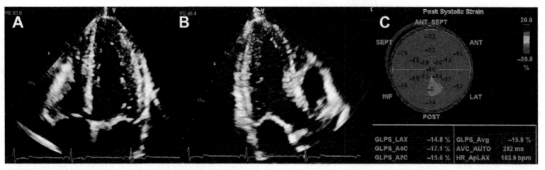

Fig. 8. Anderson-Fabry disease; 2-dimensional echocardiography and strain. (A, B) 2-dimensional echocardiography images (apical 4- and 3-chamber) demonstrate concentric LV hypertrophy and binary appearance of myocardium with hyperechogenic (thickened endocardium) and hypoechogenic components (middle and outer layers of myocardium). (C) Bull's eye strain map demonstrates typical reduction of longitudinal strain in the inferior lateral wall.

stages of AFD demonstrate lack of longitudinal systolic deformation in basal and mid inferolateral segments due to thinning of the myocardium (caused by replacement fibrosis) thus causing a reduction in strain values in this territory (see **Fig. 8**).[47]

Cardiovascular magnetic resonance

CMR is also of diagnostic utility in AFD, owing in particular to its ability to assess patterns of LV wall thickening and presence/distribution of myocardial LGE. The most common manifestations of AFD on CMR are concentric wall thickening and inferolateral midmyocardial LGE (**Fig. 9**). However, distribution of wall thickening

is widely varied and can include patterns morphologically identical to apical and asymmetric septal hypertrophy types of HCM. The LGE in AFD can also present in atypical distributions in one-fifth of cases.[44] The overlap in patterns of wall thickness and scar between AFD and HCM demonstrates that it is inadequate to rely on imaging alone and that genetic testing to confirm or rule out AFD diagnosis is indicated when there is clinical suspicion.

Iron overload cardiomyopathy

Iron overload cardiomyopathy results from the accumulation of excess iron in the myocardium. It predominantly affects patients with genetic

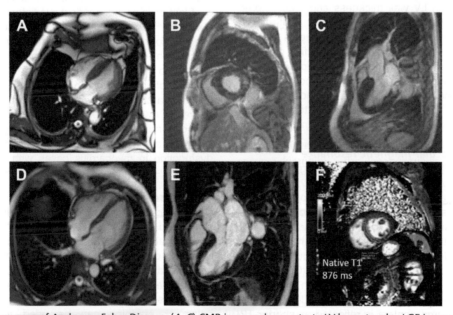

Fig. 9. Two cases of Anderson-Fabry Disease. (A–C) CMR images demonstrate LV hypertrophy. LGE images demonstrate LGE with typical distribution in the basal inferolateral wall. (D–F) In a second case, CMR images demonstrate an increase in LV mass 96 g/m2. No enhancement was seen on LGE images, but T1 values were reduced (876 ms on 1.5 T, Siemens, magnet) as seen in AFD.

disorders of iron metabolism or recipients of multiple transfusions.[49] Early diagnosis of iron overload cardiomyopathy is essential, as medical therapy can reverse myocardial dysfunction if instituted before onset of end-stage heart failure.[50] Diagnosis can be challenging in the early stages of disease. Identification of iron overload with biochemical markers and tissue biopsy are the mainstays of diagnosis; however, iron deposition in the heart tends to be patchy, and therefore biopsy may give false negative result.[49]

Echocardiography

Common features noted on 2-dimensional echocardiography include: biventricular dilation, systolic dysfunction, and diastolic dysfunction with restrictive filling pattern. Diastolic dysfunction can be detected before systolic dysfunction occurs on echocardiography.[49] Findings specifically described in patients with hereditary hemochromatosis include a decrease in peak systolic and diastolic early filling mitral annular velocity as well as prolongation of atrial reversal wave duration in the context of normal LV systolic function.[51] Overall, a thorough assessment of LV diastolic function should be performed in any patient at risk of iron overload regardless of presence of biochemical evidence of iron overload and should be repeated every 1 to 2 years.[49] Serial echocardiography can monitor and assess response to therapy in this patient cohort. In combination with iron-depleting therapies, echocardiography can demonstrate a decrease in LV wall thickness and mass, correlating with reversal of myocardial infiltration.[52] Global longitudinal strain is reduced in patients myocardial iron overload and identifies presence of myocardial iron overload with high specificity but low sensitivity.[53] Although echocardiography can detect early myocardial pathology in the setting of iron overload, it lacks the ability to demonstrate actual iron deposition in tissues.

Cardiovascular magnetic resonance

CMR is the only noninvasive imaging method capable of quantitatively assessing the degree of myocardial overload in addition to providing accurate measures of LV systolic function, volumes, and mass.[49] Myocardial iron quantification is possible through measurements of the time constant of decay for spin echo (SE)-induced relaxation time (T2) or gradient echo (GE)-induced relaxation time (T2*). Increased iron in tissues progressively shortens relaxation times; thus, increased iron content is reflected as shorter T2/T2*.[49] T2* less than 10 ms identifies those at high risk of cardiac decompensation, while T2* greater than 20 ms is consistent with a low risk for

imminent development of heart failure syndrome (**Fig. 10**).[54] Cardiac MRI with T2* assessment should be performed in any patient at risk of iron overload cardiomyopathy.[49] Changes in myocardial T2* over time demonstrate myocardial iron removal and can be used to monitor response to iron chelation therapy.[55]

Inflammatory Cardiomyopathy/Myocarditis

Myocardial inflammation is a nonspecific response to various triggers including bacterial or viral infection, cardiotoxic agents, catecholamines, or mechanical injury. Myocarditis can present with a wide spectrum of symptoms from chest pain and arrhythmias to cardiogenic shock and sudden cardiac death. Endomyocardial biopsy is still considered by many to be the gold standard; however, it is significantly limited by patchy myocardial involvement in this condition.[56] Therefore, noninvasive imaging also plays an essential role.

Echocardiography

Echocardiographic features of myocarditis are varied and nonspecific, ranging from dilated to hypertrophic to restrictive patterns depending on the timing of presentation.[57] Segmental wall motion abnormalities (WMAs) in the acute setting are common.[57] Acute myocarditis is associated with increased sphericity and LV volumes.[58] Wall thickness can be increased in the acute phase consistent with myocardial edema.[56] Pericardial effusion may be present.[57] The presence of RV systolic dysfunction is an independent predictor of adverse outcome.[59] Unfortunately, the diagnostic value of echocardiography is limited by this highly varied distribution of findings in myocarditis and the inability to reliably differentiate from CAD in the absence of anatomic coronary assessment. Global longitudinal strain is reduced and correlates with the degree of myocardial edema in acute myocarditis and can add valuable information, especially in diagnosis and assessment of degree of myocardial dysfunction in myocarditis cases with preserved LVEF on 2-dimensional echocardiography.[60]

Cardiovascular magnetic resonance

CMR is recommended in clinically stable patients suspected of having myocarditis prior to endomyocardial biopsy.[61] Its major strength is for the diagnosis of acute myocarditis. Active myocarditis demonstrates intracellular/interstitial edema, capillary leakage, hyperemia, and cellular necrosis/fibrosis in more severe cases. T2 weighted imaging or mapping can be used to identify myocardial edema (**Fig. 11**).[62] Contrast-enhanced T1 weighted imaging is used to measure early gadolinium enhancement ratio (EGEr),

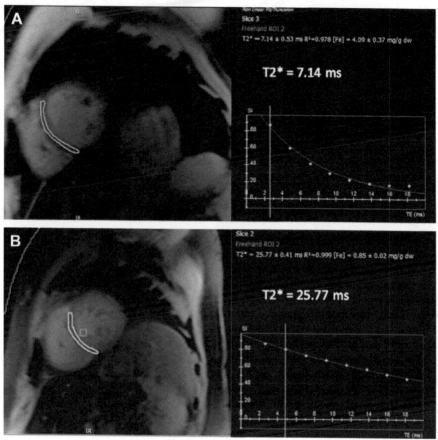

Fig. 10. Two cases of T2* measurement. Top panel (*A*) demonstrates a patient with significant iron overload with T2* values measured in the interventricular septum at 7.14 ms. Bottom panel (*B*) demonstrates a patient with repeated transfusions but no signs of iron overload, with a T2* value at the septum of 25.77 ms.

reflective of hyperemia/capillary leak and inflammation.[63] Finally, myocardial LGE reflects myocardial injury/fibrosis and is most commonly subepicardial in distribution in myocarditis, differentiating it from ischemic LGE (subendocardial) (see **Fig. 11**).[64] The combined application of these 3 CMR imaging methods has been termed the "Lake Louise Criteria." Presence of 2 of the 3 CMR characteristics provides high specificity but relatively low sensitivity for the diagnosis of biopsy-proven myocarditis.[63]

Nuclear/positron emission tomography
FDG-PET can also be used in the diagnosis of myocardial inflammation and acute myocarditis. Findings correlate well with CMR, although FDG-PET is less commonly used in this clinic setting.[65]

Cancer Therapeutics-Related Cardiac Dysfunction

Cardiotoxicity from chemotherapy, targeted therapy, or immune therapy in patients with malignancies can be identified because of a change in cardiac function or new clinical cardiac symptoms compared with baseline. The most commonly used definition of cancer therapeutics-related cardiac dysfunction (CTRCD) pertains to a reduction in LVEF in the context of anthracyclines or trastuzumab therapy and has been recently defined in the American Society of Echocardiography (ASE) expert consensus document as a reduction in LVEF by greater than 10% and to less than 53%.[66] However, other definitions exist.[67] Given this definition, accurate and reproducible measurements of LVEF are vital, particularly as findings may impact decisions to alter cancer treatment.[68]

Echocardiography
Echocardiography is the primary method for sequential assessment of LVEF. Because of the superior reproducibility of 3-dimensional LVEF, it is the suggested method to sequentially follow patients during cancer therapy (**Fig. 12**).[68] Regardless of the technique used, however, LVEF does not appear to be a robust marker to identify early myocardial dysfunction. Existing literature suggests

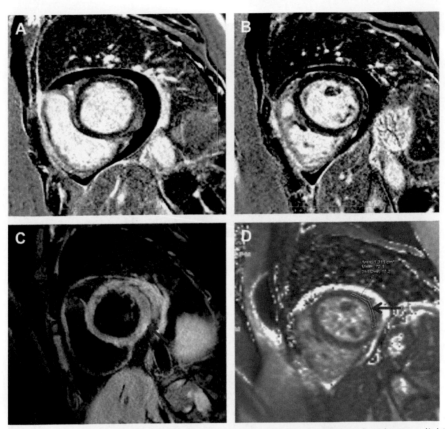

Fig. 11. Acute myocarditis. (*A, B*) CMR LGE images, demonstrating subepicardial and midmyocardial LGE in the same patient. Also pericardial effusion is shown. (*C*) T2 weighted imaging shows increased signal in the inferior lateral wall (*arrow*). (*D*) Elevated T2 values on T2 mapping consistent with myocardial edema (*arrow*).

that once a reduction in LVEF occurs, most patients will not have complete recovery of cardiac dysfunction despite appropriate heart failure therapy.[69]

Myocardial strain is highly sensitive for detecting early myocardial changes during cancer therapy compared with LVEF.[70] The ASE suggests that a relative decrease in GLS greater than 15% from baseline is indicative of subclinical LV dysfunction (see **Fig. 12**).[66] Change in GLS should be confirmed with repeat strain imaging 2 to 3 weeks later.[70] Despite the enthusiasm about strain, data on whether a strain-based approach to initiation of cardiac medications changes cardiovascular outcomes remain to be seen. Also, most existing literature has focused on patients receiving anthracyclines and trastuzumab therapy, and hence the value of strain in a plethora of other potentially cardiotoxic cancer therapies is not known.

Multiple-gated radionuclide angiography

Multiple-gated radionuclide angiography (MUGA) scans are an alternative to monitor LVEF during cancer therapy. However, their use is limited by recent data demonstrating concerns about reproducibility,[71] inability to identify early cardiac

dysfunction, and the need for repeated radiation exposure.[72]

Cardiovascular magnetic resonance

CMR is considered the gold standard for measurement of LV function and volumes, provides myocardial tissue characterization, and is ideally suited to assess for subclinical CTCRD. Myocardial inflammation (EGE) and edema (T1/T2 weighted imaging or mapping) detected on CMR and increased LV end-systolic volume may reflect early changes of CTCRD. Quantification of ECV may also be helpful in detection of late cardiotoxicity and has been associated with decreased cardiopulmonary fitness in pediatric cancer survivors.[73]

Regardless of the method used to monitor LVEF during cancer therapy, it should be stressed that the same initial imaging method should be repeated in an individual patient on serial testing to allow for accurate comparison over time.

Takotsubo Cardiomyopathy

Takotsubo cardiomyopathy (TTC), stress cardiomyopathy, or apical ballooning syndrome is a transient form of LV dysfunction that on clinical

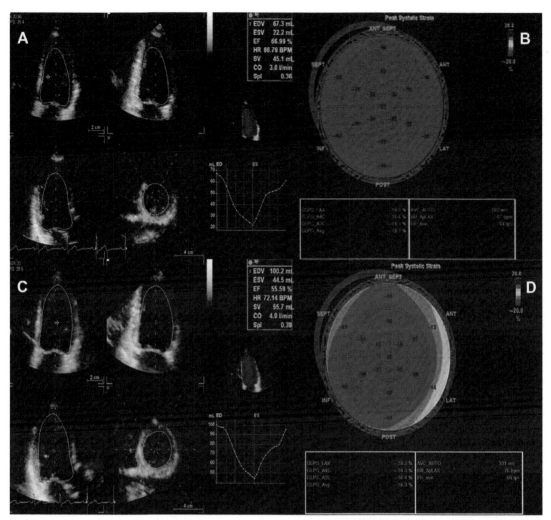

Fig. 12. Chemotherapy-related subclinical LV dysfunction. (*A, B*) Echocardiography performed prior to commencement of trastuzumab therapy and (*C, D*) subsequent echocardiography 6 months into trastuzumab therapy demonstrating development of subclinical LV dysfunction as evidenced by reduction in GLS greater than 15% (−19.7% to −16.3%), although reduction in 3-dimensional LVEF does not meet criteria for cardiotoxicity.

presentation is often indistinguishable from an acute coronary syndrome. The pathophysiology of this condition remains uncertain.[74] It commonly presents in menopausal women after an emotional or physical stress with chest pain, electrocardiogram (ECG) changes (ST segment elevation or T wave inversion), and modestly elevated cardiac biomarkers. As this is indistinguishable clinically from an acute coronary syndrome due to epicardial coronary stenosis, imaging characteristics are critical for diagnosis after ruling out CAD.

Echocardiography
The typical WMAs seen in TTC are symmetric and extend beyond the territory of a single coronary artery. Apical akinesis with preserved or hypercontractile basal segments (apical type) is the classic presentation. However, WMAs may affect midventricular (midventricular type) or basal (inverted type) wall segments. Important factors associated with adverse events assessed with echocardiography include LVEF, wall motion score index, reversible moderate-to-severe MR and E/e' ratio.[75] The right ventricle is involved in 13% of cases of Takotsubo and is also associated with poor prognosis.[76] Other complications of acute presentations of TTC readily identified on echocardiography include dynamic LV outflow tract obstruction-associated SAM and acute MR, pericardial effusion, and thrombus formation.[77]

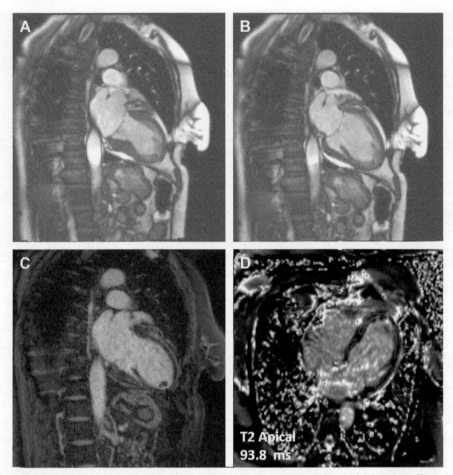

Fig. 13. Takotsubo cardiomyopathy. Two-chamber image in systole (*A*) and diastole (*B*) with wall motion abnormality involving the LV apex. (*C*) No enhancement on LGE images with presence of LV apical thrombus (*arrow*). (*D*) T2 map demonstrates high T2 values at apex consistent with myocardial edema. On follow-up imaging in same patient, all findings completely resolved.

Cardiovascular magnetic resonance

CMR has the ability to demonstrate myocardial edema, which may be present as a result of an inflammatory process (**Fig. 13**).[62] Edema usually corresponds to the area of WMA and is an important hallmark of inflammatory cell injury. However, the presence of edema alone cannot differentiate TTC from alternate diagnoses such as myocarditis. LGE can help in the diagnosis as it is usually absent in TTC and is commonly present in myocarditis (see **Fig. 13**).[74]

Left Ventricular Noncompaction

LV noncompaction (LVNC) is characterized by trabeculated myocardium with adjacent deep intertrabecular recesses communicating with the LV cavity.[78] LVNC has been associated infrequently with fatal complications such as embolic events, arrhythmia, and sudden cardiac death. Early diagnosis and the prompt initiation of treatment can avoid such complications. Noninvasive imaging techniques are essential to delineation of morphologic appearance of the myocardium in LVNC and screening for complications such as LV thrombus.[79]

Echocardiography

Echocardiography is the first-line imaging technique for the diagnosis of LVNC. In general, an end-systolic ratio of noncompacted-to-compacted myocardium greater than 2 in the parasternal short axis view is considered diagnostic (**Fig. 14**). This was proposed along with other criteria by Jenni and colleagues[80] in 2001. It is essential to demonstrate a 2-layered myocardium with thinning of the compacted segments. This is best accomplished using echocardiography-enhancing agents (see **Fig. 14**). Stollberger and colleagues[81] redefined echocardiographic criteria in 2012, making the presence of more than three trabeculations and 2-layered myocardium both requirements, to avoid

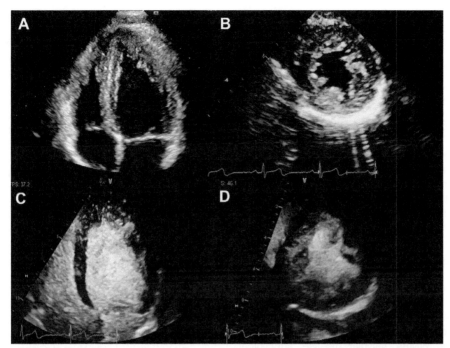

Fig. 14. LV noncompaction. (*A, B*) Two-dimensional echocardiography images (apical 4-chamber view and para-sternal short axis view) prior to echo-enhancing agent and (*C, D*) after echo-enhancing agent, delineating non-compacted myocardium with ratio greater than 2 at end systole in short axis view. Echo-enhancing agent allows improved appreciation of trabeculated myocardium and deep intertrabecular recesses, which fill with contrast.

possible overdiagnosis. The presence of an LV twist pattern with basal and apical rotation in the same direction, known as LV rigid body rotation, has a good predictive value for the diagnosis of LVNC[82] and is associated with worse functional status.[83]

Cardiovascular magnetic resonance

CMR can also demonstrate prominent trabeculations and provide an assessment of extent of non-compacted myocardium.[84,85] MRI diagnostic criteria proposed by Petersen and colleagues[86] include: visual appearance of 2 distinct myocardial layers – compacted epicardial and noncompacted endocardial, presence of marked trabeculations and deep intertrabecular recesses within a non-compacted layer, and noncompacted to com-pacted myocardial ratio greater than 2.3 measured at end-diastole in a plane perpendicular to the compacted myocardium (**Fig. 15**).[79,86] Other CMR diagnostic criteria have also been proposed,

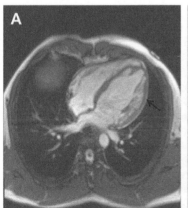
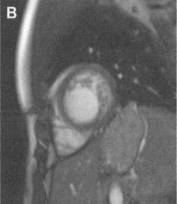
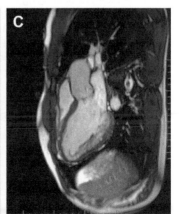

Fig. 15. Patient with LV noncompaction. (*A–C*) All 3 views demonstrate prominent trabeculations involving the mid- to distal anterior and inferior lateral walls. Particularly in the 4-chamber view, the addition of thinning of the compacted myocardium (*arrow*) can also be seen. The ratio of noncompacted-to-compacted myocardial seg-ments was greater than 2.3:1.

although less commonly used clinically.[84] Additionally, CMR LGE imaging may help identify areas of fibrosis in noncompacted myocardium, which could be a substrate for potential arrhythmias. CMR can also assess for coexisting congenital heart defects and complications of LVNC including LV thrombus.[79]

Cardiac computed tomography

Cardiac CT can delineate the compacted and non-compacted layers of the left ventricle and prominent trabeculations typical of LVNC. MDCT is less commonly used than MRI as it lacks the ability to characterize tissue and identify areas of fibrosis compared with MRI and exposes the patient to radiation.[87]

SUMMARY

Cardiovascular imaging plays an essential role in the diagnosis, management, and prognosis of cardiomyopathies. Echocardiography remains the primary modality for the initial assessment with strengths in determining WMAs, valvular disease, subclinical myocardial dysfunction, and diastolic function. Its major limitation is in the inter- and intraobserver variability of the measurements. CMR has excellent reproducibility in the measurement of myocardial function, but, its major strength is in tissue characterization with specific strength in the assessment of infiltrative cardiomyopathies, myocarditis, iron overload, and hypertrophic cardiomyopathy. The primary role of cardiac CT in cardiomyopathies is to rule out CAD as the potential cause. Nuclear imaging, and in particular PET imaging, is useful in the assessment of myocardial perfusion and metabolism. Its primary clinical application today is in the assessment of sarcoidosis and myocarditis. Given the plethora of imaging modalities available, the choice of imaging modality in the workup of cardiomyopathy should be based on the specific clinical question and the knowledge of the strengths and limitations of each imaging modality.

ACKNOWLEDGEMENT

We would like to acknowledge Dr. R. Iwanochko for providing the PET images included in this manuscript.

REFERENCES

1. Yancy CW, Jessup M, Bozkurt B, et al. 2013 ACCF/AHA guideline for the management of heart failure: a report of the American College of Cardiology Foundation/American Heart Association Task Force on practice guidelines. J Am Coll Cardiol 2013;62(16):e147–239.

2. Doltra A, Amundsen BH, Gebker R, et al. Emerging concepts for myocardial late gadolinium enhancement MRI. Curr Cardiol Rev 2013;9(3):185–90.

3. Nakazato R, Berman DS, Alexanderson E, et al. Myocardial perfusion imaging with PET. Imaging Med 2013;5(1):35–46.

4. Siontis KC, Chareonthaitawee P. Prognostic value of positron emission tomography myocardial perfusion imaging beyond traditional cardiovascular risk factors: Systematic review and meta-analysis. Int J Cardiol Heart Vasc 2015;6:54–9.

5. Nagueh SF, Bierig SM, Budoff MJ, et al. American Society of Echocardiography clinical recommendations for multimodality cardiovascular imaging of patients with hypertrophic cardiomyopathy: Endorsed by the American Society of Nuclear Cardiology, Society for Cardiovascular Magnetic Resonance, and Society of Cardiovascular Computed Tomography. J Am Soc Echocardiogr 2011;24(5):473–98.

6. Maron BJ, Seidman JG, Seidman CE. Proposal for contemporary screening strategies in families with hypertrophic cardiomyopathy. J Am Coll Cardiol 2004;44(11):2125–32.

7. Serri K, Reant P, Lafitte M, et al. Global and regional myocardial function quantification by two-dimensional strain: application in hypertrophic cardiomyopathy. J Am Coll Cardiol 2006;47(6):1175–81.

8. Liu D, Hu K, Nordbeck P, et al. Longitudinal strain bull's eye plot patterns in patients with cardiomyopathy and concentric left ventricular hypertrophy. Eur J Med Res 2016;21(1):21.

9. Smiseth OA, Torp H, Opdahl A, et al. Myocardial strain imaging: how useful is it in clinical decision making? Eur Heart J 2016;37(15):1196–207.

10. Chun S, Woo A. Echocardiography in hypertrophic cardiomyopathy: in with strain, out with straining? J Am Soc Echocardiogr 2015;28(2):204–9.

11. Gersh BJ, Maron BJ, Bonow RO, et al. 2011 ACCF/AHA guideline for the diagnosis and treatment of hypertrophic cardiomyopathy: a report of the American College of Cardiology Foundation/American Heart Association Task Force on Practice Guidelines. Developed in collaboration with the American Association for Thoracic Surgery, American Society of Echocardiography, American Society of Nuclear Cardiology, Heart Failure Society of America, Heart Rhythm Society, Society for Cardiovascular Angiography and Interventions, and Society of Thoracic Surgeons. J Am Coll Cardiol 2011;58(25):e212–60.

12. Ommen SR, Park SH, Click RL, et al. Impact of intraoperative transesophageal echocardiography in the surgical management of hypertrophic cardiomyopathy. Am J Cardiol 2002;90(9):1022–4.

13. Smedira NG, Lytle BW, Lever HM, et al. Current effectiveness and risks of isolated septal myectomy for hypertrophic obstructive cardiomyopathy. Ann Thorac Surg 2008;85(1):127–33.

14. Moon JC, McKenna WJ, McCrohon JA, et al. Toward clinical risk assessment in hypertrophic cardiomyopathy with gadolinium cardiovascular magnetic resonance. J Am Coll Cardiol 2003;41(9):1561–7.

15. Haaf P, Garg P, Messroghli DR, et al. Cardiac T1 mapping and extracellular volume (ECV) in clinical practice: a comprehensive review. J Cardiovasc Magn Reson 2016;18(1):89.

16. Nihoyannopoulos P, Dawson D. Restrictive cardiomyopathies. Eur J Echocardiogr 2009;10(8):iii23–33.

17. Selvanayagam JB, Hawkins PN, Paul B, et al. Evaluation and management of the cardiac amyloidosis. J Am Coll Cardiol 2007;50(22):2101–10.

18. Liu D, Niemann M, Hu K, et al. Echocardiographic evaluation of systolic and diastolic function in patients with cardiac amyloidosis. Am J Cardiol 2011; 108(4):591–8.

19. Falk RH, Quarta CC, Dorbala S. How to image cardiac amyloidosis. Circ Cardiovasc Imaging 2014; 7(3):552–62.

20. Koyama J, Ray-Sequin PA, Falk RH. Longitudinal myocardial function assessed by tissue velocity, strain, and strain rate tissue Doppler echocardiography in patients with AL (primary) cardiac amyloidosis. Circulation 2003;107(19):2446–52.

21. Phelan D, Collier P, Thavendiranathan P, et al. Relative apical sparing of longitudinal strain using two-dimensional speckle-tracking echocardiography is both sensitive and specific for the diagnosis of cardiac amyloidosis. Heart 2012;98(19):1442–8.

22. Phelan D, Thavendiranathan P, Popovic Z, et al. Application of a parametric display of two-dimensional speckle-tracking longitudinal strain to improve the etiologic diagnosis of mild to moderate left ventricular hypertrophy. J Am Soc Echocardiogr 2014;27(8):888–95.

23. Senapati A, Sperry BW, Grodin JL, et al. Prognostic implication of relative regional strain ratio in cardiac amyloidosis. Heart 2016;102(10):748–54.

24. Syed IS, Glockner JF, Feng D, et al. Role of cardiac magnetic resonance imaging in the detection of cardiac amyloidosis. JACC Cardiovasc Imaging 2010; 3(2):155–64.

25. Maceira AM, Prasad SK, Hawkins PN, et al. Cardiovascular magnetic resonance and prognosis in cardiac amyloidosis. J Cardiovasc Magn Reson 2008;10:54.

26. Mongeon FP, Jerosch-Herold M, Coelho-Filho OR, et al. Quantification of extracellular matrix expansion by CMR in infiltrative heart disease. JACC Cardiovasc Imaging 2012;5(9):897–907.

27. Rapezzi C, Guidalotti P, Salvi F, et al. Usefulness of 99mTc-DPD scintigraphy in cardiac amyloidosis. J Am Coll Cardiol 2008;51(15):1509–10 [author reply: 1510].

28. Bokhari S, Castaño A, Pozniakoff T, et al. (99m)Tc-pyrophosphate scintigraphy for differentiating light-chain cardiac amyloidosis from the transthyretin-related familial and senile cardiac amyloidoses. Circ Cardiovasc Imaging 2013;6(2):195–201.

29. Hulten E, Aslam S, Osborne M, et al. Cardiac sarcoidosis-state of the art review. Cardiovasc Diagn Ther 2016;6(1):50–63.

30. Aggarwal NR, Snipelisky D, Young PM, et al. Advances in imaging for diagnosis and management of cardiac sarcoidosis. Eur Heart J Cardiovasc Imaging 2015;16(9):949–58.

31. Schouver ED, Moceri P, Doyen D, et al. Early detection of cardiac involvement in sarcoidosis with 2-dimensional speckle-tracking echocardiography. Int J Cardiol 2017;227:711–6.

32. Murtagh G, Laffin LJ, Patel KV, et al. Improved detection of myocardial damage in sarcoidosis using longitudinal strain in patients with preserved left ventricular ejection fraction. Echocardiography 2016;33(9):1344–52.

33. Patel MR, Cawley PJ, Heitner JF, et al. Detection of myocardial damage in patients with sarcoidosis. Circulation 2009;120(20):1969–77.

34. Parsai C, O'Hanlon R, Prasad SK, et al. Diagnostic and prognostic value of cardiovascular magnetic resonance in non-ischaemic cardiomyopathies. J Cardiovasc Magn Reson 2012;14:54.

35. Shimada T, Shimada K, Sakane T, et al. Diagnosis of cardiac sarcoidosis and evaluation of the effects of steroid therapy by gadolinium-DTPA-enhanced magnetic resonance imaging. Am J Med 2001; 110(7):520–7.

36. Greulich S, Deluigi CC, Gloekler S, et al. CMR imaging predicts death and other adverse events in suspected cardiac sarcoidosis. JACC Cardiovasc Imaging 2013;6(4):501–11.

37. Ise T, Hasegawa T, Morita Y, et al. Extensive late gadolinium enhancement on cardiovascular magnetic resonance predicts adverse outcomes and lack of improvement in LV function after steroid therapy in cardiac sarcoidosis. Heart 2014;100(15): 1165–72.

38. Crouser ED, Ruden E, Julian MW, et al. Resolution of abnormal cardiac MRI T2 signal following immune suppression for cardiac sarcoidosis. J Investig Med 2016;64(6):1148–50.

39. Osborne MT, Hulten EA, Singh A, et al. Reduction in 18F-fluorodeoxyglucose uptake on serial cardiac positron emission tomography is associated with improved left ventricular ejection fraction in patients with cardiac sarcoidosis. J Nucl Cardiol 2014;21(1): 166–74.

40. Tahara N, Tahara A, Nitta Y, et al. Heterogeneous myocardial FDG uptake and the disease activity in cardiac sarcoidosis. JACC Cardiovasc Imaging 2010;3(12):1219–28.

41. Okumura W, Iwasaki T, Toyama T, et al. Usefulness of fasting 18F-FDG PET in identification of cardiac sarcoidosis. J Nucl Med 2004;45(12):1989–98.

42. Ahmadian A, Pawar S, Govender P, et al. The response of FDG uptake to immunosuppressive treatment on FDG PET/CT imaging for cardiac sarcoidosis. J Nucl Cardiol 2017;24(2):413–24.

43. Osborne MT, Hulten EA, Murthy VL, et al. Patient preparation for cardiac fluorine-18 fluorodeoxyglucose positron emission tomography imaging of inflammation. J Nucl Cardiol 2017;24(1):86–99.

44. Deva DP, Hanneman K, Li Q, et al. Cardiovascular magnetic resonance demonstration of the spectrum of morphological phenotypes and patterns of myocardial scarring in Anderson-Fabry disease. J Cardiovasc Magn Reson 2016;18:14.

45. Yeung DF, Sirrs S, Tsang MYC, et al. Echocardiographic assessment of patients with Fabry disease. J Am Soc Echocardiogr 2018;31(6):639–49.e2.

46. Niemann M, Liu D, Hu K, et al. Prominent papillary muscles in Fabry disease: a diagnostic marker? Ultrasound Med Biol 2011;37(1):37–43.

47. Krämer J, Niemann M, Liu D, et al. Two-dimensional speckle tracking as a non-invasive tool for identification of myocardial fibrosis in Fabry disease. Eur Heart J 2013;34(21):1587–96.

48. Liu D, Hu K, Niemann M, et al. Effect of combined systolic and diastolic functional parameter assessment for differentiation of cardiac amyloidosis from other causes of concentric left ventricular hypertrophy. Circ Cardiovasc Imaging 2013;6(6):1066–72.

49. Gujja P, Rosing DR, Tripodi DJ, et al. Iron overload cardiomyopathy: better understanding of an increasing disorder. J Am Coll Cardiol 2010;56(13):1001–12.

50. Hahalis G, Alexopoulos D, Kremastinos DT, et al. Heart failure in beta-thalassemia syndromes: a decade of progress. Am J Med 2005;118(9):957–67.

51. Palka P, Macdonald G, Lange A, et al. The role of Doppler left ventricular filling indexes and Doppler tissue echocardiography in the assessment of cardiac involvement in hereditary hemochromatosis. J Am Soc Echocardiogr 2002;15(9):884–90.

52. Cecchetti G, Binda A, Piperno A, et al. Cardiac alterations in 36 consecutive patients with idiopathic haemochromatosis: polygraphic and echocardiographic evaluation. Eur Heart J 1991;12(2):224–30.

53. Poorzand H, Manzari TS, Vakilian F, et al. Longitudinal strain in beta thalassemia major and its relation to the extent of myocardial iron overload in cardiovascular magnetic resonance. Arch Cardiovasc Imaging 2018 [Epub ahead of print]. Available at: http://www.cardiovascimaging.com/preprintarticle.asp?id=238934. Accessed September 9, 2018.

54. Wood JC. Magnetic resonance imaging measurement of iron overload. Curr Opin Hematol 2007;14(3):183–90.

55. Pennell DJ, Porter JB, Piga A, et al. A 1-year randomized controlled trial of deferasirox vs deferoxamine for myocardial iron removal in β-thalassemia major (CORDELIA). Blood 2014;123(10):1447–54.

56. Skouri HN, Dec GW, Friedrich MG, et al. Noninvasive imaging in myocarditis. J Am Coll Cardiol 2006;48(10):2085–93.

57. Pinamonti B, Alberti E, Cigalotto A, et al. Echocardiographic findings in myocarditis. Am J Cardiol 1988;62(4):285–91.

58. Mendes LA, Picard MH, Dec GW, et al. Ventricular remodeling in active myocarditis. Myocarditis treatment trial. Am Heart J 1999;138(2 Pt 1):303–8.

59. Mendes LA, Dec GW, Picard MH, et al. Right ventricular dysfunction: an independent predictor of adverse outcome in patients with myocarditis. Am Heart J 1994;128(2):301–7.

60. Løgstrup BB, Nielsen JM, Kim WY, et al. Myocardial oedema in acute myocarditis detected by echocardiographic 2D myocardial deformation analysis. Eur Heart J Cardiovasc Imaging 2016;17(9):1018–26.

61. Caforio AL, Pankuweit S, Arbustini E, et al. Current state of knowledge on aetiology, diagnosis, management, and therapy of myocarditis: a position statement of the European Society of Cardiology Working Group on Myocardial and Pericardial Diseases. Eur Heart J 2013;34(33):2636–48.

62. Thavendiranathan P, Walls M, Giri S, et al. Improved detection of myocardial involvement in acute inflammatory cardiomyopathies using T2 mapping. Circ Cardiovasc Imaging 2012;5(1):102–10.

63. Friedrich MG, Sechtem U, Schulz-Menger J, et al. Cardiovascular magnetic resonance in myocarditis: a JACC white paper. J Am Coll Cardiol 2009;53(17):1475–87.

64. Codreanu A, Djaballah W, Angioi M, et al. Detection of myocarditis by contrast-enhanced MRI in patients presenting with acute coronary syndrome but no coronary stenosis. J Magn Reson Imaging 2007;25(5):957–64.

65. Nensa F, Kloth J, Tezgah E, et al. Feasibility of FDG-PET in myocarditis: Comparison to CMR using integrated PET/MRI. J Nucl Cardiol 2018;25(3):785–94.

66. Plana JC, Galderisi M, Barac A, et al. Expert consensus for multimodality imaging evaluation of adult patients during and after cancer therapy: a report from the American Society of Echocardiography and the European Association of Cardiovascular Imaging. J Am Soc Echocardiogr 2014;27(9):911–39.

67. Seidman A, Hudis C, Pierri MK, et al. Cardiac dysfunction in the trastuzumab clinical trials experience. J Clin Oncol 2002;20(5):1215–21.

68. Thavendiranathan P, Grant AD, Negishi T, et al. Reproducibility of echocardiographic techniques for sequential assessment of left ventricular ejection fraction and volumes: application to patients undergoing cancer chemotherapy. J Am Coll Cardiol 2013;61(1):77–84.

69. Cardinale D, Colombo A, Bacchiani G, et al. Early detection of anthracycline cardiotoxicity and improvement with heart failure therapy. Circulation 2015;131(22):1981–8.

70. Thavendiranathan P, Poulin F, Lim KD, et al. Use of myocardial strain imaging by echocardiography for the early detection of cardiotoxicity in patients during and after cancer chemotherapy: a systematic review. J Am Coll Cardiol 2014;63(25PA):2751–68.

71. Huang H, Nijjar PS, Misialek JR, et al. Accuracy of left ventricular ejection fraction by contemporary multiple gated acquisition scanning in patients with cancer: comparison with cardiovascular magnetic resonance. J Cardiovasc Magn Reson 2017;19(1): 34.

72. D'Amore C, Gargiulo P, Paolillo S, et al. Nuclear imaging in detection and monitoring of cardiotoxicity. World J Radiol 2014;6(7):486–92.

73. Thavendiranathan P, Wintersperger BJ, Flamm SD, et al. Cardiac MRI in the assessment of cardiac injury and toxicity from cancer chemotherapy: a systematic review. Circ Cardiovasc Imaging 2013;6(6): 1080–91.

74. Kohan AA, Levy Yeyati E, De Stefano L, et al. Usefulness of MRI in Takotsubo cardiomyopathy: a review of the literature. Cardiovasc Diagn Ther 2014;4(2): 138–46.

75. Citro R, Rigo F, D'Andrea A, et al. Echocardiographic correlates of acute heart failure, cardiogenic shock, and in-hospital mortality in Takotsubo cardiomyopathy. JACC Cardiovasc Imaging 2014;7(2): 119–29.

76. Citro R, Bossone E, Parodi G, et al. Clinical profile and in-hospital outcome of Caucasian patients with Takotsubo syndrome and right ventricular involvement. Int J Cardiol 2016;219:455–61.

77. Izumo M, Akashi YJ. Role of echocardiography for Takotsubo cardiomyopathy: clinical and prognostic implications. Cardiovasc Diagn Ther 2018;8(1): 90–100.

78. Weiford BC, Subbarao VD, Mulhern KM. Noncompaction of the ventricular myocardium. Circulation 2004;109(24):2965–71.

79. Zuccarino F, Vollmer I, Sanchez G, et al. Left ventricular noncompaction: imaging findings and diagnostic criteria. AJR Am J Roentgenol 2015;204(5): W519–30.

80. Jenni R, Oechslin E, Schneider J, et al. Echocardiographic and pathoanatomical characteristics of isolated left ventricular non-compaction: a step towards classification as a distinct cardiomyopathy. Heart 2001;86(6):666–71.

81. Stöllberger C, Gerecke B, Finsterer J, et al. Refinement of echocardiographic criteria for left ventricular noncompaction. Int J Cardiol 2013;165:463–7.

82. van Dalen BM, Caliskan K, Soliman OI, et al. Diagnostic value of rigid body rotation in noncompaction cardiomyopathy. J Am Soc Echocardiogr 2011; 24(5):548–55.

83. Peters F, Khandheria BK, Libhaber E, et al. Left ventricular twist in left ventricular noncompaction. Eur Heart J Cardiovasc Imaging 2014;15(1):48–55.

84. Thavendiranathan P, Dahiya A, Phelan D, et al. Isolated left ventricular non-compaction controversies in diagnostic criteria, adverse outcomes and management. Heart 2013;99(10):681–9.

85. Thuny F, Jacquier A, Jop B, et al. Assessment of left ventricular non-compaction in adults: side-by-side comparison of cardiac magnetic resonance imaging with echocardiography. Arch Cardiovasc Dis 2010; 103(3):150–9.

86. Petersen SE, Selvanayagam JB, Wiesmann F, et al. Left ventricular non-compaction: insights from cardiovascular magnetic resonance imaging. J Am Coll Cardiol 2005;46(1):101–5.

87. Goo HW, Park IS. Left ventricular noncompaction in an infant: use of non-ECG-gated cardiac CT. Pediatr Radiol 2007;37(2):217–20.

Ultrasound of the Lungs
More than a Room with a View

Luna Gargani, MD, PhD

KEYWORDS

• Lung ultrasound • B-lines • Pulmonary congestion • Ultrasound lung comets • Heart failure

KEY POINTS

- B-lines are the sonographic sign of pulmonary edema.
- In patients with acute heart failure they can help in the diagnosis, monitoring, and prognosis.
- Persistent pulmonary congestion after a hospitalization for acute heart failure increases the risk of being rehospitalized soon.
- An integrated cardiopulmonary ultrasound allows establishing in a few minutes the degree of cardiac impairment, and the degree of decompensation.

LUNG ULTRASOUND: HOW IT WORKS

Ultrasound of the lung has not been used in clinical practice since about the last 15 years. It is common knowledge that air is a foe to ultrasound, therefore imaging an organ full of air was considered not feasible.[1] It is true that in a normally aerated lung, ultrasound can only convey an indirect image of the pulmonary parenchyma, which is still informative. If the lung is normally aerated or overaerated, one can only visualize the pleura as a hyperechoic horizontal line, which moves synchronously with respiration (**Fig. 1**A). This movement is called "lung sliding" and is the sonographic depiction of the respiratory movement.

Below the pleural line it is impossible to visualize any other structure, because the high acoustic interface between air and the surrounding tissues is so high that the ultrasound beam is completely reflected back. When the air content decreases because the pulmonary interstitium or alveolar space is occupied by transudate, essudate, blood, or other tissues, the acoustic mismatch also decreases and the ultrasound beam can partially penetrate below the pleura. One can now visualize some hyperechoic vertical reverberation artifacts called B-lines (previously also called "ultrasound lung comets").[2] Although the physical basis of ultrasound is not clearly elucidated,[3] the main hypothesis is that, on a general basis, the less air in the lung, the more B-lines seen (**Fig. 1**B, C). When the air content is completely lost, as in a consolidation, one can then directly visualize the pulmonary parenchyma, which appears as a solid organ, with an echogenity similar to the liver (**Fig. 1**D).

Accordingly, one should consider lung ultrasound (LUS) as a kind of "densitometer" of the pulmonary parenchyma, resulting in the following patterns:

- The normal or overaerated lung, imaged as the pleural line without significant B-lines or consolidations below (see **Fig. 1**A)
- The partially deaerated lung, imaged as a variable number of multiple B-lines (usually at least three in a scanning site) (see **Fig. 1**B, C)
- The completely deaerated lung, imaged as a consolidation (see **Fig. 1**D)

Similarly, to what happens with chest radiograph and sometimes even with computed tomography, these different levels of aeration are not characteristic for a single condition; this makes LUS patterns nonspecific, underlining the need of interpreting these images in the context of the

Disclosure: The author receives speaker honoraria from Glaxo-Smith-Kline and General Electric.
Institute of Clinical Physiology, National Research Council, Via Moruzzi, 1, Pisa 56124, Italy
E-mail address: gargani@ifc.cnr.it

Heart Failure Clin 15 (2019) 297–303
https://doi.org/10.1016/j.hfc.2018.12.010

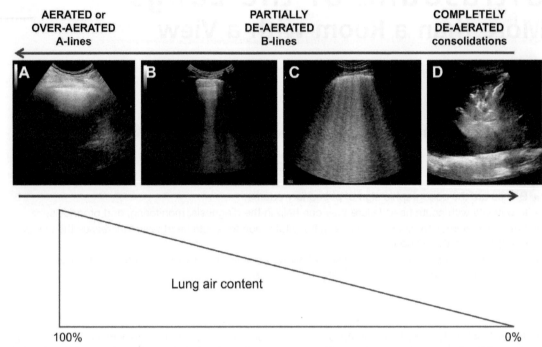

| AERATED or OVER-AERATED A-lines | PARTIALLY DE-AERATED B-lines | COMPLETELY DE-AERATED consolidations |

Fig. 1. (A–D) The concept of lung ultrasound as a densitometer: different ultrasound patterns for different levels of lung aeration.

patient's clinical picture, which is advisable for any kind of examination.

LUNG ULTRASOUND IN HEART FAILURE: THE TECHNIQUE

To assess B-lines one has to place the ultrasound probe in the intercostal spaces. There are two main scanning approaches: the longitudinal and the transverse (oblique) scan. In the longitudinal scan the ribs and their shadow are usually part of the image (Fig. 2A), whereas the transverse approach allows visualizing a larger part of the pleural line, which is not interrupted by the rib shadows (Fig. 2B). The reference point to refer to is the pleural line with its lung sliding: without a clear visualization of the lung sliding, it is impossible to infer reliable information about the lung aeration.

Different clinical settings may need different scanning approaches. If LUS is done to help in the differential diagnosis of acute dyspnea, a simple scanning scheme can be used, including eight thoracic areas (Fig. 3A). In each area the B-lines should be searched for and, if possible, enumerated. With this approach, a region is considered "positive" for B-lines when three or more B-lines are visible in a longitudinal plane between two ribs, and an examination is considered positive when at least two regions bilaterally are positive.

In patients with heart failure (HF), where LUS can be used not only for the diagnosis but also for monitoring and prognostic stratification, a more complete scanning scheme has been often used (Fig. 3B). This scheme includes 28 scanning sites, 16 on the right and 12 on the left side (where the presence of the heart usually prevents the assessment of a few scanning sites). When B-lines are clearly distinguishable (usually when they are one, two, or three in a scanning site), they are easily counted. When they are more numerous, they tend to be confluent and overlapping, so counting them one by one is less easy. It is possible to obtain a semiquantification of the sign, using an easy rule of thumb: consider the percentage of the scanning site occupied by B-lines (ie, the percentage of white screen compared with black screen below the pleural line) and then divide it by 10 (ie, 30% of "B-lines hyperechogenicity" corresponds to about three B-lines, 70% corresponds to about seven B-lines, and so on [Fig. 4]).[2]

This counting method, although apparently not so precise, allows at least a semiquantification of B-lines, and has shown to be correlated to dyspnea severity,[4] chest radiograph congestion score,[5] lung density on high-resolution computed tomography,[6] echocardiographic parameters,[4] extravascular lung water (EVLW) and PCWP as assessed invasively,[7] and postmortem lung gravimetric wet/dry ratio,[8] and to convey prognostic

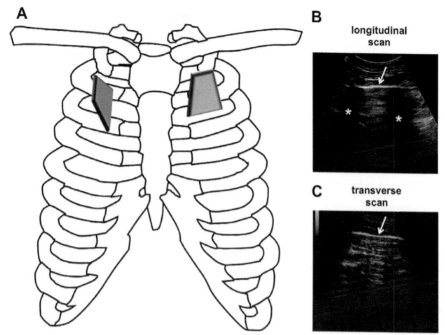

longitudinal
scan

transverse
scan

Fig. 2. Different probe positions to scan the lung. (*A*) The lungs shown with probes. (*B*) The longitudinal approach. (*C*) The transverse approach. The *asterisks* indicate the ribs' shadows. The *white arrows* indicate the pleural line.

information.[9–12] The method has been usually applied to B-lines imaged by cardiac probes, but is also applied to B-lines imaged by convex probes.

LUNG ULTRASOUND IN HEART FAILURE: DIAGNOSIS

LUS is useful to support the diagnosis of acute HF (AHF), especially in the differential diagnosis of acute dyspnea. If the dyspnea is caused, at least in part, by EVLW inducing pulmonary interstitial edema, diffuse, bilateral multiple B-lines must be visible. "Multiple" means that at least three B-lines must be visualized in a scanning area; "diffuse" means that multiple B-lines should be present in at least two adjacent scanning areas; "bilateral" means that a pattern of diffuse B-lines should be visible on the right and left hemithorax.

When multiple B-lines are detected only in one hemithorax, the situation is defined as "focal interstitial syndrome."[13] A focal interstitial syndrome is the first sonographic sign of the perilesional interstitial edema around a consolidation that is being formed. Focal interstitial edema can also be present in healthy subjects, as the sonographic sign of a small deaerated area possibly linked to previous pulmonary parenchymal involvement. The correlation with the clinical picture is crucial and the presence or absence of symptoms helps to interpret these imaging findings.

The look of the pleural line is also important in the differential diagnosis of acute dyspnea. In patients with AHF, multiple diffuse bilateral B-lines arise from a pleural line with a normal sonographic appearance, which means a hyperechoic, thin, regular line (**Fig. 5**A). If multiple bilateral B-lines arise from an irregular pleural line, the diagnosis of AHF is less likely. A frankly irregular pleural line is typical of noncardiogenic pulmonary edema, such as in acute lung injury/acute respiratory distress syndrome, as the sonographic pattern of essudate edema (**Fig. 5**B).[14] An irregular pleural line with multiple B-lines can also be detected in interstitial pulmonary fibrosis, where the subpleural interlobular septa is thickened by collagen tissue deposition (**Fig. 5**C).[15] In acute lung injury/acute respiratory distress syndrome the irregular appearance of the pleural line is usually linked to small subpleural consolidations; one can somehow consider this pattern as the sign of a more "alveolar" involvement compared with the typical interstitial involvement in early phases of AHF. However, the sonographic picture looks similar. From a practical point of view, finding diffuse bilateral B-lines arising from a distinctly irregular pleural line in a patient with a suspicion of AHF should raise the doubt that the condition determining dyspnea is not (at least not only) cardiogenic.

In a large multicentric prospective study on 2683 patients admitted to the emergency department with acute dyspnea, LUS added to the standard

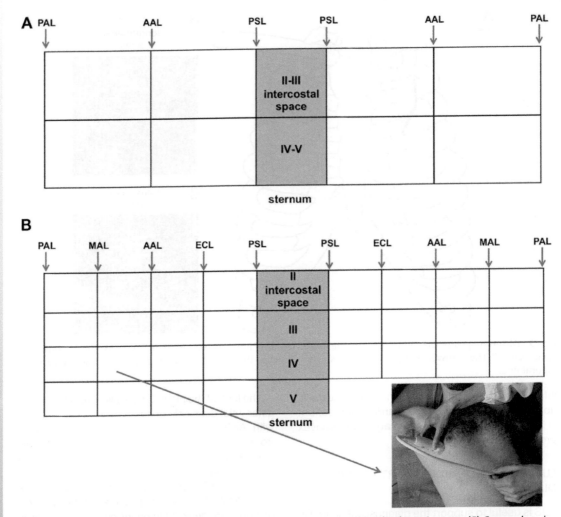

Fig. 3. Different ultrasound scanning scheme. (*A*) Simplified scheme with eight thoracic areas. (*B*) Comprehensive scheme with 28 scanning sites. AAL, anterior axillary line; ECL, midclavicular line; MAL, medium axillary line; PAL, posterior axillary line; PSL, parasternal line.

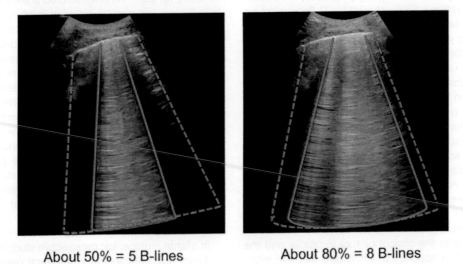

About 50% = 5 B-lines   About 80% = 8 B-lines

Fig. 4. How to quantify B-lines.

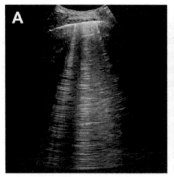 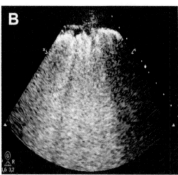 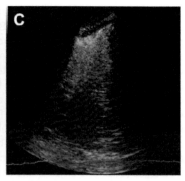

Fig. 5. Different etiologies of B-lines. (*A*) Cardiogenic pulmonary edema. (*B*) Noncardiogenic pulmonary edema. (*C*) Pulmonary fibrosis.

clinical evaluation improved the accuracy of AHF diagnosis (sensitivity and specificity = 97%), with a net reclassification index of the LUS-implemented approach compared with the standard work-up of 19.1%.[16] LUS integrated in a point-of-care ultrasound approach to acute dyspnea/acute chest pain determines a significant reduction in the time needed for the correct diagnosis; in another large study, adding the presence of multiple, bilateral B-lines increases the sensitivity of the diagnosis of AHF from 77% (standard evaluation) to 88% (*P*<.001), with a slight reduction in specificity (98 vs 96%; *P*<.001).[17]

LUNG ULTRASOUND IN HEART FAILURE: MONITORING

LUS is a promising tool to monitor changes in pulmonary congestion in AHF.[9,18,19] The sign is dynamic, because significant changes in B-lines number have been reported even only 1 to 2 hours after diuretic therapy,[19] and before and after a dialysis session[20] or, on the contrary, after a few minutes exercise.

LUS is particularly suitable for monitoring decongestion, being a noninvasive, bedside, user-friendly examination, and therefore convenient to assess even rapid changes of EVLW. The tool seems promising also to guide diuretic therapy, but no study has specifically addressed this issues.[21] Some preliminary data have shown that using LUS during AHF hospitalization to monitor decongestion led to a shorter discharge time compared with patients with standard care, including chest radiograph at admission and at discharge.[22]

The advantage of using LUS for monitoring pulmonary congestion in AHF is also linked to the possibility of reducing ionizing radiation exposure caused by serial chest radiograph, although the dose of a single chest radiograph is small, about 0.02 mSv for a single posteroanterior film.[23]

LUNG ULTRASOUND IN HEART FAILURE: PROGNOSIS

LUS B-lines have a prognostic role in patients with HF, both in inpatients and in outpatients. Persistent B-lines at discharge after a hospitalization for AHF predict readmission for decompensated HF at 3 and 6 months.[9,10,24,25] Similarly, outpatients with a higher number of B-lines during routine ambulatory office visit are more prone to be readmitted for decompensated HF in the following months.[12,26] This underlines the importance of recognizing those patients that may be "flying under the radar" after discharge, that is, patients without clinical congestion but with elevated left ventricular filling pressures often reflected by the high levels of natriuretic peptides, who may start accumulating EVLW.[27] In these patients assessment of B-lines can be performed alone, as an extension of the physical examination, or combined in an integrated cardiopulmonary assessment when the HF patient is referred to routine echocardiography.

LUNG ULTRASOUND: NOT ONLY B-LINES

LUS offers the possibility to detect other sonographic pulmonary patterns that are useful to the cardiologist. In the differential diagnosis of acute dyspnea, LUS can display a lung consolidation that may help define the correct diagnosis. If the patient has pneumonia and the consolidation reaches the pleura at some point, the "hepatized" pulmonary parenchyma is easily visible and orients the diagnosis. Typical pneumonic consolidations have blurred margins, irregular shape, and usually display an air bronchogram (the sonographic appearance of the "tree-like" bronchial branches inside the consolidation).[13] Pulmonary infarction caused by pulmonary embolism also yields a consolidation, which is, however, more regularly shaped and with more defined margins.

Acute chest pain is another situation where the cardiologist may benefit from LUS. If the chest pain is not of ischemic origin, LUS can visualize a small pleural effusion or a consolidation. In particular, if the pain has pleuritic characteristics and no LUS abnormalities are visualized in the area of the chest pain, a consolidation as the cause of pleuritic pain is practically excluded.[28] Pneumothorax is another cause of acute chest pain or hemodynamic instability and is detected by LUS as an absence of lung sliding and absence of any other LUS signs (even one small B-line or consolidation) below the area of pneumothorax.[29]

INTEGRATED CARDIOPULMONARY ULTRASOUND

Point-of-care echo is by definition a multiorgan approach, when feasible. Having the chance to scan the lung at the end of an echocardiogram is of great value to understand the ongoing cardiac issues and the degree of compensation of a patient. Adding LUS even to the simple inferior vena cava assessment significantly increases the accuracy of the diagnosis of AHF.[30]

Patients with the same degree of systolic and diastolic dysfunction may exhibit different degrees of EVLW, related to the complex interaction between the Starling forces, the alveolar capillary membrane status, and the lymphatic drainage. Completing the echocardiographic assessment with a lung scan can provide unique information on the hemodynamic consequences of a myocardial or valvular impairment in the same examination.[31] In specific clinical settings multiorgan point-of-care echo is of great value to fasten the appropriate diagnosis, sometimes even just helping in excluding life-threatening conditions.[32]

In patients with a clinical suspicion of acute pulmonary embolism, the point-of-care integration of a focused assessment of the heart (to assess the presence of a significant dilation/dysfunction of the right ventricle), of the lung (to detect a pulmonary infarction or focal interstitial syndrome), and of the leg veins (to detect a thrombus) can convey a good sensitivity and specificity.[33]

SUMMARY

LUS is one of the main revolutions in imaging in the last few years. Its versatility and user-friendly approach[34] make this tool appealing as a valuable integration to the stethoscope, as part of the fifth pillar of physical examination.[35] B-lines, the sonographic pattern of partial deaeration of the lung, are used at any stage of the management of patients with HF: from diagnosis to differentiate

AHF from other causes of dyspnea, to monitor decongestion during treatment, and for prognostic stratification. Integrating B-lines assessment to echocardiography as a cardiopulmonary ultrasound assessment is helpful in establishing not only the kind and degree of cardiac impairment, but also the hemodynamic consequences as pulmonary edema.

REFERENCES

1. Lichtenstein D, Meziere G, Biderman P, et al. The comet-tail artifact. An ultrasound sign of alveolar-interstitial syndrome. Am J Respir Crit Care Med 1997;156:1640–6.
2. Gargani L, Volpicelli G. How I do it: lung ultrasound. Cardiovasc Ultrasound 2014;12:25.
3. Soldati G, Demi M, Inchingolo R, et al. On the physical basis of pulmonary sonographic interstitial syndrome. J Ultrasound Med 2016;35:2075–86.
4. Frassi F, Gargani L, Gligorova S, et al. Clinical and echocardiographic determinants of ultrasound lung comets. Eur J Echocardiogr 2007;8:474–9.
5. Jambrik Z, Monti S, Coppola V, et al. Usefulness of ultrasound lung comets as a nonradiologic sign of extravascular lung water. Am J Cardiol 2004;93:1265–70.
6. Baldi G, Gargani L, Abramo A, et al. Lung water assessment by lung ultrasonography in intensive care: a pilot study. Intensive Care Med 2013;39:74–84.
7. Agricola E, Bove T, Oppizzi M, et al. "Ultrasound comet-tail images": a marker of pulmonary edema: a comparative study with wedge pressure and extravascular lung water. Chest 2005;127:1690–5.
8. Jambrik Z, Gargani L, Adamicza A, et al. B-lines quantify the lung water content: a lung ultrasound versus lung gravimetry study in acute lung injury. Ultrasound Med Biol 2010;36:2004–10.
9. Gargani L, Pang PS, Frassi F, et al. Persistent pulmonary congestion before discharge predicts rehospitalization in heart failure: a lung ultrasound study. Cardiovasc Ultrasound 2015;13:40.
10. Coiro S, Rossignol P, Ambrosio G, et al. Prognostic value of residual pulmonary congestion at discharge assessed by lung ultrasound imaging in heart failure. Eur J Heart Fail 2015;17:1172–81.
11. Miglioranza MH, Gargani L, Sant'anna RT, et al. Pulmonary congestion evaluated by lung ultrasound predicts admission in patients with heart failure. Eur Heart J 2013;34:P665.
12. Platz E, Lewis EF, Uno H, et al. Detection and prognostic value of pulmonary congestion by lung ultrasound in ambulatory heart failure patients. Eur Heart J 2016;37:1244–51.
13. Volpicelli G, Elbarbary M, Blaivas M, et al. International evidence-based recommendations for point-

of-care lung ultrasound. Intensive Care Med 2012; 38:577–91.

14. Copetti R, Soldati G, Copetti P. Chest sonography: a useful tool to differentiate acute cardiogenic pulmonary edema from acute respiratory distress syndrome. Cardiovasc Ultrasound 2008;6:16.

15. Gargani L, Doveri M, D'Errico L, et al. Ultrasound lung comets in systemic sclerosis: a chest sonography hallmark of pulmonary interstitial fibrosis. Rheumatology (Oxford) 2009;48:1382–7.

16. Pivetta E, Goffi A, Lupia E, et al. Lung ultrasound-implemented diagnosis of acute decompensated heart failure in the ED: a SIMEU multicenter study. Chest 2015;148:202–10.

17. Zanobetti M. Point-of-care ultrasonography for evaluation of acute dyspnea in the emergency department. Chest 2017;151:1295–301.

18. Volpicelli G, Caramello V, Cardinale L, et al. Bedside ultrasound of the lung for the monitoring of acute decompensated heart failure. Am J Emerg Med 2008; 26:585–91.

19. Martindale JL, Secko M, Kilpatrick JF, et al. Serial sonographic assessment of pulmonary edema in patients with hypertensive acute heart failure. J Ultrasound Med 2018;37(2):337–45.

20. Donadio C, Bozzoli L, Colombini E, et al. Effective and timely evaluation of pulmonary congestion: qualitative comparison between lung ultrasound and thoracic bioelectrical impedance in maintenance hemodialysis patients. Medicine (Baltimore) 2015;94:e473.

21. Agricola E, Marini C. Lung ultrasound predicts decompensation in heart failure outpatients: another piece to the puzzle but still an incomplete picture. Int J Cardiol 2017;240:324–5.

22. Mozzini C, Di Dio Perna M, Pesce G, et al. Lung ultrasound in internal medicine efficiently drives the management of patients with heart failure and speeds up the discharge time. Intern Emerg Med 2018;13(1):27–33.

23. Gargani L, Picano E. The risk of cumulative radiation exposure in chest imaging and the advantage of bedside ultrasound. Crit Ultrasound J 2015;7:4.

24. Cogliati C, Casazza G, Ceriani E, et al. Lung ultrasound and short-term prognosis in heart failure patients. Int J Cardiol 2016;218:104–8.

25. Gargani L. Prognosis in heart failure: look at the lungs. Eur J Heart Fail 2015;17:1086–8.

26. Miglioranza MH, Picano E, Badano LP, et al. Pulmonary congestion evaluated by lung ultrasound predicts decompensation in heart failure outpatients. Int J Cardiol 2017;240:271–8.

27. Gheorghiade M, Vaduganathan M, Fonarow GC, et al. Rehospitalization for heart failure. J Am Coll Cardiol 2013;61:391–403.

28. Volpicelli G, Cardinale L, Berchialla P, et al. A comparison of different diagnostic tests in the bedside evaluation of pleuritic pain in the ED. Am J Emerg Med 2012;30:317–24.

29. Lichtenstein D, Meziere G, Biderman P, et al. The comet-tail artifact: an ultrasound sign ruling out pneumothorax. Intensive Care Med 1999;25:383–8.

30. Kajimoto K, Madeen K, Nakayama T, et al. Rapid evaluation by lung-cardiac-inferior vena cava (LCI) integrated ultrasound for differentiating heart failure from pulmonary disease as the cause of acute dyspnea in the emergency setting. Cardiovasc Ultrasound 2012;10:49.

31. Gargani L. Lung ultrasound: a new tool for the cardiologist. Cardiovasc Ultrasound 2011;9:6.

32. Volpicelli G, Lamorte A, Tullio M, et al. Point-of-care multiorgan ultrasonography for the evaluation of undifferentiated hypotension in the emergency department. Intensive Care Med 2013;39:1290–8.

33. Nazerian P, Vanni S, Volpicelli G, et al. Accuracy of point-of-care multiorgan ultrasonography for the diagnosis of pulmonary embolism. Chest 2014;145:950–7.

34. McBeth PB, Crawford I, Blaivas M, et al. Simple, almost anywhere, with almost anyone: remote low-cost telementored resuscitative lung ultrasound. J Trauma 2011;71:1528–35.

35. Narula J, Chandrashekhar Y, Braunwald E. Time to add a fifth pillar to bedside physical examination: inspection, palpation, percussion, auscultation, and insonation. JAMA Cardiol 2018;3:346–50.

Imaging Device Therapy
Essentials for the Imager

Thura T. Harfi, MD, MPH*, Michael Wesley Milks, MD, David A. Orsinelli, MD, Subha V. Raman, MD, William T. Abraham, MD, Rami Kahwash, MD

KEYWORDS

- Interventional imaging • Left ventricular assist device • Mechanical circulatory support
- Extracorporeal membrane oxygenation • InterAtrial Shunt Device • Corvia

KEY POINTS

- There has been a rapid increase in the number of mechanical devices used for management of patients with heart failure, such as devices intended to provide short- or long-term mechanical circulatory support (Impella, extracorporeal membrane oxygenation, and left ventricular assist devices), monitoring surrogates of left ventricle filling pressure (PA pressure Sensors), or unloading the left ventricle (eg, interatrial shunt devices).
- Imaging is essential for the appropriate use of these devices, including for patient selection, intraoperative guidance, and postoperative surveillance and complication detection. Echocardiography (transthoracic and transesophageal) is the predominant imaging modality during these phases. Cardiac imaging specialists with knowledge and experience in the intended function and potential complications associated with these devices are essential to any successful advanced heart failure program in the current era.

 Video content accompanies this article at http://www.heartfailure.theclinics.com.

INTRODUCTION

Heart failure (HF) is an epidemic that is increasing in prevalence and is associated with high mortality, morbidity and hospital readmission rate. Recent advances in therapies for HF with reduced ejection fraction (HFrEF) include neurohormonal modulators and device-based treatments aimed at preventing sudden cardiac death and restoring cardiac synchrony. Despite these, many patients remain symptomatic and gradually succumb to end-stage pump failure (stage D), requiring heart transplantation in highly selected candidates or implantation of partial or complete mechanical circulatory support devices. Although several strategies to detect early signs of HF decompensation have been studied, direct measurement of the pulmonary artery pressure by an implantable hemodynamic sensor is the only strategy that is currently proven to reduce HF readmissions. HF with preserved EF (HFpEF) is a challenging condition and a growing epidemic manifested by backward failure caused by delayed relaxation and decreased ventricular compliance, which lead to increased left-sided filling pressures. Although medical therapy has been disappointing in treating this condition, several investigational devices have recently been proposed with the goal of reducing left-sided filling pressures by creating a small interatrial shunt. Because elevated left-sided filling pressure is also present in HFrEF, this strategy is also being investigated in the HFrEF population.

Because of the recent surge in the number of devices used in HF management and

Disclosure: The authors have nothing to disclose.
Division of Cardiology, Department of Medicine, The Ohio State University Wexner Medical Center, The Ohio State University, 473 West 12th Avenue, Suite 200, Columbus, OH 43210, USA
* Corresponding author.
E-mail address: thura.harfi@osumc.edu

Heart Failure Clin 15 (2019) 305–320
https://doi.org/10.1016/j.hfc.2018.12.011
1551-7136/19/© 2018 Elsevier Inc. All rights reserved.

hemodynamic monitoring, cardiologists are increasingly faced with the challenges of performing and interpreting diagnostic testing on patients who receive such devices. This article summarizes key aspects of interpreting cardiac imaging of patients who received partial or complete circulatory support devices, pulmonary artery hemodynamic sensors, or interatrial septal devices.

LEFT VENTRICULAR ASSIST DEVICES

Left ventricular assist devices (LVADs) have become a vital part of therapies for patients with advanced HF. LVADs can be used as a bridge to transplantation, destination therapy, or bridge to transplant candidacy or myocardial recovery. Transthoracic echocardiography (TTE) and transesophageal echocardiography (TEE) play essential roles in the clinical care of LVAD patients at multiple stages, including preoperative patient selection, perioperative imaging and postoperative surveillance, optimization of LVAD function, and complication and LVAD alarm management.[1] Computed tomography (CT) has also proven critical in selected LVAD complications such as thrombosis.

There are 2 main types of LVADs that are approved by the US Food and Drug Administration (FDA) and commonly used for surgical implantation in adults: the HeartMate II (Thoratec Corporation, Pleasanton, California) and the HeartWare HVAD (HeartWare Incorporated, Framingham, Massachusetts). All LVAD types have 3 main components: the inflow cannula located in the left ventricle, a mechanical impeller, and an outflow cannula that is anastomosed to the ascending aorta (Fig. 1).

Role of Echocardiography in Left Ventricular Assist Device Candidate Selection

A complete transthoracic echocardiogram is mandatory for evaluation of LVAD candidacy. TTE is used to evaluate LVEF, LV size, presence of intracardiac thrombi, right ventricular (RV) systolic function, and presence of any significant valvular disease. The American Society of Echocardiography has identified several echocardiographic parameters that are identified as preimplantation red flag findings (Box 1). These findings are not contraindications for LVAD therapy, but rather they indicate that special attention and consideration are needed during the LVAD candidate selection.

Patients who are candidates for LVAD therapy generally have severely reduced LVEF and high risk of LV thrombus. TTE is the initial step in the diagnosis of LV thrombus. However, TTE and

TEE, even with the use of echocardiographic contrast agents, have limited sensitivity for the detection of LV thrombi.[2] In these patients, cardiac MRI (CMR) or cardiac CT, especially when CMR is not possible because of the presence of an implantable cardioverter defibrillator (ICD), can help detect LV thrombus with much higher sensitivity (Fig. 2, Video 1).

Evaluation of Right Ventricular Function Prior to Left Ventricular Assist Device Implantation

RV failure (RVF) following LVAD implantation remains a common clinical problem in LVAD patients, occurring in about 10% to 44% of cases[3] and associated with poor outcome.[4,5]

The echocardiographic report before LVAD implantation should include, at minimum, a qualitative assessment of the RV size and systolic function and tricuspid regurgitation severity. Other measures of RV systolic function can be reported whenever possible, such as RV fractional area change, tricuspid annular-plane systolic excursion (TAPSE), tricuspid valve annulus systolic velocity (S'), and RV free wall peak longitudinal strain[6] (Fig. 3).

Some studies suggest that several preoperative echocardiographic parameters are predictive of severe postoperative RV dysfunction, such as absolute RV peak longitudinal strain of less than

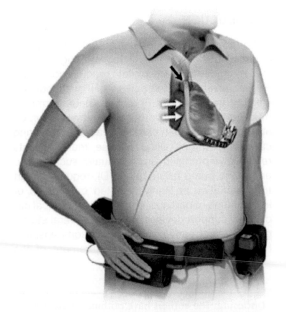

: HeartWare

Fig. 1. Illustration of the HVAD demonstrating the intrapericardial pump location, outflow graft position, and outflow graft-to-ascending aorta anastomosis. (*Reproduced with permission* of Medtronic, Inc.)

<table>
<tr><td>

Box 1
Preimplantation transthoracic/ transesophageal echocardiographic "red flag" findings

Left ventricle and interventricular septum

  Small LV size, particularly with increased LV trabeculation

  LV thrombus

  LV apical aneurysm

  Ventricular septal defect

Right ventricle

  RV dilatation

  RV systolic dysfunction

Atria, interatrial septum, and inferior vena cava

  Left atrial appendage thrombus

  PFO or atrial septal defect

Valvular abnormalities

  Any prosthetic valve (especially mechanical AV or MV)

  > mild AR

  ≥ moderate MS

  ≥ moderate TR or > mild TS

  > mild PS; ≥ moderate PR

Other

  Any congenital heart disease

  Aortic pathology: aneurysm, dissection, atheroma, coarctation

  Mobile mass lesion

  Other shunts: patent ductus arteriosus, intrapulmonary

Abbreviations: AR, aortic regurgitation; AV, aortic valve; MS, mitral stenosis; MV, mitral valve; PFO, patent foramen ovale; PR, pulmonary regurgitation; PS, pulmonary stenosis; TR, tricuspid regurgitation; TS, tricuspid regurgitation.

From Stainback RF, Estep JD, Agler DA, et al. Echocardiography in the management of patients with left ventricular assist devices: recommendations from the American Society of Echocardiography. J Am Soc Echocardiogr 2015;28(8):857; with permission.

</td></tr>
</table>

9.6% and an RV:LV end diastolic diameter ratio of greater than 0.75.[7] However, in general, there is no single variable that reliably identifies patients who will develop RVF after LVAD. Therefore, multiple echocardiographic parameters, in combination with hemodynamic and clinical data, should be used to form a comprehensive evaluation of RV systolic function.[8]

Perioperative Left Ventricular Assist Device Imaging

TEE plays a critical role in the perioperative management of LVAD patients. The role of TEE in peri-implantation LVAD management can be divided into preimplantation and immediate postimplantation phases.

Preimplantation phase

Comprehensive TEE should be performed in the operating room before LVAD implantation. It is an important examination to confirm the TTE findings and to identify potentially undiagnosed or underappreciated pathologic conditions. Careful reevaluation of aortic regurgitation, RV function, tricuspid regurgitation (TR) severity, intracardiac shunts such as Patent Foramen Ovale (PFO), and presence of intracardiac thrombi should be performed.

Acute postimplantation phase

The role of TEE in the immediate postimplantation period is to confirm the appropriate placement of inflow and outflow cannulas and to detect early specific LVAD-related complications or echocardiographic changes (**Figs. 4** and **5**, Videos 2–4). Certain caveats are important to recognize in LVAD imaging during the immediate postimplantation period:

1. Detection of PFO: careful re-examination for PFO is necessary, as the presence of PFO can in some cases be unmasked after implantation, because of the accompanying decrease in the left atrial (LA) pressure.
2. Aortic regurgitation: the degree of any preexisting aortic regurgitation usually worsens after LVAD implantation because of the reduction the LV filling pressures and the increase in central aortic pressure (**Fig. 6**).
3. Detection of RVF, which can be caused by underlying RV dysfunction, cardiopulmonary bypass (CPB) related factors, or high LVAD speed. RVF is usually seen concurrent with worsening TR (Videos 5 and 6).
4. Detection of inflow cannula location, orientation, and flow: normal position of the inflow cannula should be near the apex facing the mitral valve inflow. Slight, but not severe, deviation toward the septum is acceptable. Normal flow should be less than 1.5 m/s and laminar (see **Fig. 4**, Videos 2 and 3). Measurement of HVAD inflow velocity is obscured by a typical Doppler artifact (**Figs. 7** and **8**).
5. Detection of outflow cannula location and flow: flow should also be laminar and unidirectional with some systolic augmentation. An outflow

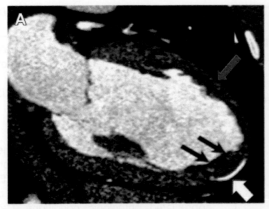
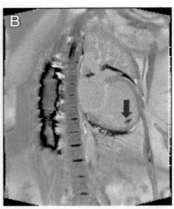

Fig. 2. (A) contrast-enhanced cardiac CT showing the heart in typical 2-chamber view with a layered thrombus in the apex and distal inferior wall (*black arrows*). Note also the thinning of the mid and distal anterior wall and distal inferior walls (*red arrow*) with calcific changes in the necrotic apical myocardium (*white arrow*). The patient had a prior large infarction with resultant severe cardiomyopathy. (B) Late gadolinium-enhanced (LGE) image showing no LGE uptake by the mass (*red arrow*), supporting the diagnosis of LV thrombus.

graft peak systolic velocity of greater than 2 m/s is usually abnormal and warrants further investigation or monitoring, as it can suggest obstruction (see **Fig. 5**, Video 4).

Cardiac Imaging After Left Ventricular Assist Device Implantation

Similar to perioperative LVAD management, TTE is the cornerstone of cardiac imaging in patients with LVADs in the postimplantation period. All patients with LVADs should undergo routine TTE surveillance. This should be done at either 2 weeks after implantation or prior to hospital discharge (if earlier than 2 weeks). The American Society of Echocardiography recommends LVAD surveillance TTE at 1, 3, 6, and 12 months, then every 6 to 12 months thereafter.[1] Surveillance TTE should include a general TTE and also certain LVAD-specific images, with special attention to LV and

RV size and systolic function, valvular function (especially aortic regurgitation), frequency and duration of AV opening, interventricular septal position, and inflow cannula and outflow graft interrogation.

Typically, TEE of a normally functioning LVAD should show the interventricular septum in a midline position and the aortic valve opening intermittently. A leftward shift can be caused by elevated RV end diastolic pressures, reduced LV preload, or LV overdecompression resulting from excessive LVAD speed.

A rightward shift is generally caused by elevated LV end-diastolic pressures resulting from an inadequate LVAD speed setting, pump dysfunction, severe aortic regurgitation, or increased LV afterload such as systemic hypertension. New moderate mitral regurgitation might suggest insufficient unloading of the LV while moderate or severe TR

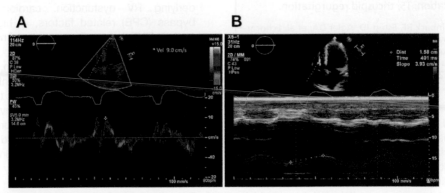

Fig. 3. Quantitative parameters for RV function in an LVAD candidate. (A) shows that the tricuspid valve annulus velocity S prime is reduced (normal >10 cm/s). (B) tricuspid annular-plane systolic excursion (TAPSE) is also reduced at 1.6 (normal >1.6 cm). Both parameters suggest mild RV systolic dysfunction.

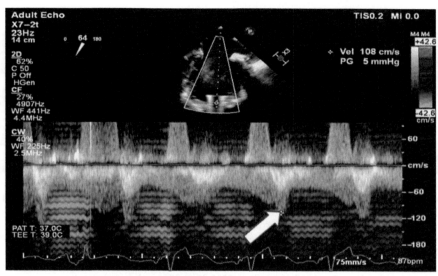

Fig. 4. Continuous-wave spectral Doppler interrogation of the inflow cannula (to screen for inflow obstruction) shows normal inflow-cannula systolic flow (*white arrow*).

might suggest RVF or high LVAD speed, especially if associated with rightward septal deviation. Inflow cannula velocity should remain less than 1.5 m/s. Fluctuation of inflow velocities that tracks with the cardiac cycle is expected because of intrinsic LV function. Higher velocities suggest possible inflow cannula obstruction. HVAD inflow cannula velocities cannot be accurately measured because of a characteristic Doppler artifact caused by the direct connection of the inflow cannula to the adjacent impeller housing (see **Fig. 7**).

Visualizing the outflow graft anastomosis to the aorta is usually challenging and requires the use of atypical echocardiographic windows such as high left parasternal views. Outflow graft velocities of greater than 2 m/s at any level may be abnormal

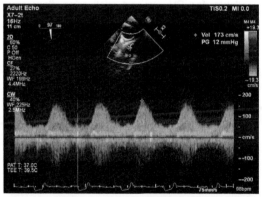

Fig. 5. Continuous wave Doppler signal of the outflow cannula on TEE showing normal peak systolic velocity of less than 200 cm/s suggesting unobstructed flow.

and warrant further consideration for possible obstruction, although benchmark data are lacking. The outflow graft flow velocity of the HVAD exceeds that of the HM II because of graft size, with outflow grafts measuring 1.0 cm (HVAD) and 1.6 cm (HM II) (See **Fig. 8**).

Left Ventricular Outflow Tract Optimization Echocardiography (Speed Ramp Test)

LVAD optimization echocardiography can be performed in asymptomatic patients with no device alarms or other clinical indicators of abnormal LVAD or cardiac function. It includes routine comprehensive TTE at the baseline speed setting followed by stepwise incremental adjustments to the LVAD speed in revolutions per minute (RPM). Several echo parameters are collected at each new speed, such as LV internal dimension in diastole (LVIDd), interventricular septal position, AV opening frequency/duration, and TR or MR severity. A typical optimization protocol (speed ramp test) as suggested by the American Society of Echocardiography is shown (**Box 2, Fig. 9**).[1]

Left Ventricular Assist Device Problem-Focused Echocardiographic Examination

A problem-focused echocardiographic examination should be obtained whenever there is a new or abnormally persistent symptom, LVAD alarm, or clinical findings concerning for LVAD dysfunction, such as hemolysis, unexplained hypotension, or arrhythmia. An LVAD problem-focused examination consists of a routine LVAD surveillance examination

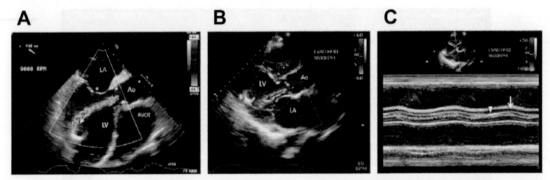

Fig. 6. Assessment of aortic regurgitation (AR). (*A*) TEE shows at least moderate and likely severe continuous AR during LVAD support. The AR vena contracta is >3 mm, and the jet width/LVOT width is greater than 46%. Color-flow Doppler reveals inflow cannula systolic entrainment of the AR jet (*arrow*). Also note that the closed mitral valve and trace MR are indicative of marked systolic AR. (*B, C*) During LVAD support, at least moderate continuous AR (*arrow*) is seen in the transthoracic parasternal long-axis view with color Doppler (*B*) and color M-mode imaging (*C*). The inflow cannula is denoted by an asterisk. (*From* Stainback RF, Estep JD, Agler DA, et al. Echocardiography in the management of patients with left ventricular assist devices: recommendations from the American Society of Echocardiography. J Am Soc Echocardiogr 2015;28(8):866; with permission.)

with or without a speed ramp test (**Fig. 10**). Generally, LVAD alarms can be divided into 2 types: low-flow and high-flow alarms. **Tables 1** and **2** summarize the differential diagnosis and echocardiographic findings of these alarms.

Role of Computed Tomography in Evaluation of Left Ventricular Assist Device Patients

CT has been increasingly used in the evaluation of LVAD patients. The high spatial resolution and 3-dimensional imaging capabilities of CT allow for the effective evaluation of inflow and outflow cannula patency, outflow graft kinking, and inflow cannula position or malposition.[9] Given the presence of significant metallic artifact when imaging the main LVAD rotor, CT is not able to evaluate for rotor thrombosis with adequate sensitivity. Therefore, it is important to note that absence of CT evidence of graft thrombus does not rule out

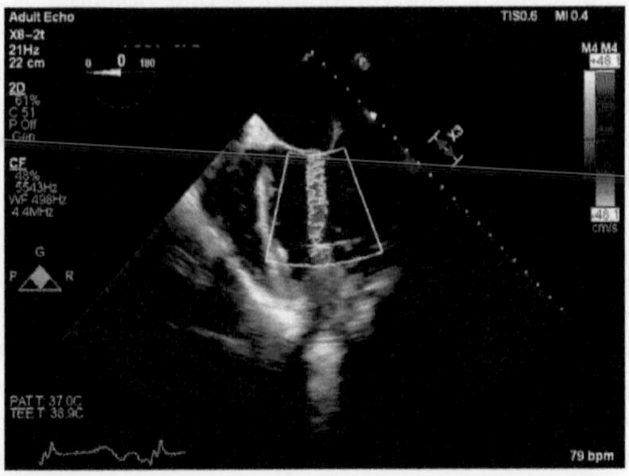

Fig. 7. Typical Doppler artifact seen in the HVAD, prohibiting accurate inflow cannula Doppler assessment.

thrombosis within the LVAD rotor when the clinical presentation suggests it (**Figs. 11** and **12**).

PERCUTANEOUS MECHANICAL CIRCULATORY SUPPORT DEVICES

Certain temporary mechanical circulatory support devices can fill an essential role when circulatory augmentation needs to occur acutely in a patient for whom a surgical option is not feasible. The range of devices available include intra-aortic balloon counterpulsation, a left atrial-to-femoral artery assist device (TandemHeart, Cardiac Assist Incorporated), and left ventricle-to-aortic assist devices, which can be placed surgically or percutaneously. The Impella (Abiomed Incorporated, Danvers, Massachusetts) 2.5 left percutaneous (LP, 12 Fr) and cardiac power (CP, 14 Fr, offering up to 4 L/min of support) devices are the focus of this section. However, an Impella RP is also available for RV support, delivering flow from the inferior vena cava to the pulmonary artery.

Imaging to Guide the Use of Percutaneously Placed Impella Devices

Prior to retrograde aortic Impella deployment, echocardiography is necessary to assess the extent of valvular disease, as severe aortic stenosis, aortic regurgitation, and mitral stenosis are relative contraindications to use.[1] A flexible pigtail tip at the distal end provides stability of the device within the LV but can result in entanglement within the submitral apparatus.[10] The inflow port is generally placed 3.5 to 4 cm from the aortic annulus,[1] often guided by fluoroscopy in the catheterization laboratory, with ongoing confirmatory imaging of correct placement by subsequent echocardiography.

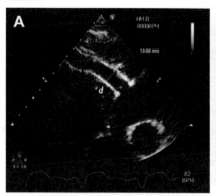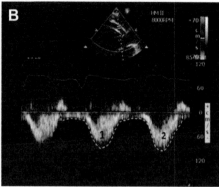

Fig. 8. (*A*) LVAD outflow cannula to ascending aorta anastomosis from high left parasternal long axis view at seen by TTE. (*B*) pulse Doppler examination of the outflow graft just proximal to the anastomosis site. LVAD outflow can be calculated by multiplying the VTI of the pulse wave Doppler signal by with outflow graft area. (*From* Stainback RF, Estep JD, Agler DA, et al. Echocardiography in the management of patients with left ventricular assist devices: recommendations from the American Society of Echocardiography. J Am Soc Echocardiogr 2015;28(8):878; with permission.)

Intracardiac echocardiography is occasionally employed.[3] Generally, 2-dimensional echocardiography is sufficient to confirm the maintenance of proper placement, but in some cases 3-dimensional echocardiography can better demonstrate partial inflow obstruction, such as caused by papillary muscle impingement.[11,12]

Complications

Exacerbation of existing or creation of new significant aortic regurgitation is possible after Impella deployment, sometimes requiring intervention.[13] Iatrogenic mitral regurgitation has also been described,[14] often caused by entanglement of the pigtail within the submitral apparatus; low-flow alarms may result if the mitral leaflets or submitral structures impede inflow.[1] Echocardiography is the primary method of determining new or worsening valvular dysfunction after Impella deployment.

EXTRACORPOREAL MEMBRANE OXYGENATION
Background and Indications

Extracorporeal membrane oxygenation (ECMO) is a widely utilized technique of providing oxygen delivery to the blood via an external system.[15] The essential elements in modern ECMO systems include, in general order of circulatory flow: a drainage cannula that removes blood from the body, pump, membrane-oxygenator, blender, temperature control element, and return cannula that reintroduces oxygenated blood into the circulation.[16] Use of venovenous (VV) ECMO corrects hypoxemia, with the assumption that cardiac output is sufficient. Venoarterial (VA) ECMO offers both oxygenation and circulatory support, the primary

indications for which include cardiogenic shock and weaning from cardiopulmonary bypass after cardiac surgery. Given that VA ECMO completely bypasses the heart, the reduction in cardiac preload may be helpful in support of ventricular function, whereas the marked increase in afterload may be detrimental to ventricular recovery.

Imaging in Venoarterial Extracorporeal Oxygenation Implementation

Venoarterial ECMO necessitates aortic valvular competency, as aortic-LV regurgitant flow is worsened when VA ECMO is employed in the presence of significant aortic insufficiency.[17] Detection of aortic dissection is also essential, as cannulation could lead to extension of a localized dissection.[18] (**Table 3**). Ongoing imaging should assess cannulae, pericardial effusion, cardiac chamber size, frequency of aortic valvular opening, degree of aortic regurgitation, and cardiac output (CO). Ultrasonic enhancing agents (eg, Definity, Optison) have mixed reports of safety, as the imaging agent can potentially trigger the bubble detector alarm, leading to engagement of zero-flow mode.[19]

Imaging of Extracorporeal Oxygenation Complications

Abrupt decreases in ECMO flows can result from patient movement and cannula repositioning, which highlights the importance of visualizing the cannula and any significant inflow acceleration.[20] The comparative attention to pericardial imaging before and during ECMO implementation is critical, as a rapidly expanding pericardial collection during or after cannulation is suggestive of hemopericardium.

Box 2
Left ventricular assist device optimization (speed ramp) echo protocol

Perform baseline LVAD surveillance study (annotate BP, pump type, baseline pump speed)

At baseline pump speed, acquire the following:

- LVIDd in the parasternal long-axis view
- RV VTI (to calculate cardiac output) in the parasternal short-axis view
- AV opening by 2-dimensional and M-mode in the parasternal long-axis view (color Doppler M-mode if needed)
- 2-dimensional imaging In the parasternal tong- and short-axis views
- Color Doppler examination of AR and MR in the parasternal long-axis and apical views
- Color Doppler examination of TR in the RV inflow and apical tour-chamber view
- Standard mitral valve PW Doppler inflow parameters
- Positioning of the interventricular and interatrial septa

Decrease pump speed to as low as 8000 rpm (for HM-II)

 or

Decrease pump speed to as low as 2400 rpm (for HVAD)

- Wait 2 minutes
- Repeat data acquisition

Increase pump speed by 400 rpm (for HM-II)

 or

Increase pump speed by 20 to 40 rpm (for HVAD)

- Wait 2 minutes
- Repeat data acquisition

HM-II:

   Continue to increase pump speed in 400 rpm increments to a pump speed of up to 12,000 rpm or until endpoint, acquiring data at each stage

HVAD:

   Continue to increase pump speed in 20 to 40 rpm increments to a pump speed of up to 3200 rpm, or until end point, acquiring data at each stage

Endpoints

- Completion of test
- Suction event: decrease in LV size (typically <3 cm), +/− ventricular ectopy, +/− inflow-cannula intermittent obstruction, leftward ventricular septal shift worsening TR
- Symptoms including, but not limited to palpitations, dizziness, chest pain, shortness of breath, or headache
- Hypertension (eg, MAP >100 mm Hg or symptoms)
- Hypotension (eg, MAP <60 mm Hg or symptoms)

Abbreviations: AR, aortic regurgitation; AV, aortic valve; BP, blood pressure; HM-II, HeartMate II; HVAD, HeartWare ventricular assist system; LVIDd, LV internal diameter at end-diastole; MAP, mean arterial pressure; MR, mitral regurgitation; PLAX, parasternal long-axis; PW, pulsed Doppler; TR, tricuspid regurgitation; TV, tricuspid valve; VTI, velocity-time integral.

From Stainback RF, Estep JD, Agler DA, et al. Echocardiography in the management of patients with left ventricular assist devices: recommendations from the American Society of Echocardiography. J Am Soc Echocardiogr 2015;28(8):907; with permission.

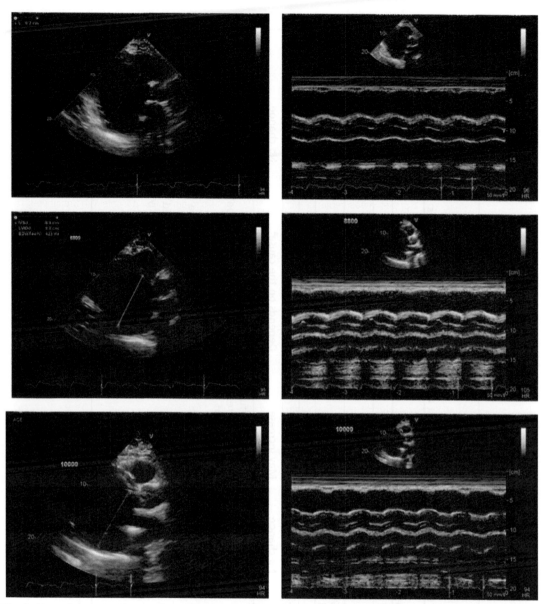

Fig. 9. Normal ramp test in a patient with LVAD. TTE images of parasternal long axis showing sequential images of the LV along with M-mode images of the aortic valve at 3 different speeds of HeartMate II. There is progressive decreasing in the LV end diastolic dimension with increasing LVAD speed from 8000 to 8800 to 10,000 rpm. Additionally, aortic valve opening also responding normally from opening with every cardiac cycle at 8000 rpm to opening intermittent at 8800 rpm to remaining closed at 10,000 rpm speed.

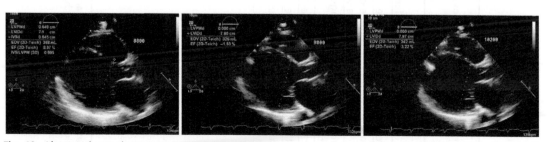

Fig. 10. Abnormal speed ramp test. TTE images with parasternal long axis view showing the LV end diastolic dimension unchanged with increasing LVAD HeartMate II speed. This confirms the presence of LVAD dysfunction. Additionally, the aortic valve continues to open with every heart beat despite speed increases (not shown).

Table 1
Left ventricular assist device low-flow alarms

	Major Causes of LVAD Low Flow Alarms with Most Common Echocardiographic Findings					
	Hyopvolemia	RV Failure	Severe Hypertension	Tamponade	Suction Event	Inflow Thrombus or Outflow Obstruction
Left ventricle size	Decrease	Decrease	Increase	Decrease	Decrease	Increase
Right ventricle Size	Decrease or no change	Increase	No change	Decrease	Depends on the cause[a]	No change
Interventricular septal shift	No change	Septal shift toward left	No change	No change	Depends on the cause[a]	No change
Aortic valve opening	Decrease	Decrease	Decrease	No change	Depends on the cause[a]	Increase
Mitral regurgitation	Decrease	No change	Increase	No change	Depends on the cause[a]	Increase
Tricuspid regurgitation	Decrease	Increase	No change	May increase	Depends on the cause[a]	No change
Others			Increase outflow cannula peak systolic velocity	Pericardial effusion with compressed left and/or right atrium	Inflow cannula abutting endocardium and position off-axis There will be also increased inflow -cannula peak velocity Also, there will be increased ventricular ectopy or arrhythmia on electrocardiogram	Elevated peak outflow cannula velocity >2 m/s Also blunted change in the following parameters with pump-speed augmentation: LV dimension reduction Aortic valve opening reduction RVOT VTI increase

Abbreviations: RVOT, right ventricular outflow; VTI, velocity time integral.
[a] Suction events can be caused by hypovolemia, RV failure, tamponade, inflow cannula malposition or arrhythmia.

Table 2
Left ventricular assist device high-flow alarms

	Major Causes of LVAD High-Flow Alarms with Most Common Echocardiographic Findings		
	LVAD (Rotor) Thrombosis with Pump Malfunction	Vasodilatation of Sepsis	Significant Aortic Regurgitation
Left ventricle size	Increase	No change	Increase
Right ventricle size	No change	No change	No change
Interventricular septal shift	No change	No change	No change
Aortic valve opening	Increase	Increase	Increase
Mitral regurgitation	Increase	No change or decrease	Might increase
Tricuspid regurgitation	No change	No change	No change
Others	Blunting changes in the following parameters with pump-speed augmentation: LVEDd reduction. AV opening time reduction, RVOT VTI increase	Clinical findings of infection or vasodilatory medication exposure	Signs of severe aortic regurgitation with AR seen on color Doppler during systole and diastole and ≥0.3 cm vena contracta and jet width/LVOT width ≥46%
	Increase in the inflow cannula systolic to diastolic peak velocity ratio (increase systolic peak and decrease diastolic nadir)		
	Usually associated with significant hemolysis		

Abbreviations: AV, aortic valve; AR, Aortic regurgitation; LVEDd, left ventricular end diastolic dimension; LVOT, left ventricular outflow; RVOT, right ventricular outflow; VTI, velocity time integral.

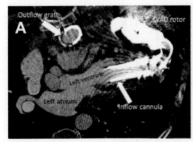 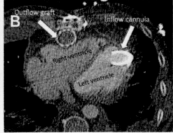 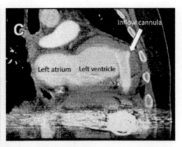

Fig. 11. (*A*) Ideal positioning of the inflow cannula directed toward the mitral valve away from the myocardial walls. There is fill opacification of the inflow cannula with contrast suggesting no thrombosis. (*B*) Inflow cannula position in the apex, directed slightly toward with septum without abutting it. This is generally accepted position assuming no signs of low LVAD flow are present. Note also that the outflow graft is not filled with contrast, suggesting outflow graft thrombosis. (*C*) Severe malalignment of the LVAD inflow abutting the anteroseptal wall. Such severe malalignment resulted in flow obstruction and required surgical correction.

Visualization of thrombus is common, either in association with a cannula or a result of hemostasis. Infrequent or absent aortic valvular opening and spontaneous echo contrast are markers of static blood flow in the aortic root and ascending aorta, and the duration of aortic hemostasis is associated with risk of thrombosis (Video 8).

INVESTIGATIONAL DEVICE-BASED THERAPIES FOR HEART FAILURE

HFpEF is a growing health epidemic with high rates of mortality, morbidity, and hospitalizations. It is estimated that acute diastolic HF is responsible for approximately 40% to 50% of all HF admissions, and this number is expected to rise to 60% by the year 2020,[21] with a projected health care cost of $47 billion by 2030.[22] HFpEF is associated with similar mortality as HFrEF, with annual mortality rate ranging from 10% to 30%[23] and 5-year mortality rates as high as 50% to 60%.[24] Symptomatically, patients with HFpEF express the same degree of functional decline as their counterparts with HFrEF.[25] Although many classes of drugs and device-based therapies have been proven to reduce morbidity and mortality in HFrEF, studies on medical treatment for HFpEF have been disappointing. Thus, published HF guidelines have primarily focused on the generalized approach of treating symptoms of volume overload and addressing the underlying risk factors such as hypertension and atrial fibrillation. Because of the absence of established benefits from medical therapies for HFpEF, several device-based therapies aimed to reduce left atrial pressure (LAP) have been proposed.

InterAtrial Shunt Device

The InterAtrial Shunt Device (IASD, Corvia Medical, Tewkesbury, Massachusetts) is an innovative device-based therapy for HFpEF that has completed a phase II clinical trial (REDUCE LAP-HF I)[23] showing adequate safety and efficacy.

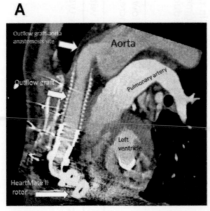 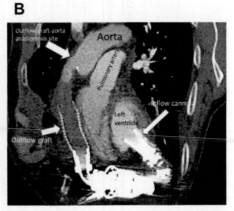

Fig. 12. (*A*) Normal outflow graft of HeartMate II. The graft has normal anastomosis to the ascending aorta without any kinking. There is good and complete opacification of the graft consistent with no thrombosis. (*B*) Almost complete lack of contrast filling in the outflow graft consistent with thrombosis (confirmed after LVAD explanation). The graft-aorta anastomosis is normal. The contrast filling at the distal part of the graft is secondary to retrograde filling.

Table 3
Common use of imaging modalities throughout the spectrum of extracorporeal membrane oxygenation therapy

Time Period	Left Ventricle/Right Ventricle Size and Functional Assessment	Valvular Disease and PA Pressure Estimation	Pericardial Imaging, Detection of Effusion	Aortic and Aortic Valvular Assessment	Guidewire and Cannula Positioning
Preimplantation and choice of support technique (VV vs VA ECMO)	TTE, CECT[a]	TTE	TTE	TTE	TEE
During implantation			TTE, TEE[b]	TTE, TEE[b]	Fluoroscopy, TTE, TEE[b]
Monitoring on ECMO support	TTE	TTE	TTE, NCCT[a]	TTE, TEE[a]	CXR, TEE[a], NCCT[a]
Surveillance for potential complications	TTE	TTE	TTE, NCCT[a]	TTE, TEE[a], CECT[a]	CXR, TEE[a], NCCT[a]

Abbreviations: CXR, chest X-ray; CECT, contrast-enhanced CT; NCCT, noncontrast CT; PA, pulmonary arterial.
[a] Denotes "as indicated".
[b] Denotes "often intraoperatively".

The device is currently being investigated in a randomized, multicenter phase III trial (REDUCE LAP-HF II)[26] aimed at assessing clinical endpoints. The IASD is implanted percutaneously via a femoral approach into the atrial septum and functions as a pop off valve between the left and right atria to decompress the left atrium dynamically, at rest and with exercise. It is well established that LAP is strongly associated with exertional dyspnea and functional limitations. By reducing LAP, IASD can potentially improve symptoms and functional capacity in the HFpEF population. The IASD has a dual-disc design that extends through the atrial septum with a small opening located in the center (**Figs. 13** and **14**).[26] The device is advanced to the desired location through a 16 Fr sheath over a 0.035 in guidewire and implanted using a conventional trans-septal puncture technique. Deployment of the IASD is performed under fluoroscopic and intracardiac echocardiographic guidance. After performing trans-septal puncture, the IASD is advanced over a guidewire, followed by exposing the left atrial disc. This is followed by withdrawing the right atrial disk from the sheath, which leads to complete device release (**Fig. 15**).[26] The device is radiopaque and is visible under fluoroscopy. Echocardiographic color Doppler imaging will demonstrate left-to-right atrial flow (**Fig. 16**).

V Wave Technology

The V-Wave Shunt (V-Wave Ltd., Or Akiva, Israel) is another novel device-based therapy that is being developed for the treatment of both HFpEF and HFrEF. The V-Wave Shunt device (http://www.vwavemedical.com) follows a similar concept to the IASD in its design and is implanted in the interatrial septum to decompress the LAP. Early designs included a built-in 1-way valve to guarantee a

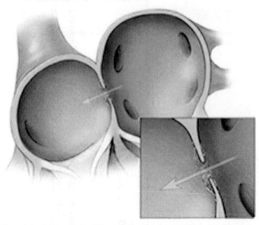

Fig. 14. Schematic illustration of IASD in position in the atrial septum. The arrow indicates shunt direction and flow over the device. (*From* Hasenfuss G, Gustafsson F, Kaye D, et al. Rationale and design of the reduce elevated left atrial pressure in patients with heart failure (Reduce LAP-HF) trial. J Card Fail 2015;21(7):595; with permission.)

unidirectional left-to-right shunt; however, this valve was removed from subsequent designs because of a high rate of obstruction. This device demonstrated a good safety profile in early studies that tested its use in symptomatic New York Heart Association (NYHA) functional class III patients.[27,28] A prospective, multi-center, 1:1 randomized trial will be initiated soon that will explore the clinical effectiveness of this device in NYHA functional class III or ambulatory class IV HF patients,

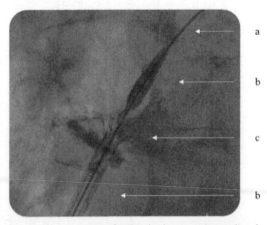

Fig. 15. Fluoroscopy of IASD deployment immediately after the release of the right atrial part of the device. (*A*) Guidewire. (*B*) Advance delivery system. (*C*) Engaged left atrial legs of the IASD against the septal wall. (*From* Hasenfuss G, Gustafsson F, Kaye D, et al. Rationale and design of the reduce elevated left atrial pressure in patients with heart failure (Reduce LAP-HF) trial. J Card Fail 2015;21(7):598; with permission.)

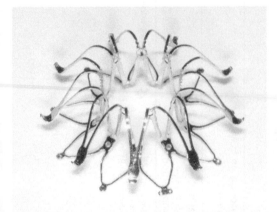

Fig. 13. The InterAtrial Shunt Device. (*Courtesy of* Corvia Medical, Tewkesbury, Massachusetts.)

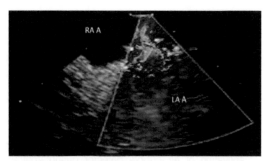

Fig. 16. Echogradiographic image at time of implant. Color Doppler demonstrates left-to-right atrial flow. LA, left atrium; RA, right atrium.

irrespective of LVEF, who at baseline are treated with guideline-directed medical treatments.

PULMONARY ARTERY HEMODYNAMIC SENSOR

Chronic HF management has traditionally relied on clinical parameters and indirect surrogates of congestion such daily weight measurements, vital signs, peripheral edema, and patients' self-assessment of symptoms. Although these strategies can be beneficial, they are generally unreliable, and patient adherence remains a significant limiting factor.

The CardioMEMS HF system is a fully implantable wireless pulmonary artery pressure (PAP) monitoring system that consists of a PAP sensor, external electronic measuring device, and a secure Web site that can be easily accessed by physicians. The sensor is implanted percutaneously using a right heart catheterization technique via a femoral venous approach. The sensor is loaded on a specialized delivery catheter that is advanced over a guidewire into a suitable segment (7–15 mm in diameter) of the pulmonary artery tree. Placement can be confirmed by pulmonary angiography (Fig. 18). Counterclockwise rotation of the tethering knob located at the delivery catheter handle will release the sensor and allow the nitinol hoops to expand and meet with the walls of adjacent pulmonary artery branch. The delivery catheter and guidewire are then withdrawn slowly under fluoroscopy to avoid traction on the fully implanted sensor (Videos 11–12). The sensor does not have a battery and never needs to be replaced. Patients are instructed to take daily measurements, which can be securely transmitted to clinicians.

The CardioMEMS-guided management of chronic HF was evaluated in the CHAMPION trial.[29] Compared with the control group, patients with PAP-guided management had a significant 28% reduction in HF-related hospitalizations at 6 months and 37% reduction in HF

hospitalizations at 15 months. The FDA approved the CardioMEMS system for NYHA class III patients on May 28, 2014.

SUMMARY AND FUTURE DIRECTIONS

A significant surge in the number of devices used for the treatment and remote monitoring of HF has taken place in the last few years. With the limited number of donor hearts, durable mechanical circulatory assist devices have gained popularity in the management algorithm of end-stage HFrEF and are routinely offered to appropriate candidates. Short-term assist devices are commonly used in the management of cardiogenic shock. Cardiac imaging, specifically echocardiography, is essential in the selection process, intraoperative guidance, speed optimization, and postoperative surveillance for thrombotic and infectious complications associated with mechanical circulatory support devices. Furthermore, implantable hemodynamic sensors have become the standard of care in preventing HF readmissions, and they have a distinct radiographic appearance on chest imaging. Newer, novel devices that work by creating a left-to-right shunting to unload the left atrium, such as the atrial septal shunt devices, are currently being investigated to improve HF symptoms.

Practicing cardiologists are facing a rapidly evolving field with newer technologies and devices with distinct imaging features. Cardiac imaging specialists with good knowledge of these devices, and vast experience in assessing their intended function and complications, are now essential to any successful advanced HF program in the current era.

SUPPLEMENTARY DATA

Supplementary data related to this article can be found online at https://doi.org/10.1016/j.hfc.2018.12.011.

REFERENCES

1. Stainback RF, Estep JD, Agler DA, et al. Echocardiography in the management of patients with left ventricular assist devices: recommendations from the American Society of Echocardiography. J Am Soc Echocardiogr 2015;28(8):853–909.
2. Porter TR, Mulvagh SL, Abdelmoneim SS, et al. Clinical applications of ultrasonic enhancing agents in echocardiography: 2018 American Society of Echocardiography guidelines update. J Am Soc Echocardiogr 2018;31(3):241–74.
3. Hayek S, Sims DB, Markham DW, et al. Assessment of right ventricular function in left ventricular assist

device candidates. Circ Cardiovasc Imaging 2014; 7(2):379–89.

4. Genovese EA, Dew MA, Teuteberg JJ, et al. Incidence and patterns of adverse event onset during the first 60 days after ventricular assist device implantation. Ann Thorac Surg 2009;88(4):1162–70.

5. Kormos RL, Teuteberg JJ, Pagani FD, et al. Right ventricular failure in patients with the HeartMate II continuous-flow left ventricular assist device: incidence, risk factors, and effect on outcomes. J Thorac Cardiovasc Surg 2010;139(5):1316–24.

6. Puwanant S, Hamilton KK, Klodell CT, et al. Tricuspid annular motion as a predictor of severe right ventricular failure after left ventricular assist device implantation. J Heart Lung Transplant 2008;27(10):1102–7.

7. Grant AD, Smedira NG, Starling RC, et al. Independent and incremental role of quantitative right ventricular evaluation for the prediction of right ventricular failure after left ventricular assist device implantation. J Am Coll Cardiol 2012;60(6):521–8.

8. Lampert BC, Teuteberg JJ. Right ventricular failure after left ventricular assist devices. J Heart Lung Transplant 2015;34(9):1123–30.

9. Raman SV, Sahu A, Merchant AZ, et al. Noninvasive assessment of left ventricular assist devices with cardiovascular computed tomography and impact on management. J Heart Lung Transplant 2010; 29(1):79–85.

10. Rihal CS, Naidu SS, Givertz MM, et al. 2015 SCAI/ACC/HFSA/STS clinical expert consensus statement on the use of percutaneous mechanical circulatory support devices in cardiovascular care: endorsed by the American Heart Association, the Cardiological Society of India, and Sociedad Latino Americana de Cardiologia Intervencion; affirmation of value by the Canadian Association of Interventional Cardiology-Association Canadienne de Cardiologie d'Intervention. J Am Coll Cardiol 2015;65(19):e7–26.

11. Abusaid GH, Ahmad M. Transthoracic real time three-dimensional echocardiography in Impella placement. Echocardiography 2012;29(4):E105–6.

12. Revilla MI, Amado MG, Sasse M, et al. The 3D transoesophageal echocardiography role in the Impella 3.5 placement. Eur Heart J Cardiovasc Imaging 2014;15(11):1212.

13. Chandola R, Cusimano R, Osten M, et al. Postcardiac transplant transcatheter core valve implantation for aortic insufficiency secondary to Impella device placement. Ann Thorac Surg 2012;93(6): e155–7.

14. Bhatia N, Richardson TD, Coffin ST, et al. Acute mitral regurgitation after removal of an Impella device. Am J Cardiol 2017;119(8):1290–1.

15. Stretch R, Sauer CM, Yuh DD, et al. National trends in the utilization of short-term mechanical circulatory support: incidence, outcomes, and cost analysis. J Am Coll Cardiol 2014;64(14):1407–15.

16. Lee S, Chaturvedi A. Imaging adults on extracorporeal membrane oxygenation (ECMO). Insights Imaging 2014;5(6):731–42.

17. Kapoor PM. Echocardiography in extracorporeal membrane oxygenation. Ann Card Anaesth 2017; 20(Supplement):S1–3.

18. Baliga RR, Nienaber CA, Bossone E, et al. The role of imaging in aortic dissection and related syndromes. JACC Cardiovasc Imaging 2014;7(4):406–24.

19. Grecu L, Fishman MA. Beware of life-threatening activation of air bubble detector during contrast echocardiography in patients on venoarterial extracorporeal membrane oxygenator support. J Am Soc Echocardiogr 2014;27(10):1130–1.

20. Douflé G, Roscoe A, Billia F, et al. Echocardiography for adult patients supported with extracorporeal membrane oxygenation. Crit Care 2015;19(1): 326.

21. Oktay AA, Rich JD, Shah SJ. The emerging epidemic of heart failure with preserved ejection fraction. Curr Heart Fail Rep 2013;10(4):401–10.

22. Mozaffarian D. Heart disease and stroke statistics-2015 update: a report from the American Heart Association (vol 131, pg e29, 2015). Circulation 2015; 131(24):E535.

23. Feldman T, Mauri L, Kahwash R, et al. Transcatheter interatrial shunt device for the treatment of heart failure with preserved ejection fraction (REDUCE LAP-HF I [reduce elevated left atrial pressure in patients with heart failure]). A phase 2, randomized, sham-controlled trial. Circulation 2018;137(4):364–75.

24. Shah SJ, Gheorghiade M. Heart failure with preserved ejection fraction: treat now by treating comorbidities. JAMA 2008;300(4):431–3.

25. Ingle L, Cleland JG, Clark AL. Perception of symptoms is out of proportion to cardiac pathology in patients with "diastolic heart failure.". Heart 2008;94(6): 748–53.

26. Hasenfuss G, Gustafsson F, Kaye D, et al. Rationale and design of the reduce elevated left atrial pressure in patients with heart failure (reduce LAP-HF) trial. J Card Fail 2015;21(7):594–600.

27. Amat-Santos IJ, Del Trigo M, Bergeron S, et al. Left atrial decompression using unidirectional left-to-right interatrial shunt: Initial experience in treating symptomatic heart failure with preserved ejection fraction with the W-wave device. JACC Cardiovasc Interv 2015;8(6):870–2.

28. Del Trigo M, Bergeron S, Bernier M, et al. Unidirectional left-to-right interatrial shunting for treatment of patients with heart failure with reduced ejection fraction: a safety and proof-of-principle cohort study. Lancet 2016;387(10025):1290–7.

29. Abraham WT, Adamson PB, Bourge RC, et al. Wireless pulmonary artery haemodynamic monitoring in chronic heart failure: a randomised controlled trial. Lancet 2011;377(9766):658–66.

Biomarkers and Imaging
Complementary or Subtractive?

Andrea Salzano, MD[a,b], Alberto M. Marra, MD[c], Roberta D'Assante, PhD[c], Michele Arcopinto, MD[d], Eduardo Bossone, MD, PhD[e], Toru Suzuki, MD, PhD[a], Antonio Cittadini, MD[b,f],*

KEYWORDS

- Heart failure • Biomarkers • Imaging • Cardiovascular disease • Prognosis

KEY POINTS

- The development of novel biomarkers is one of the most productive field of research in heart failure.
- Biomarkers are used in routine clinical care for diagnosis, monitoring (response to treatment), and risk stratification of patients with heart failure.
- Natriuretic peptides represent the gold standard circulating biomarkers in heart failure, and transthoracic echocardiography is an indispensable tool in the management of patients with heart failure.
- A multibiomarker approach might grant broader information, which in turn might be helpful for the daily clinical management of this clinical condition.
- The multibiomarker strategy, in particular if circulating and imaging biomarkers are combined and information from different pathophysiological pathways are provided, seems to be the most promising strategy that goes beyond the limits of the current management of heart failure.

INTRODUCTION

An unacceptably high mortality rate, worse than that for many cancers, and a slow but steady increase in its prevalence, represent ominous peculiarities of heart failure (HF),[1] leading to a huge economic and social burden.[2,3] The scientific community is trying to modify this trend, and one of the most active field is the development of novel biomarkers. Indeed, in the last years, the level of interest in the search and discovery of new cardiovascular biomarkers has progressively grown.[4]

Currently, biomarkers are routinely used in clinical care for the diagnosis, monitoring (response to treatment), and risk stratification of patients with HF.[5] However, to date none of the novel biomarkers has demonstrated enough prognostic power when used alone. Thus, it is commonly recognized that, rather than a single biomarker, it is the integration of multiple biomarkers that yields the best strategy, although few studies have tested this hypothesis.[6]

Circulating biomarkers are the most commonly used in clinical scenarios, although emerging novel categories are actively tested in several trials. Among these, imaging biomarkers hold great promise, thanks to the impressive advances in imaging techniques.

Disclosure Statement: Dr A. Salzano receives research grant support from Cardiopath. The other authors have nothing to disclose.

[a] Department of Cardiovascular Sciences, NIHR Leicester Biomedical Research Centre, University of Leicester, Glenfield Hospital, Groby Road, Leicester LE3 9QP, UK; [b] Department of Translational Medical Sciences, Federico II University, Via Pansini 5, Naples 80138, Italy; [c] IRCCS SDN, Naples, Italy; [d] Emergency Department, A Cardarelli Hospital, Via Cardarelli 9, Naples 80131, Italy; [e] Cardiology Division, A Cardarelli Hospital, Via Cardarelli 9, Naples 80131, Italy; [f] Interdisciplinary Research Centre in Biomedical Materials (CRIB), Piazzale Tecchio 80, Naples 80125, Italy
* Corresponding author. Department of Translational Medical Sciences, "Federico II" University-School of Medicine, Via Pansini 5, Naples 80131, Italy.
E-mail address: antonio.cittadini@unina.it

Heart Failure Clin 15 (2019) 321–331
https://doi.org/10.1016/j.hfc.2018.12.008
1551-7136/19/© 2018 Elsevier Inc. All rights reserved.

In this review, we dwell on blood-derived and imaging biomarkers in 2 different sections. We then discuss the potential combination of these 2 categories of biomarkers available in HF, aiming at understanding whether their role is complementary or subtractive in HF.

BIOMARKERS: DEFINITION AND THE IDEAL BIOMARKER

Nowadays, the word biomarker is commonly used, and in some cases misused, to describe a number of emerging tools, technologies, and strategies widely aimed to improve knowledge about several diseases.

In 2001, translating the necessity of reaching an agreement on a proper definition and classification of biomarkers, being the discover of the ideal biomarker a main goal of the research community, the Biomarkers and Surrogate End Point Working Group proposed the following definition: "a characteristic that is, objectively measured and evaluated as an indicator of normal biological processes, pathogenic processes, or pharmacologic responses to a therapeutic intervention."[7] In this context, biomarkers have also been categorized in 3 different types[8]:

- Type 0: biomarkers related to a specific disease correlated with clinical indices that can be monitored longitudinally;
- Type I: biomarkers used to evaluate in parallel the effects of a pharmacologic intervention associated with the mechanism of action of a therapeutic drug; and
- Type II: biomarkers considered surrogate end points that are able to predict clinical benefit.

A surrogate biomarker is used in therapeutic trials and is representative of the patient clinical status/outcome. It is supposed to predict the effect of pharmacologic therapy, being an indicator of disease prognosis and progression benefit.[8] However, before using a biomarkers as a surrogate end point, several fundamental pieces of information are needed. First, it is necessary to have a strong correlation between the impact of an intervention on the biomarker and the impact of the intervention on a clinical meaningful end point; second, the outcome of interest should be modifiable through the therapeutic intervention; third, a biomarker should reflect both benefits and risks related to the intervention; and finally, the sampling strategies and relative risk related should be well-known, as well as the time course between the change in biomarker and the outcome.[9,10]

In particular, the search for the ideal biomarker is focused on the improvement in disease treatment and the reduction of health care costs.[11] Moreover, a biomarker should be specific for a particular disease, easy to detect, cost effective, and able to provide accurate results.[12] It should be taken into account that, although many studies report the identification of new disease biomarkers, some of them do not satisfy the analytical validation based on well-established criteria of sensitivity and specificity that must be fulfilled to take a step toward for market applications.[13] For this reason, it is necessary to implement appropriate strategies starting from an accurate selection of patients, sample preparation, improvement of laboratory assays, to the final steps of statistical/analytical validation.[12]

In addition, Morrow and de Lemos have recently defined 3 criteria a biomarker should have to be useful in clinic context[14]: (i) it has to be an accurate, repeated measurement that must be possible to measure with a reasonable cost and in short time; (ii) the biomarker must provide information that is not already available from a careful clinical assessment; and (iii) the measurement of the biomarker should support clinician in medical decision making.

According to this definition, biomarkers may derive from the blood, the urine, a genetic study, imaging, a physiologic test, and tissue specimen biopsies.[15] In addition, further than prognosis, an ideal biomarker should be suited for a precision medicine approach to target specific interventions, and should provide biological plausibility for characterization of HF phenotype[16] and in patient selection.[17]

CIRCULATING BIOMARKERS

Considering that an impressive number of circulating biomarkers has been studied,[5,15,18] the purpose of this section is to provide a brief overview of the best characterized and promising of them. For this reason, we first discuss the classical HF biomarkers, used in everyday clinical practice worldwide and then emerging biomarkers separately.

Classical Biomarkers

Circulating biomarkers are undeniable tools in HF management for several reasons: (1) they are essential for HF diagnosis, (2) they are helpful in assessing prognosis of patients with HF, and (3) they are potentially useful in guiding therapy.[19]

The most studied and useful biomarkers in HF are the natriuretic peptides, namely B-type natriuretic peptide, N-terminal pro-brain natriuretic peptide (NT-proBNP) and the mid-regional precursor of the atrial natriuretic peptide (MR-proANP). Natriuretic peptides mirror the volume/pressure overload, being secreted in response to end-diastolic wall stress.[20,21] According to the European Society of Cardiology guidelines, the presence of serum BNP of less than 35 pg/mL and NT-proBNP of less than 100 pg/mL is enough to rule out HF, even when signs symptoms highly suggestive of HF are present.[22] Furthermore, in the acute setting, higher cutoffs (BNP of <100 pg/mL or NT-proBNP of <300 pg/mL) yield a 99% negative predictive value of excluding a HF diagnosis.[23] MR-proANP has a lower diagnostic power when compared with BNP and NT-proBNP.[24] Besides their relevance for HF diagnosis, natriuretic peptides are powerful biomarkers with regard to prognosis in patients with HF. According to the Acute Decompensated Heart Failure National Registry (ADHERE), BNP levels at the admission are strongly predictive of in-hospital mortality regardless of any other clinical and laboratory variables, both in HF with reduced ejection fraction (EF) as well as HF with preserved EF.[25] Both BNP[26] and NT-proBNP[27] levels are able to predict accurately outcomes in HF, whereas with regard to therapy guidance conflicting results were reported.[28–31] Although useless in HF-diagnosis, an increase in MR-proANP levels is strongly associated with outcomes in HF.[32]

Serum troponins (TnI/TnT) are often elevated in patients with HF, but their specificity for HF diagnosis is questionable. Of note, because the clinical presentation of HF and acute coronary syndrome may be quite similar, the assessment of TnI and TnT is useful in differentiating the 2 clinical syndromes. Specifically, during acute coronary syndrome troponins usually increase after 6 hours, whereas they remain stable in HF in a similar timeframe.[19] In contrast, elevated serum troponins are able to predict the decline of systolic function[33] and survival in patients with HF.[34]

Emerging Biomarkers in Heart Failure

In the last decade, enormous attention was paid to the role of micro-RNAs in cardiovascular diseases. Micro-RNAs regulate protein translation and there is evidence to suggest their role in facilitating the diagnosis of HF.[35] However, their prognostic role in HF is questionable.[36,37]

Inflammation plays an active role in HF. Bowel hypoperfusion may lead to bacterial and endotoxin translocation into the bloodstream.[38] In this regard, C-reactive protein is associated with the severity of HF[39] and related mortality.[40,41] Other markers of inflammatory activation are able to predict survival in HF such as IL-9[42] or source of tumorigenicity 2,[43,44] a member of the IL-1 receptor family. Interestingly, source of tumorigenicity 2

also showed a correlation with right ventricular size and function.[44] Galectin-3 is associated with macrophages activation and cardiac fibroblast proliferation which ultimately lead to left ventricular (LV) stiffness[45] and predicts outcome in HF with reduced EF as well as in HF with preserved EF.[46] Likewise, growth differentiation factor 15 may predict all-cause mortality in patients with HF with reduced EF.[47] Taken together, inflammatory activation is an important feature of HF and is strictly associated with prognosis. However, because inflammation belongs to a broad spectrum of diseases, inflammatory biomarkers lack specificity.

Strictly related to the inflammation burst, a robust body of evidence suggests the importance of hormonal deficiencies in HF.[48–55] This finding is not surprising, considering the well-known relationship between cardiovascular diseases and hormonal pathways.[56–60] The most studied hormonal abnormality in HF is the deficiency of the growth hormone/insulin-like growth factor 1 axis, which is independently correlated with all-cause mortality in HF.[61–63] Interestingly, growth hormone deficiency replacement has demonstrated in some preliminary studies to be a potential therapeutic target in patients with HF.[64–67]

Another intriguing features of HF pathophysiology is the interplay between the gut and the cardiovascular system. Recently, in the context of the gut hypothesis of HF,[68] trimethylamine N-oxide, a gut microbiome-mediated metabolite, has been shown to be a strong prognostic biomarker in both acute and chronic (stable) HF.[69–74]

Taken together, natriuretic peptides represent the cornerstone of HF diagnosis, management, and prognosis. However, a multibiomarker approach might grant broader information, which in turn might be helpful for the daily clinical management of this clinical condition. **Table 1** summarizes the evidence regarding biomarkers in HF.

IMAGING BIOMARKERS

Along with established circulating biomarkers, findings from different imaging techniques are extremely useful in prognosis estimation and in guiding therapy in HF. Three specific role have been identified for cardiac imaging in HF[75]: it identifies HF phenotype, assesses severity of heart dysfunction, and monitors responses to interventions. In the future, another important role for imaging will likely be the selection of appropriate patients for cardiac devices (**Fig. 1**).

Transthoracic Echocardiography

Transthoracic echocardiography (TTE) is the indispensable tool in the management of patients with

Table 1
Circulating biomarkers and their role in the management of heart failure

Biomarkers	Pathophysiological Background	Diagnosis	Prognosis Assessment	Therapy Guidance
Natriuretic peptides (BNP, NT-proBNP, MR-proANP)	Reflect pressure/volume overload owing to increased filling pressures	+++	+++	++ (MR-proANP useless)
Troponins	Myocardial damage	− (Lack of specificity)	++	−−
CRP	Inflammation	−− (Lack of Specificity)	++	+
ST2, G-3 and GDF-15	Cardiac fibrosis	−−	++	−
Hormones (GH, IGF-1, testosterone)	Reflect the anabolic imbalance	+	++	+
TMAO	Gut microbiota involvement in HF	+	++	−
MiRNAs	Remodeling of heart chambers	−−	+	+

Abbreviations: −, maybe not useful (small or lack of evidences); −−, not useful; + possibly useful (small or lack of evidences); ++, very useful; +++, use recommended; BNP, brain natriuretic peptide; CRP, C-reactive protein; G-3, galectin-3; GDF-15, growth differentiation factor 15; GH, growth hormone; HF, heart failure; IGF-1, insulin-like growth factor-1; MiRNAs, microribonucleic acids; MR-proANP, mid-regional precursor of the atrial natriuretic peptide; NT-proBNP, amino terminal fragment of the pro-hormone brain type natriuretic peptide; ST2, source of tumorigenicity 2; TMAO, trimethylamine N-oxide.

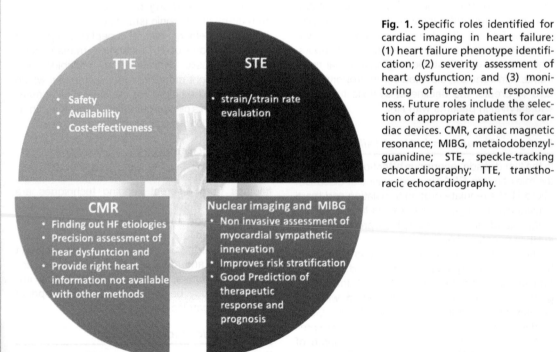

Fig. 1. Specific roles identified for cardiac imaging in heart failure: (1) heart failure phenotype identification; (2) severity assessment of heart dysfunction; and (3) monitoring of treatment responsiveness. Future roles include the selection of appropriate patients for cardiac devices. CMR, cardiac magnetic resonance; MIBG, metaiodobenzylguanidine; STE, speckle-tracking echocardiography; TTE, transthoracic echocardiography.

HF for its safety and availability.[2] The main TTE parameters in HF include those strictly related to LV dysfunction and remodeling (eg, LV EF, LV volumes and sphericity, and LV deformation pattern) and those related to other cardiac abnormalities (eg, left atrial [LA] volume and contractile function, right chambers dimensions and function, pulmonary artery pressures, and signs of congestion). All of them carry prognostic information.

The LVEF is best measured with the biplane Simpson method and it is one of the most important parameters in assessing HF.[76] Further, it has an important role in guiding device therapy (ie, implantable cardioverter defibrillator/cardiac resynchronization therapy in patients with an EF of <35%).[2] LV mass (truncated ellipsoid method) and LV sphericity (LV diameter/length ratio) are easy available secondary prognostic measures.[77]

Furthermore, recent technologies shed novel lights on LV systolic mechanics by imaging its deformation pattern during ejection (longitudinal and circumferential shortening and radial thickening). Such deformation can be estimated by strain (change in the length of a myocardial segment relative to its resting length) and strain rate (strain divided by time) by speckle-tracking echocardiography. These speckles are stable acoustic markers in the ultrasound images that can be tracked to generate myocardial deformation curves.[78] Among such measures, global longitudinal strain adds prognostic value to LVEF and is independent predictor of major adverse cardiac events in large trials.[79]

LA enlargement (biplane area–length method) is common in patients with HF and represents an adverse prognostic marker because it is associated with atrial fibrillation and major adverse cardiac events.[80] LA contractile function, possibly estimated with speckle-tracking echocardiography, is gaining importance to better elucidate LA physiology although less robust evidence is available as a prognostic marker in HF.[81]

A glimpse of the right heart is of paramount importance to properly evaluate patients with HF.[82–85] Elevated systolic pulmonary artery pressures, estimated by peak velocity of the tricuspid regurgitation jet and right atrium estimated pressure, is widely prevalent in patients with HF and represents an established prognostic marker.[86] Independent of systolic pulmonary artery pressures, the presence of right ventricular systolic dysfunction also has prognostic implications in HF.[87] Although TTE is not the gold standard technique for RV quantification, several parameters are available for this purpose, including tricuspid annular plane systolic excursion, fractional area change, and RV free wall strain (speckle-tracking echocardiography).[88] Moreover, an increased inferior vena cava diameter, reflecting congestion,[89] identifies patients with an adverse outcome.[90]

Finally, with regard to hospitalized patients, a recent study suggested that patients who had an echocardiogram had a lower in-hospital mortality.[91]

Cardiac Magnetic Resonance

Unlike echocardiography, cardiac magnetic resonance (CMR) can image any plane, eliminating one of the limitations of TTE. Indeed, with CMR use, geometric assumptions are not needed, warranting more precision than TTE. The tradeoff is that the CMR has a higher cost, lesser availability, and is more time consuming than TTE. To date, CMR should be proposed only to selected patients for whom there is a specific clinical question to answer. Indeed, CMR has decisive relevance, for example, to strengthen the clinical suspicion of rare HF etiologies such as myocarditis, arrhythmogenic right ventricular cardiomyopathy, iron overload cardiomyopathy, amyloidosis, sarcoidosis, and Fabry disease.[92]

Apart from rare etiologies, the differentiation between ischemic and nonischemic causes of HF is a common challenge not always resolved by coronary angiography; in this regard, gadolinium-chelated contrast agents are used in CMR for infarct/fibrosis imaging. Of note, the physiologic basis of late gadolinium enhancement (LGE) are the increase in its volume of distribution within areas of scarring or fibrosis and a prolonged washout in the irreversibly injured myocardium.[93] Patients who had LGE of any pattern showed an 8-fold higher risk of major adverse cardiac events and appropriate implantable defibrillator discharges compared with patients without LGE.[94] In addition, the presence of scarring on LGE CMR in patients with nonischemic HF is predictive of inducible ventricular tachycardia, even after adjustment for LVEF.[95] In addition, it has been demonstrated that the presence of LGE is the best independent predictor of CMR-derived indexes in patients with HF.[96] Moreover, dedicated protocols for the quantification of the RVEF and volume are available in CMR and are significantly more accurate than TTE estimation, thus allowing for a more precise prognostication.[97] Further, CMR has a specific protocol to evaluate the epicardial fat. This process has been associated with the presence of comorbidities and seems to be very useful in particular in the setting of HF with preserved and mid-range reduced EF.[98,99]

Recently, Arvidsson and colleagues[100] suggested a possible use of intracardiac hemodynamic forces analysis for risk stratification and cardiac resynchronization therapy implantation guidance. Indeed, the assessment of intracardiac hemodynamic forces computed from 4-dimensional flow CMR could provide independent biomarkers of cardiac function, in particular in patients with LV dyssynchrony.

Taken together, these findings support the idea that CMR makes a substantial contribution to both diagnosis and management in patients with HF over and above standard echocardiography.[101] Further studies are needed to clarify the role of CMR in the management of HF.

Nuclear Imaging

Cardiac sympathetic nervous system is a key pathophysiological player and a primary therapeutic target in HF.[102] Metaiodobenzylguanidine (^{123}I-MIBG), an iodine-radiolabeled norepinephrine analogue used in nuclear imaging for scintigraphy and single photon emission computed tomography/PET imaging, is retained within myocardial nerve endings and can be imaged to characterize myocardial uptake and thus obtain a noninvasive assessment of cardiac sympathetic innervation (cardiac adrenergic receptor density).[103]

In general, healthy individuals have high cardiac uptake of ^{123}I-MIBG, whereas those with HF have lower myocardial uptake, reflecting decreased receptor density. The heart-to-mediastinum ratio (HMR) is the main measure of ^{123}I-MIBG uptake. In the ADMIRE-HF trial, the risk of major cardiac events was significantly lower for participants with higher HMR than for those with a lower HMR (using a cutoff 1.6)[104]; other researchers found that the addition of the ^{123}I-MIBG HMR to validated HF score (eg, Seattle Heart Failure Model) improved risk stratification with a net reclassification improvement of more than 20%.[105]

Moreover, it has been postulated that the MIBG pattern and its modification after therapy can predict therapeutic response and further improve the prognosis prediction and may have role in therapy tailoring in the future.[106] Further, recently cardiac ^{123}I-MIBG scintigraphy was demonstrated to be helpful in the selection of patients with HF who might not benefit from an implantable cardioverter defibrillator.[107] To date, although PET imaging has superior quantitative capabilities, ^{123}I-MIBG single photon emission computed tomography imaging is the only widely available nuclear imaging method for assessing regional myocardial sympathetic innervation.[108] Recently, in the BETTER-HF trial, the investigators demonstrated that myocardial contractility as assessed by global longitudinal strain is correlated with autonomic denervation assessed by ^{123}I-mIBG scintigraphy, and was able to discriminate severe cardiac denervation.[109]

COMBINING BIOMARKERS

Although the number of biomarkers studied in the past decades has increased dramatically,[15,18] relatively few of them may change our decision making in the clinical arena. To date, even if they are influenced by a number of cardiac and noncardiac conditions, natriuretic peptides (BNP and NT-proBNP) represent the gold standard biomarkers in HF.[2,110–112] An interesting matter of debate, considering the improvement in the field of biomarkers, is whether circulating and imaging biomarkers could be considered subtractive or complementary.

On the one hand, it is important to highlight that circulating biomarkers have an important role in risk prediction models.[113] Indeed, the single biomarker or more often a combination of different circulating biomarkers are combined with clinical variables to predict mortality or hospitalization or both in patients with HF. In addition, the most promising models are made by a combination of biomarkers related to different pathophysiological pathways.[114] Of note, it has been reported recently that only a few of the published models have been validated in independent cohorts and not all of them have been adequately validated in their original population.[115] On the other hand, in the last year, even more study have been published with regard to the role of novel imaging biomarkers in HF.[75]

To date, most of the data available are based on 2-dimensional TTE.[116] Even if interesting information derived from 3-dimensional TTE, from CMR and from other imaging techniques, for its worldwide diffusion and for its availability and cost-effectiveness, TTE remains the most used technique in all the stage of HF. For this reason, almost all the studies in which circulating and imaging biomarkers have been combined are confined to TTE.

In this context, in the Cardiovascular Health Study, the investigators demonstrated that the combination of echocardiography and NT-proBNP significantly reclassifies 5-year risk of HF in older adults when added to a clinical model, in particular in intermediate-risk individuals.[117] Further, Lupon and colleagues[118] demonstrated that a multimarker strategy combining circulating and imaging biomarkers was useful for risk stratification in HF.

The combination strategy is endowed with a good performance not only in HF with reduced

EF; recently, in HF with preserved EF, it has been demonstrated that a 2-step algorithm combining imaging and circulating biomarkers (ie, echocardiographic evaluation followed by the assessment of galectin-3) improves the diagnosis and prognostic assessment of patients with suspected HF with preserved EF.[119]

As reported recently,[120] the management and assessment of HF extend beyond basic clinical evaluations, and the currently available numerous tools need to be applied in a coherent and effective manner within each phase of the patient management cycle. In modern medicine, these tools are a combination of clinical information and circulating and imaging biomarkers. In the future, even more tools will be available to clinicians.

SUMMARY

Although the number of biomarkers investigated in HF in the past decades has increased dramatically, to date relatively few of them modify our decision making in the clinical arena and may therefore be termed "clinically useful." Natriuretic peptides (BNP and NT-proBNP) represent the gold standard circulating biomarkers in HF, whereas TTE represents the indispensable tool in the management of patients with HF for its safety, low cost, and availability. A multibiomarker strategy, in particular if circulating and imaging biomarkers are combined and information from different pathophysiological pathways are provided, seems to be the most promising strategy that goes beyond the limits of the current management of HF. In the near future, we can expect the development of an ever-increasing number of novel blood-derived and imaging biomarkers capable of better predict HF prognosis, at the same time providing innovative pathophysiological mechanisms and guiding HF therapy. Major challenges remain particularly the definition of an optimal multibiomarker strategy, but patients with heart diseases are likely to benefit from these efforts.

REFERENCES

1. Benjamin EJ, Virani SS, Callaway CW, et al, American Heart Association Council on Epidemiology and Prevention Statistics Committee and Stroke Statistics Subcommittee. Heart disease and stroke statistics-2018 update: a report from the American Heart Association. Circulation 2018;137:e67–492.

2. Ponikowski P, Voors AA, Anker SD, et al. 2016 ESC guidelines for the diagnosis and treatment of acute and chronic heart failure: the Task Force for the diagnosis and treatment of acute and chronic heart failure of the European Society of Cardiology (ESC). Developed with the special contribution of the Heart Failure Association (HFA) of the ESC. Eur J Heart Fail 2016;18:891–975.

3. Braunwald E. Heart failure. JACC Heart Fail 2013; 1:1–20.

4. Suzuki T. Cardiovascular diagnostic biomarkers: the past, present and future. Circ J 2009;73:806–9.

5. Suzuki T, Bossone E. Biomarkers of heart failure: past, present, and future. Heart Fail Clin 2018;14:ix–x.

6. Nymo SH, Aukrust P, Kjekshus J, et al. Limited added value of circulating inflammatory biomarkers in chronic heart failure. JACC Heart Fail 2017;5:256–64.

7. Biomarkers Definitions Working Group. Biomarkers and surrogate endpoints: preferred definitions and conceptual framework. Clin Pharmacol Ther 2001; 69:89–95.

8. Naylor S. Biomarkers: current perspectives and future prospects. Expert Rev Mol Diagn 2003;3: 525–9.

9. Ibrahim NE, Gaggin HK, Konstam MA, et al. Established and emerging roles of biomarkers in heart failure clinical trials. Circ Heart Fail 2016;9 [pii: e002528].

10. Januzzi JL Jr. Will biomarkers succeed as a surrogate endpoint in heart failure trials? JACC Heart Fail 2018;6:570–2.

11. Ghashghaei R, Arbit B, Maisel AS. Current and novel biomarkers in heart failure: bench to bedside. Curr Opin Cardiol 2016;31:191–5.

12. Drucker E, Krapfenbauer K. Pitfalls and limitations in translation from biomarker discovery to clinical utility in predictive and personalised medicine. EPMA J 2013;4:7.

13. Mayeux R. Biomarkers: potential uses and limitations. NeuroRx 2004;1:182–8.

14. Morrow DA, de Lemos JA. Benchmarks for the assessment of novel cardiovascular biomarkers. Circulation 2007;115:949–52.

15. Braunwald E. Biomarkers in heart failure. N Engl J Med 2008;358:2148–59.

16. Sinning C, Kempf T, Schwarzl M, et al. Biomarkers for characterization of heart failure - distinction of heart failure with preserved and reduced ejection fraction. Int J Cardiol 2017;227:272–7.

17. deFilippi CR, Seliger SL. A multibiomarker approach to heart failure prognostication: a work in progress. JACC Heart Fail 2017;5:265–7.

18. Ahmad T, Fiuzat M, Felker GM, et al. Novel biomarkers in chronic heart failure. Nat Rev Cardiol 2012;9:347–59.

19. Magnussen C, Blankenberg S. Biomarkers for heart failure: small molecules with high clinical relevance. J Intern Med 2018;283:530–43.

20. Yasue H, Yoshimura M, Sumida H, et al. Localization and mechanism of secretion of B-type

natriuretic peptide in comparison with those of A-type natriuretic peptide in normal subjects and patients with heart failure. Circulation 1994;90: 195–203.

21. Iwanaga Y, Nishi I, Furuichi S, et al. B-type natriuretic peptide strongly reflects diastolic wall stress in patients with chronic heart failure: comparison between systolic and diastolic heart failure. J Am Coll Cardiol 2006;47:742–8.

22. Ponikowski P, Voors AA, Anker SD, et al, ESC Scientific Document Group. 2016 ESC guidelines for the diagnosis and treatment of acute and chronic heart failure: the Task Force for the Diagnosis and Treatment of Acute and Chronic Heart Failure of the European Society of Cardiology (ESC). Developed with the special contribution of the Heart Failure Association (HFA) of the ESC. Eur Heart J 2016;37:2129–200.

23. Januzzi JL Jr, Camargo CA, Anwaruddin S, et al. The N-terminal Pro-BNP investigation of dyspnea in the emergency department (PRIDE) study. Am J Cardiol 2005;95:948–54.

24. Seronde MF, Gayat E, Logeart D, et al, Great network. Comparison of the diagnostic and prognostic values of B-type and atrial-type natriuretic peptides in acute heart failure. Int J Cardiol 2013; 168:3404–11.

25. Fonarow GC, Peacock WF, Phillips CO, et al, ADHERE Scientific Advisory Committee and Investigators. Admission B-type natriuretic peptide levels and in-hospital mortality in acute decompensated heart failure. J Am Coll Cardiol 2007;49: 1943–50.

26. Cheng V, Kazanagra R, Garcia A, et al. A rapid bedside test for B-type peptide predicts treatment outcomes in patients admitted for decompensated heart failure: a pilot study. J Am Coll Cardiol 2001; 37:386–91.

27. O'Brien RJ, Squire IB, Demme B, et al. Pre-discharge, but not admission, levels of NT-proBNP predict adverse prognosis following acute LVF. Eur J Heart Fail 2003;5:499–506.

28. Januzzi JL Jr, Rehman SU, Mohammed AA, et al. Use of amino-terminal pro-B-type natriuretic peptide to guide outpatient therapy of patients with chronic left ventricular systolic dysfunction. J Am Coll Cardiol 2011;58:1881–9.

29. Felker GM, Anstrom KJ, Adams KF, et al. Effect of natriuretic peptide-guided therapy on hospitalization or cardiovascular mortality in high-risk patients with heart failure and reduced ejection fraction: a randomized clinical trial. JAMA 2017;318:713–20.

30. Pfisterer M, Buser P, Rickli H, et al, TIME-CHF Investigators. BNP-guided vs symptom-guided heart failure therapy: the Trial of Intensified vs Standard Medical Therapy in Elderly Patients With Congestive Heart Failure (TIME-CHF) randomized trial. JAMA 2009;301:383–92.

31. Sanders-van Wijk S, van Asselt AD, Rickli H, et al, TIME-CHF Investigators. Cost-effectiveness of N-terminal pro-B-type natriuretic-guided therapy in elderly heart failure patients: results from TIME-CHF (Trial of Intensified versus Standard Medical Therapy in Elderly Patients with Congestive Heart Failure). JACC Heart Fail 2013;1:64–71.

32. Masson S, Anand I, Favero C, et al, Valsartan Heart Failure Trial (Val-HeFT) and Gruppo Italiano per lo Studio della Sopravvivenza nell'Insufficienza Cardiaca–Heart Failure (GISSI-HF) Investigators. Serial measurement of cardiac troponin T using a highly sensitive assay in patients with chronic heart failure: data from 2 large randomized clinical trials. Circulation 2012;125:280–8.

33. Horwich TB, Patel J, MacLellan WR, et al. Cardiac troponin I is associated with impaired hemodynamics, progressive left ventricular dysfunction, and increased mortality rates in advanced heart failure. Circulation 2003;108:833–8.

34. Omland T, de Lemos JA, Sabatine MS, et al. Prevention of events with angiotensin converting enzyme inhibition trial I: a sensitive cardiac troponin T assay in stable coronary artery disease. N Engl J Med 2009;361:2538–47.

35. Watson CJ, Gupta SK, O'Connell E, et al. MicroRNA signatures differentiate preserved from reduced ejection fraction heart failure. Eur J Heart Fail 2015;17:405–15.

36. Masson S, Batkai S, Beermann J, et al. Circulating microRNA-132 levels improve risk prediction for heart failure hospitalization in patients with chronic heart failure. Eur J Heart Fail 2018;20:78–85.

37. Bayes-Genis A, Lanfear DE, de Ronde MWJ, et al. Prognostic value of circulating microRNAs on heart failure-related morbidity and mortality in two large diverse cohorts of general heart failure patients. Eur J Heart Fail 2018;20:67–75.

38. Krack A, Sharma R, Figulla HR, et al. The importance of the gastrointestinal system in the pathogenesis of heart failure. Eur Heart J 2005;26:2368–74.

39. Anand IS, Latini R, Florea VG, et al. C-reactive protein in heart failure: prognostic value and the effect of valsartan. Circulation 2005;112:1428–34.

40. Alonso-Martinez JL, Llorente-Diez B, Echegaray-Agara M, et al. C-reactive protein as a predictor of improvement and readmission in heart failure. Eur J Heart Fail 2002;4:331–6.

41. Siirila-Waris K, Lassus J, Melin J, et al. Characteristics, outcomes, and predictors of 1-year mortality in patients hospitalized for acute heart failure. Eur Heart J 2006;27:3011–7.

42. Marra AM, Arcopinto M, Salzano A, et al. Detectable interleukin-9 plasma levels are associated with impaired cardiopulmonary functional capacity and all-cause mortality in patients with chronic heart failure. Int J Cardiol 2016;209:114–7.

43. Januzzi JL Jr, Peacock WF, Maisel AS, et al. Measurement of the interleukin family member ST2 in patients with acute dyspnea: results from the PRIDE (Pro-Brain Natriuretic Peptide Investigation of Dyspnea in the Emergency Department) study. J Am Coll Cardiol 2007;50:607–13.

44. Shah RV, Chen-Tournoux AA, Picard MH, et al. Serum levels of the interleukin-1 receptor family member ST2, cardiac structure and function, and long-term mortality in patients with acute dyspnea. Circ Heart Fail 2009;2:311–9.

45. Sharma UC, Pokharel S, van Brakel TJ, et al. Galectin-3 marks activated macrophages in failure-prone hypertrophied hearts and contributes to cardiac dysfunction. Circulation 2004;110:3121–8.

46. de Boer RA, Lok DJ, Jaarsma T, et al. Predictive value of plasma galectin-3 levels in heart failure with reduced and preserved ejection fraction. Ann Med 2011;43:60–8.

47. Sharma A, Stevens SR, Lucas J, et al. Utility of growth differentiation factor-15, a marker of oxidative stress and inflammation, in chronic heart failure: insights from the HF-ACTION study. JACC Heart Fail 2017;5:724–34.

48. Sacca L. Heart failure as a multiple hormonal deficiency syndrome. Circ Heart Fail 2009;2:151–6.

49. Bossone E, Arcopinto M, Iacoviello M, et al, TOSCA Investigators. Multiple hormonal and metabolic deficiency syndrome in chronic heart failure: rationale, design, and demographic characteristics of the T.O.S.CA. Registry. Intern Emerg Med 2018; 13:661–71.

50. Marra AM, Bobbio E, D'Assante R, et al. Growth hormone as biomarker in heart failure. Heart Fail Clin 2018;14:65–74.

51. Marra AM, Arcopinto M, Bobbio E, et al. An unusual case of dilated cardiomyopathy associated with partial hypopituitarism. Intern Emerg Med 2012; 7(Suppl 2):S85–7.

52. Bossone E, Limongelli G, Malizia G, et al, Investigators TOSCA. The T.O.S.CA. Project: research, education and care. Monaldi Arch Chest Dis 2011;76:198–203.

53. Jankowska EA, Biel B, Majda J, et al. Anabolic deficiency in men with chronic heart failure: prevalence and detrimental impact on survival. Circulation 2006;114:1829–37.

54. Jankowska EA, Rozentryt P, Ponikowska B, et al. Circulating estradiol and mortality in men with systolic chronic heart failure. JAMA 2009;301:1892–901.

55. Salzano A, Marra AM, Ferrara F, et al, Investigators TOSC. Multiple hormone deficiency syndrome in heart failure with preserved ejection fraction. Int J Cardiol 2016;225:1–3.

56. Pasquali D, Arcopinto M, Renzullo A, et al. Cardiovascular abnormalities in Klinefelter syndrome. Int J Cardiol 2013;168:754–9.

57. Marra AM, Improda N, Capalbo D, et al. Cardiovascular abnormalities and impaired exercise performance in adolescents with congenital adrenal hyperplasia. J Clin Endocrinol Metab 2015;100: 644–52.

58. Sacca F, Puorro G, Marsili A, et al. Long-term effect of epoetin alfa on clinical and biochemical markers in Friedreich ataxia. Mov Disord 2016;31:734–41.

59. Salzano A, Arcopinto M, Marra AM, et al. Klinefelter syndrome, cardiovascular system, and thromboembolic disease: review of literature and clinical perspectives. Eur J Endocrinol 2016;175:R27–40.

60. Salzano A, D'Assante R, Heaney LM, et al. Klinefelter syndrome, insulin resistance, metabolic syndrome, and diabetes: review of literature and clinical perspectives. Endocrine 2018;61:194–203.

61. Arcopinto M, Salzano A, Giallauria F, et al, Investigators TOSC. Growth hormone deficiency is associated with worse cardiac function, physical performance, and outcome in chronic heart failure: insights from the T.O.S.CA. GHD Study. PLoS One 2017;12:e0170058.

62. Arcopinto M, Isgaard J, Marra AM, et al. IGF-1 predicts survival in chronic heart failure. Insights from the T.O.S.CA. (Trattamento Ormonale Nello Scompenso CArdiaco) registry. Int J Cardiol 2014;176: 1006–8.

63. Arcopinto M, Salzano A, Bossone E, et al. Multiple hormone deficiencies in chronic heart failure. Int J Cardiol 2015;184:421–3.

64. Cittadini A, Saldamarco L, Marra AM, et al. Growth hormone deficiency in patients with chronic heart failure and beneficial effects of its correction. J Clin Endocrinol Metab 2009;94:3329–36.

65. Cittadini A, Marra AM, Arcopinto M, et al. Growth hormone replacement delays the progression of chronic heart failure combined with growth hormone deficiency: an extension of a randomized controlled single-blind study. JACC Heart Fail 2013;1:325–30.

66. Salzano A, Marra AM, D'Assante R, et al. Growth hormone therapy in heart failure. Heart Fail Clin 2018;14:501–15.

67. Arcopinto M, Salzano A, Isgaard J, et al. Hormone replacement therapy in heart failure. Curr Opin Cardiol 2015;30:277–84.

68. Nagatomo Y, Tang WH. Intersections between microbiome and heart failure: revisiting the gut hypothesis. J Card Fail 2015;21:973–80.

69. Troseid M, Ueland T, Hov JR, et al. Microbiota-dependent metabolite trimethylamine-N-oxide is associated with disease severity and survival of patients with chronic heart failure. J Intern Med 2015;277:717–26.

70. Suzuki T, Heaney LM, Bhandari SS, et al. Trimethylamine N-oxide and prognosis in acute heart failure. Heart 2016;102:841–8.

71. Tang WH, Wang Z, Kennedy DJ, et al. Gut microbiota-dependent trimethylamine N-oxide (TMAO) pathway contributes to both development of renal insufficiency and mortality risk in chronic kidney disease. Circ Res 2015;116:448–55.

72. Schuett K, Kleber ME, Scharnagl H, et al. Trimethylamine-N-oxide and heart failure with reduced versus preserved ejection fraction. J Am Coll Cardiol 2017;70:3202–4.

73. Tang WH, Wang Z, Fan Y, et al. Prognostic value of elevated levels of intestinal microbe-generated metabolite trimethylamine-N-oxide in patients with heart failure: refining the gut hypothesis. J Am Coll Cardiol 2014;64:1908–14.

74. Albert CL, Tang WHW. Metabolic biomarkers in heart failure. Heart Fail Clin 2018;14:109–18.

75. Sengupta PP, Kramer CM, Narula J, et al. The potential of clinical phenotyping of heart failure with imaging biomarkers for guiding therapies: a focused update. JACC Cardiovasc Imaging 2017; 10:1056–71.

76. Bristow MR, Kao DP, Breathett KK, et al. Structural and functional phenotyping of the failing heart: is the left ventricular ejection fraction obsolete? JACC Heart Fail 2017;5:772–81.

77. Tischler MD, Ashikaga T, LeWinter MM. Relation between left ventricular shape and Doppler filling parameters in patients with left ventricular dysfunction secondary to coronary artery disease. Am J Cardiol 1995;76:553–6.

78. Geyer H, Caracciolo G, Abe H, et al. Assessment of myocardial mechanics using speckle tracking echocardiography: fundamentals and clinical applications. J Am Soc Echocardiogr 2010;23: 351–69 [quiz: 453–5].

79. Hasselberg NE, Haugaa KH, Sarvari SI, et al. Left ventricular global longitudinal strain is associated with exercise capacity in failing hearts with preserved and reduced ejection fraction. Eur Heart J Cardiovasc Imaging 2015;16:217–24.

80. Tsang TS, Abhayaratna WP, Barnes ME, et al. Prediction of cardiovascular outcomes with left atrial size: is volume superior to area or diameter? J Am Coll Cardiol 2006;47:1018–23.

81. Santos AB, Kraigher-Krainer E, Gupta DK, et al, Investigators PARAMOUNT. Impaired left atrial function in heart failure with preserved ejection fraction. Eur J Heart Fail 2014;16:1096–103.

82. Marra AM, Benjamin N, Eichstaedt C, et al. Gender-related differences in pulmonary arterial hypertension targeted drugs administration. Pharmacol Res 2016;114:103–9.

83. Marra AM, Bossone E, Salzano A, et al. Biomarkers in pulmonary hypertension. Heart Fail Clin 2018;14: 393–402.

84. Ferrara F, Gargani L, Armstrong WF, et al. The Right Heart International Network (RIGHT-NET): rationale, objectives, methodology, and clinical implications. Heart Fail Clin 2018;14:443–65.

85. Pleister A, Kahwash R, Haas G, et al. Echocardiography and heart failure: a glimpse of the right heart. Echocardiography 2015;32(Suppl 1):S95–107.

86. Thenappan T, Roy SS, Duval S, et al. beta-blocker therapy is not associated with adverse outcomes in patients with pulmonary arterial hypertension: a propensity score analysis. Circ Heart Fail 2014;7: 903–10.

87. Puwanant S, Priester TC, Mookadam F, et al. Right ventricular function in patients with preserved and reduced ejection fraction heart failure. Eur J Echocardiogr 2009;10:733–7.

88. Lang RM, Badano LP, Mor-Avi V, et al. Recommendations for cardiac chamber quantification by echocardiography in adults: an update from the American Society of Echocardiography and the European Association of Cardiovascular Imaging. J Am Soc Echocardiogr 2015;28:1–39 e14.

89. Salzano A, Sirico D, Golia L, et al. The portopulmonary hypertension: an overview from diagnosis to treatment. Monaldi Arch Chest Dis 2013;80:66–8 [Italian].

90. Pellicori P, Carubelli V, Zhang J, et al. IVC diameter in patients with chronic heart failure: relationships and prognostic significance. JACC Cardiovasc Imaging 2013;6:16–28.

91. Papolos A, Narula J, Bavishi C, et al. U.S. hospital use of echocardiography: insights from the nationwide inpatient sample. J Am Coll Cardiol 2016;67: 502–11.

92. Peterzan MA, Rider OJ, Anderson LJ. The role of cardiovascular magnetic resonance imaging in heart failure. Card Fail Rev 2016;2:115–22.

93. Kim RJ, Chen EL, Lima JA, et al. Myocardial Gd-DTPA kinetics determine MRI contrast enhancement and reflect the extent and severity of myocardial injury after acute reperfused infarction. Circulation 1996;94:3318–26.

94. Assomull RG, Prasad SK, Lyne J, et al. Cardiovascular magnetic resonance, fibrosis, and prognosis in dilated cardiomyopathy. J Am Coll Cardiol 2006; 48:1977–85.

95. Bello D, Fieno DS, Kim RJ, et al. Infarct morphology identifies patients with substrate for sustained ventricular tachycardia. J Am Coll Cardiol 2005;45: 1104–8.

96. Abbasi SA, Ertel A, Shah RV, et al. Impact of cardiovascular magnetic resonance on management and clinical decision-making in heart failure patients. J Cardiovasc Magn Reson 2013;15:89.

97. Larose E, Ganz P, Reynolds HG, et al. Right ventricular dysfunction assessed by cardiovascular magnetic resonance imaging predicts poor prognosis late after myocardial infarction. J Am Coll Cardiol 2007;49:855–62.

98. Haykowsky MJ, Nicklas BJ, Brubaker PH, et al. Regional adipose distribution and its relationship to exercise intolerance in older obese patients who have heart failure with preserved ejection fraction. JACC Heart Fail 2018;6:640–9.

99. van Woerden G, Gorter TM, Westenbrink BD, et al. Epicardial fat in heart failure patients with mid-range and preserved ejection fraction. Eur J Heart Fail 2018;20(11):1559–66.

100. Arvidsson PM, Toger J, Pedrizzetti G, et al. Hemodynamic forces using 4D flow MRI: an independent biomarker of cardiac function in heart failure with left ventricular dyssynchrony? Am J Physiol Heart Circ Physiol 2018. [Epub ahead of print].

101. Lum YH, McKenzie S, Brown M, et al. Impact of cardiac MRI in heart failure patients referred to a tertiary advanced heart failure unit: improvements in diagnosis and management. Intern Med J 2018. [Epub ahead of print].

102. Cohn JN, Levine TB, Olivari MT, et al. Plasma norepinephrine as a guide to prognosis in patients with chronic congestive heart failure. N Engl J Med 1984;311:819–23.

103. Carrio I, Cowie MR, Yamazaki J, et al. Cardiac sympathetic imaging with mIBG in heart failure. JACC Cardiovasc Imaging 2010;3:92–100.

104. Al Badarin FJ, Wimmer AP, Kennedy KF, et al. The utility of ADMIRE-HF risk score in predicting serious arrhythmic events in heart failure patients: incremental prognostic benefit of cardiac 123I-mIBG scintigraphy. J Nucl Cardiol 2014;21:756–62 [quiz: 753–55, 763–5].

105. Ketchum ES, Jacobson AF, Caldwell JH, et al. Selective improvement in Seattle Heart Failure Model risk stratification using iodine-123 meta-iodobenzylguanidine imaging. J Nucl Cardiol 2012;19:1007–16.

106. Wessler BS, Udelson JE. Neuronal dysfunction and medical therapy in heart failure: can an imaging biomarker help to "personalize" therapy? J Nucl Med 2015;56(Suppl 4):20S–4S.

107. Verschure DO, de Groot JR, Mirzaei S, et al. Cardiac (123)I-mIBG scintigraphy is associated with freedom of appropriate ICD therapy in stable chronic heart failure patients. Int J Cardiol 2017;248:403–8.

108. Dimitriu-Leen AC, Scholte AJ, Jacobson AF. 123I-MIBG SPECT for evaluation of patients with heart failure. J Nucl Med 2015;56(Suppl 4):25S–30S.

109. Cruz MC, Abreu A, Portugal G, et al. Relationship of left ventricular global longitudinal strain with cardiac autonomic denervation as assessed by (123)I-mIBG scintigraphy in patients with heart failure with reduced ejection fraction submitted to cardiac resynchronization therapy: assessment of cardiac autonomic denervation by GLS in patients with heart failure with reduced ejection fraction submitted to CRT. J Nucl Cardiol 2017. [Epub ahead of print].

110. Maisel AS, Duran JM, Wettersten N. Natriuretic peptides in heart failure: atrial and B-type natriuretic peptides. Heart Fail Clin 2018;14:13–25.

111. Richards AM. N-terminal B-type natriuretic peptide in heart failure. Heart Fail Clin 2018;14:27–39.

112. McKie PM, Burnett JC Jr. NT-proBNP: the gold standard biomarker in heart failure. J Am Coll Cardiol 2016;68:2437–9.

113. Alba AC, Agoritsas T, Jankowski M, et al. Risk prediction models for mortality in ambulatory patients with heart failure: a systematic review. Circ Heart Fail 2013;6:881–9.

114. Grande D, Leone M, Rizzo C, et al. A multiparametric approach based on NT-proBNP, ST2, and Galectin3 for stratifying one year prognosis of chronic heart failure outpatients. J Cardiovasc Dev Dis 2017;4 [pii:E0009].

115. Doumouras BS, Lee DS, Levy WC, et al. An appraisal of biomarker-based risk-scoring models in chronic heart failure: which one is best? Curr Heart Fail Rep 2018;15:24–36.

116. Gong FF, Campbell DJ, Prior DL. Noninvasive cardiac imaging and the prediction of heart failure progression in preclinical stage A/B subjects. JACC Cardiovasc Imaging 2017;10:1504–19.

117. Kalogeropoulos AP, Georgiopoulou VV, deFilippi CR, et al. Echocardiography, natriuretic peptides, and risk for incident heart failure in older adults: the Cardiovascular Health Study. JACC Cardiovasc Imaging 2012;5:131–40.

118. Lupon J, de Antonio M, Galan A, et al. Combined use of the novel biomarkers high-sensitivity troponin T and ST2 for heart failure risk stratification vs conventional assessment. Mayo Clin Proc 2013;88:234–43.

119. Kosmala W, Przewlocka-Kosmala M, Rojek A, et al. Comparison of the diastolic stress test with a combined resting echocardiography and biomarker approach to patients with exertional dyspnea: diagnostic and prognostic implications. JACC Cardiovasc Imaging 2018. [Epub ahead of print].

120. Girerd N, Seronde MF, Coiro S, et al, INI-CRCT, Great Network, and the EF-HF Group. Integrative assessment of congestion in heart failure throughout the patient journey. JACC Heart Fail 2018;6:273–85.

, Croydon, CR0 4YY